IARC HANDBOOKS OF CANCER PREVENTION

Tobacco Control

International Agency for Research on Cancer
World Health Organization

Volume 13

Evaluating the Effectiveness
of Smoke-free Policies

IARC

2009

International Agency for Research on Cancer

The International Agency for Research on Cancer (IARC) was established in 1965 by the World Health Assembly, as an independently funded organisation within the framework of the World Health Organization. The headquarters of the Agency are in Lyon, France.

The Agency conducts a programme of research concentrating particularly on the epidemiology of cancer and the study of potential carcinogens in the human environment. Its field studies are supplemented by biological and chemical research carried out in the Agency's laboratories in Lyon and, through collaborative research agreements, in national research institutions in many countries. The Agency also conducts a programme for the education and training of personnel for cancer research.

The publications of the Agency contribute to the dissemination of authoritative information on different aspects of cancer research. Information about IARC publications, and how to order them, is available via the Internet at: http://www.iarc.fr/en/publications/index.php.

This publication represents the views and opinions of an IARC Working Group on Evaluating the effectiveness of smoke-free policies which met in Lyon, France, 31 March - 5 April 2008.

IARC Handbooks on Tobacco Control, Volume 13:
Evaluating the Effectiveness of Smoke-free Policies
31 March to 5 April 2008, Lyon, France

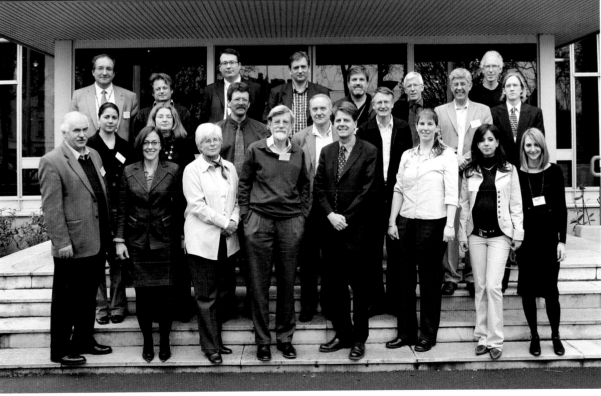

Published by the International Agency for Research on Cancer,
150 cours Albert Thomas, 69372 Lyon Cedex 08, France

© International Agency for Research on Cancer, 2009

Distributed by
WHO Press, World Health Organization, 20 Avenue Appia, 1211 Geneva 27, Switzerland (tel: +41 22 791 3264; fax: +41 22 791 4857; email: bookorders@who.int).

Format for Bibliographic Citation

IARC Handbooks of Cancer Prevention, Tobacco Control, Vol. 13: Evaluating the effectiveness of smoke-free policies (2009: Lyon, France)

IARC Library Cataloguing in Publication Data

Evaluating the effectiveness of smoke-free policies / IARC Working Group on the Evaluation of the Effectiveness of Smoke-free Policies (2008 : Lyon, France)

(IARC Handbooks of Cancer Prevention ; 13)

1. Neoplasms – prevention & control 2. Program Evaluation 3. Public Policy
4. Smoking Cessation 5. Tobacco Smoke Pollution – legislation & jurisprudence I. IARC Working Group on the Evaluation of the Effectiveness of Smoke-free Policies II. Series

ISBN   978-92-832-3013-7   (NLM Classification QZ 39)
ISSN   1027- 5622

Table of Contents

List of Participants

John P. Pierce *(Chair)*
Department of Family
and Preventive Medicine
Moores Cancer Center
University of California, San Diego
3855 Health Sciences Drive,
Room 3065
La Jolla, CA 92093-0901
USA

Douglas Bettcher
Tobacco Free Initiative
World Health Organization
20, avenue Appia
CH-1211 Geneva 27
Switzerland

Frank J. Chaloupka
University of Illinois at Chicago
National Bureau of Economic
Review
1747 W. Roosevelt,
Room 558
Chicago, IL 60608
USA

Richard A. Daynard
Northeastern University
School of Law
Public Health Advocacy Institute
400 Huntington Avenue
Boston, MA 02115
USA

Esteve Fernández
Tobacco Control Research Unit
Cancer Prevention and Control
Department
Catalan Institute of Oncology
Av. Gran Via 199-203
08907 L'Hospitalet
Barcelona
Spain

Elizabeth Gilpin
Cancer Prevention and Control
Program
Moores Cancer Center
University of California, San Diego
La Jolla, CA 92093-0901
USA

Sally Haw
Scottish Collaboration for Public
Health Research and Policy
(SCPHRP) MRC
Human Genetics Unit
Western General Hospital
Crewe Road
Edinburgh
EH4 2XU
Scotland

NHS Health Scotland
Thistle House
91 Haymarket Terrace
Edinburgh
EH12 5HE
Scotland

Andrew Hyland *(not attending)*
Department of Health Behaviour
Roswell Park Cancer Institute
Elm and Carlton Streets
Buffalo, NY 14263
USA

Jennifer K. Ibrahim
Department of Public Health
Temple University
1301 Cecil B. Moore Avenue
Ritter Annex - 9th Floor - 004-09
Philadelphia, PA 19122
USA

Giovanni Invernizzi
Tobacco Control Unit
National Cancer Institute/SIMG
Via Venezian, 1
20133 Milan
Italy

Karl E. Lund
Norwegian Institute for Alcohol
and Drug Research
PO Box 565 Centrum
0105 Oslo
Norway

Armando Peruga
Tobacco Free Initiative
World Health Organization
20, avenue Appia
CH-1211 Geneva 27
Switzerland

Krzysztof Przewozniak
WHO Collaborating Centre
Department of Cancer Epidemiology
and Prevention
Maria Sklodowska-Curie
Memorial Cancer Center
5, Roentgena Street
02-781 Warsaw
Poland

Jonathan Samet
Department of Epidemiology
Bloomberg School of Public Health
Johns Hopkins University
615 North Wolfe Street
Baltimore, MD 21205-2179
USA

Michelle Scollo *(not attending)*
School of Public Health A27
University of Sydney
NSW 2006 Sydney
Australia

Nick Wilson
Department of Public Health
University of Otago, Wellington
Box 7343 Wellington South
New Zealand

Alistair Woodward
School of Population Health
University of Auckland
Private Bag 92019
Auckland 1142
New Zealand

IARC Secretariat

Paolo Boffetta (Group Head)
Elisabeth Couto (Rapporteur)
John Daniel (Editor, Plenary Session)
Fabrizio Giannandrea (Rapporteur)
María E. León (Responsible Officer)
Kunnambath Ramadas
Nualnong Wongtongkam (Post-Meeting)

Technical/Administrative Assistance

Latifa Bouanzi (Library)
Rim Boudjema (Secretarial)
Jennifer Donaldson (Editor)
Roland Dray (Graphics)
Sharon Grant (Library)
Brigitte Kajo (Bibliography)
Georges Mollon (Photography)
Sylvia Moutinho (Secretarial)
Stéphanie Royannais (Layout)

Acknowledgements

The Working Group acknowledges the invaluable help provided in the data preparation presented in this Handbook by the following researchers: Elizabeth Khaykin (Johns Hopkins University, Baltimore, Maryland, USA), Anita Lal (The Cancer Council Victoria, Carlton, Victoria, Australia), Birgit Lehner (Tobacco Free Initiative, World Health Organization, Geneva, Switzerland), Luminita Sanda (Tobacco Free Initiative, World Health Organization, Geneva, Switzerland), Shaheen Sultana (University of Auckland, Auckland, Australia), Edward Sweda (Public Health Advocacy Institute, Boston, Massachusetts, USA), and Barbara Zolty (Tobacco Free Initiative, World Health Organization, Geneva, Switzerland).

The IARC and WHO secretariat are grateful to Sylvia Moutinho (Lifestyle and Cancer Group, IARC) and Miriamjoy Aryee-Quansah (Tobacco Free Initiative, WHO) and to the staff of the Libraries at the International Agency for Research on Cancer, Lyon, France and the World Health Organization, Geneva, Switzerland.

Preface

A key intervention in reducing the burden of disease attributable to tobacco use is protecting people from exposure to secondhand tobacco smoke (SHS). Volume 13 of the IARC Handbook series on Cancer Prevention presents the evidence on the effectiveness of measures enforced at the societal level to eliminate tobacco smoking and tobacco smoke from the environments where exposure takes place. This volume offers a critical review of the evidence on the economic effects and health benefits of smoke-free legislation and the adoption of voluntary smoke-free policies in households.

SHS contains nicotine, carcinogens, and toxins and the IARC (2004) concluded that exposure to SHS is carcinogenic to humans. Article 8 of the WHO Framework Convention on Tobacco Control (FCTC) recognises "that scientific evidence has unequivocally established that exposure to tobacco smoke causes death, disease and disability." It mandates Parties to this treaty to "adopt and implement... effective legislative, executive, administrative and/or other measures, providing for protection from exposure to tobacco smoke in indoor workplaces, public transport, indoor public places and, as appropriate, other public places." (WHO, 2005). Guidelines adopted by the Conference of the Parties to assist Parties in meeting their obligation under this article of the treaty, clearly state that this requires "the total elimination of smoking and tobacco smoke in a particular space or environment in order to create a 100% smoke-free environment." (WHO, 2007a).

Today, 164 countries have ratified the WHO FCTC and more are expected to do so in the future. As a result, countries around the world are working towards designing, implementing, and enforcing legal measures aimed at creating 100% smoke-free environments in public and workplaces. The relevant content of this Handbook will serve as guiding principles to those countries.

The literature reviewed for this Handbook was published from 1990 mostly up to April 2008, when the meeting took place to conduct the evaluation of the gathered evidence. The Working Group drafting the volume acknowledged the need to document the enforcement and reach of smoke-free policies in many developing countries where smoke-free legislation either does not exist or is not effective, translating into millions of people, particularly children, who are routinely exposed to SHS. Globally, about half of never smokers are exposed to tobacco smoke in different settings: work (including hospitality venues), home, cars, and other means of transportation. About 10-15% of lung cancers in never smokers may be attributed to SHS (Boyle & Levin, 2008). Comprehensive smoke-free legislation, as described in the guidelines of Article 8 of the WHO FCTC, will lead signing Parties towards removing this major cause of disease and death worldwide.

Chapter 1
Overview of Handbook volume 13

IARC, which is part of the World Health Organization, coordinates and conducts research on the causes of human cancer and the mechanisms of carcinogenesis, and develops scientific strategies for cancer control. In Handbook Volume 13, IARC considered, for the first time, the effectiveness of public policies in its reviews. This IARC Handbook is focused on the effectiveness of tobacco control policies implemented to protect nonsmokers from secondhand tobacco smoke (SHS). The goal of smoke-free legislation is to eliminate involuntary exposure to SHS entirely.

In 2004, IARC published Monograph 83 - a definitive review of the carcinogenicity of exposure to SHS through involuntary smoking (IARC, 2004). This Handbook does not seek to update that review, as assessment of carcinogenicity is not the domain of the Handbooks[1]. Rather, the purpose is to focus on the effectiveness of the implementation of the health policy recommended by the WHO Framework Convention for Tobacco Control (FCTC). There are two relevant components to this. The first is a consideration of the strategies and evidence that

opponents use to promote less than strict adherence to the recommended WHO FCTC legislative language. The second is consideration of the evidence for effectiveness of smoke-free legislation that has been implemented, as reported in the scientific literature and government reports. The first jurisdiction to implement a strict smoke-free policy, the US state of California, has 10 years experience with it; many others have close to five. It is timely to undertake an early review of the evidence and draw conclusions about the effectiveness of smoke-free policies. This Handbook will be useful for health professionals and policymakers in countries who are currently considering legislation to protect the population from SHS.

Secondhand smoke: the problem

SHS is defined as the smoke emitted either from the burning end of a tobacco product or by the exhalation of smoke-filled air by a smoker, both of which contain known human carcinogens (IARC, 2004). The ambient air in the immediate environment of a smoker quickly becomes contaminated with carbon monoxide; large quantities

of particulate matter, as well as nitrogen oxides; several substances recognised as human carcinogens, such as formaldehyde, acetaldehyde, benzene, and nitrosamines; and possible human carcinogens, such as hydroquinone and cresol (IARC, 2004; U.S. Department of Health and Human Services, 2006). As these contaminants are absorbed (and later released) by materials in the environment (e.g. furniture covering, curtains), the potential for SHS exposure lasts considerably longer than the act of smoking. No safe level of SHS exposure has been identified.

Nonsmokers (and smokers) become exposed to SHS when they breathe this contaminated air. In addition to carcinogens, SHS contains compounds such as pyridine that produce unpleasant odors (National Cancer Institute, 1999), and particles such as nicotine, acrolein, and formaldehyde that cause mucosal irritation (Lee et al., 1993). However, the degree to which nonsmokers will notice and respond to SHS exposure is related to the age of the exposed person, their olfactory acuity, as well as their annoyance threshold (U.S. Department of Health and Human Services, 2006). Thus, harm may

---

[1] IARC will re-visit the carcinogenicity of involuntary tobacco smoke in its forthcoming Monograph volume 100 E (Lifestyle factors) during a meeting from September 29 to October 6 2009 in Lyon, France (http://monographs.iarc.fr/ENG/Meetings/index.php).

occur whether or not the individual realises that they are exposed.

Exposure to air that is not smoke-free will lead to the uptake of SHS contaminants. The dose of SHS contaminants that reach a target organ determines the risk of disease to that organ in the nonsmoker, as well as the smoker. The amount of exposure to a nonsmoker will vary with both the concentration of SHS in the ambient air and with the time that the individual spends in contact with it. Ventilation and air cleaning have been advocated as possible ways of reducing the exposure of nonsmokers to SHS. The dose of SHS contaminants that a nonsmoker receives varies with the number of cigarettes smoked per unit of time in an area, and is inversely proportional to the intensity of ventilation and the rate of cleaning or removal of SHS components from the air (Ott, 1999).

In most homes, ventilation occurs by a natural exchange of indoor and outdoor air. However, public and commercial buildings generally have systems for ventilation and air exchange. These heating, ventilating, and air conditioning systems often distribute SHS throughout a building in the process of air exchange, thereby potentially magnifying the number of nonsmokers who are exposed to SHS (U.S. Department of Health and Human Services, 2006). Measurements of ambient nicotine concentrations have confirmed that current ventilation systems are insufficient to eliminate SHS from indoor air (Repace & Lowrey, 1993). Further, in the presence of multiple indoor smoking episodes, reducing SHS to very low levels by ventilation has generally not been considered

feasible because of the high cost of installing the necessary ventilation system and the impairment of comfort levels that implementing such a system would entail (e.g. by making the air less thermally tolerable). Given the strength of cigarettes, and other combusted tobacco products, as a source of toxic particles and gases indoors, air cleaning has also been judged to be ineffective for controlling SHS exposure (American Society of Heating, Refrigerating and Air-Conditioning Engineers, Inc., 2005; U.S. Department of Health and Human Services, 2006; WHO, 2007b).

The need for policies to protect nonsmokers

Unlike many indoor pollutants that cause disease, exposure to SHS can be completely prevented by removing the source - tobacco smoke. This requires public policy. Early steps have focused on banning smoking from areas in which smokers and nonsmokers might congregate. An example was seen in 1970 when the World Health Assembly banned smoking in meeting rooms (WHO, 1970). By 1975, a number of countries had banned smoking in hospitals and schools, public transport, libraries, theaters, and concert halls. By the end of the 1980s, some countries had even banned smoking in government offices. The first jurisdiction to mandate a smoke-free workplace was California, where most workplaces were legislated to be smoke-free by 1995, but establishments serving alcohol were not covered until 1998. However, unlike many other types of public health legislation, there

were no similar laws passed in other jurisdictions until 2002.

A landmark event for the protection of nonsmokers from SHS occurred when WHO agreed to negotiate and promote a Framework Convention for Tobacco Control (FCTC). The first big success was that this treaty was negotiated in 2003 and ratified by so many member nations. The second success was that the WHO FCTC developed evidence-based model language for smoke-free legislation, which is embodied in Article 8. WHO's FCTC marked a new epoch where tobacco control was seen as a global problem with global solutions. Since the ratification of the treaty, there has been rapid progress in countries implementing smoke-free workplaces using language similar to that recommended by Article 8. Under the FCTC, "smoke-free" air means that a nonsmoker will not be able to see, smell, or sense tobacco smoke, nor will components of tobacco smoke be able to be measured in the air.

Measurement of SHS

The issue of how exposure to SHS is measured is central to the discussion on the health consequences of SHS and the effectiveness of policies to reduce exposure among non-smokers. There are several comprehensive reviews of this field, such as that of the California Environmental Protection Agency (California Environmental Protection Agency: Air Resources Board, 2005); this Handbook does not add to this literature. The most common methods of measurement of SHS exposure are self-reported questionnaires, atmospheric markers, and biomarkers of exposure within individuals. A table listing these measures, along with identified advantages and disadvantages, is presented in Appendix 1. A summary of this literature is provided to assist readers with different chapters in this Handbook.

Self-reported questionnaires

Measuring exposure to SHS by self-reported questionnaires is a method frequently used in studies, whether the exposure data are collected retrospectively or prospectively. Self-reported measures can be useful for determining if any SHS exposure has taken place and for determining the location of exposure (Borland *et al.*, 1992; Matt *et al.*, 1999). However, they have limitations because of respondents' inability to accurately assess and then recall the duration and intensity of SHS exposure, or of ventilation or air conditioning practices in a particular environment (U.S. Department of Health and Human Services, 2006). As mentioned earlier, there is significant individual variability in sensitivity to smells and irritants that will add inconsistencies to anything more detailed than broad exposure assessment. More credibility is given to self-reported exposure in the home than to exposure in other multiple locations.

Individual biomarkers

An individual's exposure to SHS can be assessed objectively using the same biomarkers as are used for assessing active smoking. The most commonly used biomarkers are body fluid concentrations of nicotine (Benowitz, 1999), its more stable metabolite cotinine (Feyerabend & Russell, 1980; Pierce *et al.*, 1987), and urinary concentrations of 4-(N-nitrosomethylamino)-1-(3-pyridyl)-1-butanol (NNAL) - a potent tobacco specific carcinogen (Hecht & Hoffmann, 1988; Hecht, 2002). Hair and toenails also take up nicotine, and gradients in concentration across tissue have been detected allowing for an estimate of longer-term exposure to SHS (Al-Delaimy, 2002; Al-Delaimy *et al.*, 2002a,b). Levels of these biomarkers should be zero among people unexposed to tobacco smoke; any detectable level indicates exposure. The change in nicotine, cotinine, and NNAL are sensitive to even short-term exposure.

Atmospheric markers

The level of SHS in an environment is commonly measured by concentrations of either airborne nicotine or particulate matter (PM). About 95% of the nicotine in SHS is in the vapour phase (Leaderer & Hammond, 1991). Vapour-phase nicotine in the air can be passively collected in a sorbent tube or a filter treated with sodium bisulphate, and then analysed by gas chromatography. PM is defined as solid particles or liquid droplets suspended in the atmosphere. They can remain suspended for varying amounts of time depending on their properties and prevailing atmospheric conditions. PM is produced primarily from combustion processes originating from many different indoor and outdoor sources, including cooking and heating appliances and combustion engines. The rate of deposition of PM increases with the square of the particle diameter for particles >1 μm (Hinds, 1982). Therefore, larger particles (over 5 μm in diameter) tend to remain suspended for shorter periods, while smaller particles (submicrometric) can remain suspended for hours or even days (Institute of Medicine, 2001).

Although PM is not a specific marker of SHS, the amount of PM pollution generated by smoking can be extremely high in indoor environments (Repace & Lowrey, 1980). The typical metric for particulate matter is the mass concentration of particles of a given size, for example $PM_{2.5}$ (the mass of particles equal or less than 2.5 μm in diameter per unit of volume). This is the standard size measured as the majority of particles in SHS are within this diameter (Institute of Medicine, 2001). PM concentrations can be determined gravimetrically by collecting particles on a filter medium and then weighing them to provide a single integrated value for the sampling period. They can also be assessed in real time using optical or light-scattering monitors, which are capable of taking measurements every second, thus allowing exposure peaks to be recorded (Invernizzi *et al.*, 2002).

Other measures of SHS exposure have included determinations of airborne carbon monoxide and polycyclic aromatic hydrocarbons (Chuang *et al.*, 1999; Klepeis, 1999).

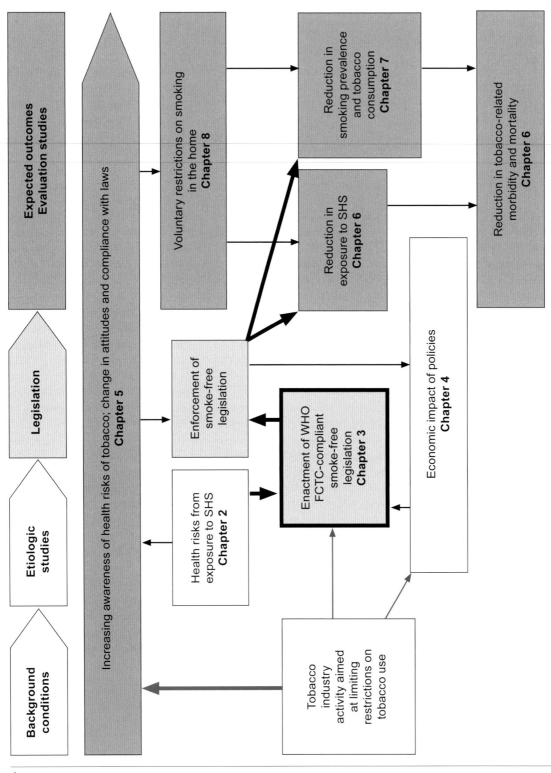

Figure 1 A logic model for SHS legislation

Outline of the Handbook

The logic model used for this Handbook is presented in Figure 1. This volume focuses on the enactment of smoke-free legislation, displayed in the middle of the figure. We consider the forces associated with the passage of such legislation, as well as the evidence for the effect of the enacted laws. Prior to consideration of public health legislation, there are a series of etiologic studies conducted which document health risks. Public awareness and acceptance of these risks will be accompanied by advocacy for protective action, which will be critical to gaining the necessary political support to enact the legislation. Meaningful restrictions on smoking will not only protect nonsmokers from the health consequences of exposure to SHS, but also may reduce the magnitude of the cigarette business within the jurisdiction. Accordingly, it is to be expected that the tobacco industry will be active in opposing the legislation in order to maintain their cigarette business. The tobacco industry strategies to oppose this legislation were uncovered in the 1990s, when the previously secret "Brown and Williamson" documents were released publicly (Glantz *et al.*, 1995; 1998). Further public releases occurred with legal discovery as part of lawsuits against the industry.

Public and legislator acceptance of the need for legislation is influenced by tobacco industry activities. One key concern prior to passing a policy is the potential economic impact on a given jurisdiction. Legislation for a policy also needs to consider the

level of necessary enforcement; oftentimes a budget for inspections and policing of the policy is not available. It is presumed that social norms alone will be sufficient to enforce the new laws.

Once legislation has been enacted, the effectiveness can be evaluated. Such effectiveness will be related to the level of compliance with the law which depends on public awareness and acceptance.

Chapter 2: The health effects of exposure to secondhand smoke

It is important to establish the scientific basis for SHS policy. Acceptance of the health consequences from exposure to SHS is central to efforts to promote legislation to protect the public's health, and, therefore, in the logic model in Figure 1, it precedes legislative efforts. Research on SHS has been ongoing for decades, with the first reviews of the evidence undertaken in the mid 1980s. Since then, authoritative scientific bodies have revisited the data at regular intervals particularly focusing on the evidence that exposure to SHS causes cancer, cardiovascular disease, and respiratory disease. These reviews have carefully considered the published epidemiological studies; they have reviewed the evidence on the suggested mechanisms for the effects of SHS and have considered potential confounding from other risk factors, as well as exposure misclassification. A summary of this body of evidence is provided in this chapter accompanied by results of both published and *de novo* meta-analyses, establishing the strong

scientific basis for urgent public health action to protect nonsmokers from exposure to SHS.

Chapter 3: The evolution of smoke-free policies

In 2003, WHO achieved consensus that a key to protecting people from the harmful consequences of exposure to SHS was legislation creating smoke-free environments - one of the pillars of the WHO FCTC. It was also recognised that such legislation can be written in a manner that appears to meet the public health goal, but contains clauses that do not protect the public from exposure to SHS as initially envisioned. Accordingly, specific model language was proposed in Article 8 of the WHO FCTC, which is presented in this chapter. Legislation is initiated by a governmental entity that has the power to both implement and enforce laws within its jurisdiction. Such an entity is a national or federal government, a sub-national government (state or province), or, in some countries, it can be a lower level of government, such as a local city or county government.

There is a long history of attempting to restrict smoking behaviour in different locations starting from the early days of the cigarette smoking epidemic. As cigarette smoking became more prevalent, nonsmokers' ability to maintain their rights disappeared. It was not until after the health consequences of smoking were accepted that restrictions on smoking began to be considered again. The Working Group briefly reviewed this history noting some of the landmarks and also noting that the diffusion was faster in some parts of the world than in others. Prominent reports concluding that exposure to SHS has serious health consequences for nonsmokers started in the mid 1980s; a paper in a major scientific journal appeared in 1992 calling for public health action to ensure a smoke-free workplace (Borland *et al.*, 1992). The first jurisdiction to implement a smoke-free workplace was the US state of California. Legislation was passed in 1994, but not fully enacted until 1998. Following WHO's initiative on the FCTC, smoke-free workplaces started to rapidly disseminate. The first country with nation-wide smoke-free workplaces was Ireland in 2004. The chapter summarises the rapidity of the diffusion of this important SHS legislation throughout this period. It also presents details of the legislation, including evidence of enforcement, for some of the key jurisdictions.

Chapter 4: Impact of smoke-free policies on businesses, the hospitality sector, and other incidental outcomes

In many jurisdictions, legislators, as well as residents, put a high value on ensuring that laws are "business friendly," meaning that enactment will not have a negative impact on business in the community (i.e. their profit margins) or on the taxation base of the community. As most community members, including legislators, will have little personal experience with which to judge the likely impact of the new policies, they will rely quite heavily on the economic reports from other places that have introduced similar legislation. Thus, research that

addresses the evidence of economic impact of smoke-free legislation can have an important impact on whether a given jurisdiction initiates SHS legislation or not, a link depicted in the logic model. The tobacco industry has generated much of this literature, disseminating reports favorable to their vested interest. However, the methodological rigor used by many of these tobacco industry-sponsored studies leaves much to be desired. Indeed, these methodologically unsound studies have often led to conclusions that are quite the opposite of those studies that used appropriate scientific methodology. Unfortunately, the findings from these studies, particularly those that focus on the hospitality industry, have been promoted widely by the tobacco industry, thus leading to the appearance of scientific controversy. This chapter lays out the methodological criteria for a study that can contribute to the science. It also discusses the consistency of the findings on the economic impact of smoke-free legislation on the hospitality industry from available scientifically-appropriate studies accessible up to April 2008.

Chapter 5: Public attitudes towards smoke-free policies - including compliance with policies

The passage of smoke-free legislation in any jurisdiction occurs within both a social and political context. It requires the multi-level support of stakeholders and potentially difficult negotiations in order to ensure enough votes for passage. A major determinant to the ease of passage of legislation will be the level of awareness and concern

in the community on the issue and the strength of support for restrictions on smoking to protect nonsmokers from exposure to SHS. Community awareness and concern will also dictate the level of compliance with legislation that has been introduced. Thus, in the logic model, community awareness and attitudes are presented as an important variable that acts across the continuum from background conditions to the outcomes following implementation and enforcement of SHS legislation (Figure 1). This chapter reviews the evidence for the level of community attitudes and support for smoke-free policies, as well as changes in these that occur after enactment of legislation.

Chapter 6: Reductions in exposure to secondhand smoke and effects on health due to restrictions on smoking

Prior to the passage of smoke-free legislation, many workplaces within a jurisdiction will already have voluntary restrictions on smoking behaviour, some of which will require smoke-free settings. Voluntary smoke-free workplaces, as well as jurisdictions that have smoke-free legislation, have been studied. There is now 10 years of follow-up for the jurisdiction with the first smoke-free legislation. Thus, there is a sufficient research base to allow an assessment of the short- and long-term effectiveness of the legislation in protecting nonsmokers from exposure to SHS, as indicated in the logic model (Figure 1).

Given that some of the health consequences of exposure to SHS have short-term onset, there has been considerable research interest in the change in prevalence of respiratory symptoms, and even acute coronary events, following reduction or elimination of SHS resulting from the implementation of smoke-free legislation. It is too early to assess any long-term health benefits, such as a change in the incidence of lung cancer. This chapter reviews the research documenting changes in exposure to SHS following smoke-free legislation and draws conclusions on the change in short-term health consequences following the implementation of a smoke-free workplace.

Chapter 7: The effect of mandated smoking restrictions on smoking behaviour

Restrictions on smoking behaviour to protect nonsmokers can also provide health benefits to smokers, by limiting their opportunity to smoke, reducing their level of consumption, and encouraging them to quit. Indeed, restrictions may also have a role in preventing young people from progressing to the same level of nicotine dependence that they may have done otherwise (Pierce et al., 1991). Reductions in population level nicotine dependence can be expected to modify both the short- and long-term health consequences of smoking in the community. These outcomes need to be considered in any assessment of the effectiveness of this public policy action (see Figure 1).

The literature is consistent that lung cancer, as a consequence of smoking, can be predicted from a power function of both the duration and intensity of smoking (Doll & Peto, 1978; Flanders et al., 2003). Thus, both cessation behaviour and consumption level of continuing smokers need to be part of the assessment of the effectiveness of smoke-free legislation. There are a number of studies that compare smoking behaviour in workplaces with total, partial, and no restrictions on smoking. In this chapter, we review these studies and draw conclusions on the role of smoke-free workplaces in modifying smoking behaviour in the community.

Chapter 8: Home smoking restrictions: effects on exposure to secondhand smoke and smoking behaviour

One key measure of the degree of acceptance of smoke-free policies is the extent to which community members implement their own voluntary restrictions in their homes, particularly smoke-free homes. In Figure 1, this relation is shown by connecting attitudes and compliance with voluntary restrictions on smoking in the home. Jurisdictions in which smokers live in smoke-free homes can be expected to require less enforcement of smoke-free policies, as the societal norms will be more aligned with the legislation. Further, a high proportion of smokers living in smoke-free homes and working in smoke-free workplaces is expected to be associated with a lower population level of nicotine dependence in continuing smokers. Smoke-free homes might also be associated with a reduction in the probability of smoking initiation by the children in the home. Finally, as

mentioned in the previous chapter, a reduction in smoking behaviour (proportion of smokers and their level of smoking intensity) should result in a reduction in tobacco-related morbidity and mortality.

This chapter reviews and draws conclusions from the available studies that report on voluntary home smoking restrictions, the protection of nonsmokers, and smoking behaviour among continuing smokers. This is a relatively new area of research; it can be expected that the scientific basis for conclusions will increase significantly over the next years.

Summary of findings of the Handbook

In each of the above chapters, the Working Group conducted a comprehensive examination of the peer-reviewed literature and publicly accessible government reports since 1990. Having completed that, the Working Group assessed the quality of the evidence in each of the areas and voted on it for a series of findings listed in the Evaluation chapter. The scale for the quality of evidence lists "sufficient" as the highest classification, indicating that the association was highly likely to be causal; a lesser classification of "strong" indicates that the association is consistent, but evidence of causality is limited. Three additional classification criteria were available when judging the strength of the evidence. Finally, the Working Group proposed several public health and research recommendations. On the basis of the evidence reviewed, an overall recommendation made by the Working Group is that governments enact and implement smoke-free policies that conform to the WHO FCTC. A short report of the Working Group's findings was published shortly after the conclusion of the Handbook meeting in Lyon. This report summarised the findings as follows: "Implementation of such policies can have a broader population effect of increasing smoke-free environments. Not only do these policies achieve their aim of protecting the health of non-smokers by decreasing exposure to secondhand smoke, they also have many effects on smoking behaviour, which compound the expected health benefits. These benefits will be greater if these policies are enacted as part of a comprehensive tobacco-control strategy that implements all of the provisions called for by the WHO FCTC." (Pierce & Leon, 2008).

Chapter 2
Health effects of exposure to secondhand smoke (SHS)

Introduction

In this chapter the Working Group summarises the major reviews that have been conducted in the last 10 years on the health effects of secondhand smoke (SHS). Where substantial new studies have been reported in the last few years, we describe these also, but do not attempt a formal assessment of the evidence overall. First, the literature on the relation between SHS and cardiovascular diseases is reviewed, since these conditions, and acute myocardial infarction (AMI) in particular, are leading contributors to the burden of disease caused by SHS. The chapter then provides an overview of effects of SHS on respiratory conditions and child health. Lastly, the link between SHS and cancer is examined, including the accumulation of evidence over time, and what is known about the relationship with cancers at particular sites. The emphasis in this chapter lies on the already answered question of whether SHS is a cause of disease, and if so, what is the relation between level of exposure and risk of disease. However, briefly we consider the related question of how much ill health may be attributed to exposures to SHS. This quantity, the burden of disease due to SHS, may be an important consideration for policy-makers and depends heavily on local circumstances, particularly the prevalence of exposure.

Non-malignant effects of SHS exposure

Overview

Exposure to SHS adversely affects the health of children and adults (Table 2.1). The inhalation of this mixture of irritant, toxic particles, and gases has respiratory effects, as well as effects on other organ systems, including causing coronary heart disease (CHD) in adults and sudden infant death syndrome (SIDS) in infants. There has been extensive research on mechanisms by which SHS causes these adverse effects; that evidence has been most recently reviewed in the 2006 report of the US Surgeon General and is not covered specifically in this chapter. However, we note the evidence was sufficient to support a major conclusion of this report, that "[c]hildren exposed to secondhand smoke are at increased risk for sudden infant death syndrome (SIDS), acute respiratory infections, ear problems and more severe asthma. Smoking by parents causes respiratory symptoms and slows lung growth in their children" (U.S. Department of Health and Human Services, 2006).

This chapter briefly reviews the findings of the various reports on the consequences of exposure to SHS (Table 2.1). The many adverse effects of SHS, beyond the causation of cancer, strengthen the rationale for achieving smoke-free environments, including not only public and workplaces, but homes, so as to ensure that children are protected from exposure to SHS. The most recent reports, particularly the 2005 California Environmental Protection Agency (EPA) report and the 2006 report of the US Surgeon General, provide comprehensive coverage of the epidemiological evidence and relevant research findings related to the plausibility of causal associations of SHS with respiratory and cardiovascular effects.

Beyond these adverse health effects, tobacco smoke, which contains numerous irritants, has long been linked to odor and annoyance (U.S. Department of Health and Human Services, 1986). Both questionnaire surveys and laboratory studies, involving exposure to SHS, have shown annoyance and irritation of the eyes and upper and lower airways from involuntary smoking. In several surveys of nonsmokers, complaints about tobacco smoke at work and in public places were common (U.S. Department of Health

Table 2.1 Adverse effects from exposure to tobacco smoke published in major reports

Health effect	SGR 1984	SGR 1986	EPA 1992	Cal EPA 1997	UK 1998/ 2004	WHO 1999	IARC 2004	Cal EPA* 2005**	SGR 2006
Increased prevalence of Chronic respiratory symptoms	Yes/a	Yes/a	Yes/c	Yes/c	Yes/c	Yes/c		Yes/c	Yes/c
Decrement in pulmonary function	Yes/a	Yes/a	Yes/a	Yes/a	Yes/a*	Yes/c		Yes/a	Yes/c
Increased occurrence of acute respiratory illnesses	Yes/a	Yes/a	Yes/a	Yes/c		Yes/c		Yes/c	Yes/c
Increased occurrence of middle ear disease		Yes/a	Yes/c	Yes/c	Yes/c	Yes/c		Yes/c	Yes/c
Increased severity of asthma episodes and symptoms			Yes/c	Yes/c		Yes/c		Yes/c	Yes/c
Risk factor for new asthma			Yes/a	Yes/c				Yes/c	Yes/c
Risk factor for SIDS				Yes/c	Yes/a	Yes/c		Yes/c	Yes/c
Risk factor for lung cancer in adults	Yes/c	Yes/c	Yes/c	Yes/c			Yes/c	Yes/c	Yes/c
Risk factor for breast cancer for younger, primarily premenopausal women								Yes/c	
Risk factor for nasal sinus cancer								Yes/c	
Risk factor for coronary heart disease in adults				Yes/c	Yes/c			Yes/c	Yes/c

SGR: US Surgeon General's report; EPA: US Environmental Protection Agency; Cal EPA: California Environmental Protection Agency; WHO: World Health Organization; IARC: International Agency for Research on Cancer; UK: United Kingdom Scientific Committee on Tobacco and Health
*Added in 2004
**Only effects causally associated with SHS exposure are included
Yes/a = association
Yes/c = cause
Table adapted from U.S. Department of Health and Human Services (2006) and from ASHRAE (Environmental Tobacco Smoke, position document, page 9, Table 1), (2005).
© American Society of Heating, Refrigerating and Air-Conditioning Engineers, Inc.

and Human Services, 1986). About 50% of respondents complained about tobacco smoke at work, and a majority were disturbed by tobacco smoke in restaurants. The experimental studies show that the rate of eye blinking is increased by SHS, as are complaints of nose and throat irritation (U.S. Department of Health and Human Services, 1986). One study suggests that there may be increasing sensitivity to SHS as the general level of exposure declines (Junker et al., 2001). The odor and irritation associated with SHS merit special consideration, because a high proportion of nonsmokers are annoyed by exposure to SHS, and control of concentrations in indoor air poses difficult problems in the management of heating, ventilating, and air-conditioning systems.

Childhood effects

Extensive epidemiological evidence has associated SHS exposure with respiratory and non-respiratory diseases and other adverse effects in children. Since the first reports in the 1960s, studies from around the world have shown that smoking by parents during pregnancy and after the child's birth causes disease, resulting in premature mortality and substantial morbidity. Extensive data on exposure, including measurements of SHS components in the air and of biomarkers, document the key role of smoking by parents in exposing their children to SHS. Studies have also addressed the mechanisms by which SHS causes its adverse effects. This evidence is not reviewed in this chapter, as it has been recently reviewed in the reports of the California EPA and US Surgeon General.

Table 2.1 lists the diseases and other adverse effects causally associated with exposure to SHS. The list includes SIDS, an important cause of death in children under a year of age (Anderson & Cook, 1997); acute lower respiratory illnesses, a major cause of morbidity and mortality in children under five years of age; and acute and chronic middle ear disease, also a leading child health problem (U.S. Department of Health and Human Services, 2006). SHS exposure worsens asthma and may contribute to its causation. It also slows the rate of lung growth during childhood and adolescence and is associated with increased prevalence of respiratory symptoms.

The epidemiological evidence on outcomes that have been causally linked to SHS exposure is substantial, and provides quantitative estimates of the risk associated with SHS. In general, risk increases with the number of adult smokers in the household, and attributable risk estimates indicate that SHS exposure is a substantial contributor to the burden of respiratory morbidity in childhood, as well as a major cause of SIDS (California Environmental Protection Agency: Air Resources

Board, 2005; U.S. Department of Health and Human Services, 2006).

Adulthood effects

Cardiovascular disease

The evidence indicating that SHS causes CHD in adults has been repeatedly reviewed since 1986. At that time, the US Surgeon General's report examined one case-control study and three cohort studies on the association of involuntary smoking and cardiovascular effects, concluding further research was needed to decide causality. A causal link between CHD and SHS was first reported in the California EPA report from 1997 (Table 2.1)

Causal associations between active smoking and fatal and nonfatal CHD outcomes have long been demonstrated (U.S. Department of Health and Human Services, 2004). Active cigarette smoking is considered to increase the risk of cardiovascular disease by promoting atherosclerosis; affecting endothelial cell functioning; increasing the tendency to thrombosis; causing spasm of the coronary arteries, which increases the likelihood of cardiac arrhythmias; and decreasing the oxygen-carrying capacity of the blood (U.S. Department of Health and Human Services, 1990). These same mechanisms have been considered to be relevant to SHS exposure and risk for CHD (Barnoya & Glantz, 2005; U.S. Department of Health and Human Services, 2006). Experimental studies support the relevance of these mechanisms (U.S. Department of Health and Human Services, 2006).

In 2005, the pathophysiological mechanisms by which SHS exposure might increase the risk of heart disease were summarised (Barnoya & Glantz, 2005). They suggested that passive smoking may promote atherogenesis; increase the tendency of platelets to aggregate, and thereby promote thrombosis; impair endothelial cell function; increase arterial stiffness leading to atherosclerosis; reduce the oxygen-carrying capacity of the blood; and alter myocardial metabolism, much as for active smoking and CHD. Several separate experiments, involving exposure of nonsmokers to SHS, have shown that passive smoking affects measures of platelet function in the direction of increased tendency toward thrombosis (Glantz & Parmley, 1995; Barnoya & Glantz, 2005). In a 2004 study, sidestream smoke was found to be 50% more potent than mainstream smoke in activating platelets (Rubenstein et al., 2004). It was also proposed that carcinogenic agents, such as polycyclic aromatic hydrocarbons found in tobacco smoke, promote atherogenesis by effects on cell proliferation (Glantz & Parmley, 1995). These mechanistic considerations support both acute and chronic effects of SHS exposure on risk for cardiovascular disease.

Exposure to SHS may also worsen the outcome of an ischemic event in the heart: animal data have demonstrated that SHS exposure increases cardiac damage following an experimental myocardial infarction. Experiments on two species of animals (rabbits and cockerels) have demonstrated that not only does exposure to SHS at doses similar to exposure to humans accelerate the growth of atherosclerotic plaques through the increase of lipid deposits, but it also induces atherosclerosis.

There is also impressive and accumulating evidence that SHS acutely affects vascular endothelial cell functioning (Celermajer et al., 1996; Sumida et al., 1998; Otsuka et al., 2001). Thirty minutes of exposure to SHS in healthy young volunteers was found to compromise coronary artery endothelial function in a manner that was indistinguishable from that of habitual smokers, suggesting that endothelial dysfunction may be an important mechanism by which exposure to SHS increases CHD risk (Otsuka et al., 2001).

In addition to its effects on platelets, SHS exposure affects the oxygen-carrying capacity of the blood through its carbon monoxide component. Even small increments, on the order of 1%, in the carboxyhemoglobin, may explain the finding that SHS exposure decreases the duration of exercise of patients with angina pectoris (Allred et al., 1989). This is supported with evidence that cigarette smoking has been shown to increase levels of carbon monoxide in the spaces where ventilation is low or smoking is particularly intense (U.S. Department of Health and Human Services, 1986).

A 1985 report, based on a cohort study in southern California, was the first epidemiologic investigation to raise concerns that exposure to SHS may increase risk for CHD (Garland et al., 1985). There are now more than 20 studies on the association between SHS and cardiovascular disease, including cohort and case-control studies. They cover a wide range of populations, both geographically and racially. One group of studies addressed the promotion of atherosclerosis and SHS exposure, using increased carotid intimal-medial thickness (IMT) as an indicator. These studies have shown both cross-sectional and longitudinal associations of IMT with SHS exposure (Howard et al., 1994, 1998; Diez-Roux et al., 1995).

As the evidence since the first report has mounted, it has been reviewed systematically by the American Heart Association (Taylor et al., 1992), the Australian National Health and Medical Research Council (1997), the California EPA (California Environmental Protection Agency, 1997; California Environmental Protection Agency: Air Resources Board, 2005), the Scientific Committee on Tobacco and Health in the United Kingdom (Scientific Committee on Tobacco and Health, 1998) and most recently by the US Surgeon General (U.S. Department of Health and Human Services, 2006). Review of the evidence has uniformly led to the conclusion that there is a causal association between exposure to SHS and risk of cardiovascular disease (California Environmental Protection Agency , 1997; Scientific Committee on Tobacco and Health, 1998). The meta-analysis prepared for the 2006 US Surgeon General's report, estimated the pooled excess risk for coronary heart disease from SHS exposure from marriage to a smoker as 27% (95% CI=19-36%) (U.S. Department of Health and Human Services, 2006).

There is increasing epidemiologic evidence suggestive of a causal association between SHS exposure and stroke. At least eight epidemiologic studies (four case-control, two cohort, and two cross-sectional) have been published exploring this association (Lee et al., 1986; Donnan et al., 1989; Sandler et al., 1989; Howard et al., 1998; Bonita et al., 1999; You et al., 1999; Zhang et al., 2005). A large cross-sectional study of 60 377 women in China, found an association between prevalent stroke in women and smoking by their husbands (Zhang et al., 2005). The prevalence of stroke increased with greater duration of smoking and with an increasing number of cigarettes smoked daily. A cohort study was conducted of 19 035 lifetime nonsmokers using census data from Washington County, MD (Sandler et al., 1989). Based on 297 cases among women exposed to SHS, a 24% increased risk of stroke was found compared with those unexposed (95% CI=3-49%). Null results were found for an association in men, but were limited to only 33 cases. A case-control study in New Zealand, which looked at 265 cases and 1336 controls, did find a two-fold increased risk of stroke in men exposed to SHS (Bonita et al., 1999). Additionally, a 2004 prospective cohort study used serum cotinine levels for exposure classification (Whincup et al., 2004). The 20 year study included 4729 men in the UK who provided baseline blood samples in 1978 to 1980. A consistent association was not found between serum cotinine concentration and stroke.

Respiratory disease

Exposure to SHS has been explored as a contributing factor

to respiratory morbidity in general, including respiratory symptoms and reduction of lung function, and also as a factor causing and exacerbating both chronic obstructive pulmonary disease (COPD) and asthma. The effects are plausible consequences of exposure to SHS, given the evidence on active smoking and respiratory health, and knowledge of the components and toxicity of SHS. To date, a range of adverse effects has been investigated. The evidence is most consistent in showing that SHS exposure of adults may contribute to respiratory symptoms, exacerbate underlying lung disease, and slightly reduce lung function (Table 2.1).

Secondhand smoke (SHS) and cancer

Historical perspective

The health effects of active smoking and the carcinogenicity of tobacco smoke became a focus of research in the first decades of the 20th century, as the first indications of the emerging lung cancer epidemic were identified. By the 1950s, substantial epidemiological and experimental research was in progress, leading to the conclusion in the 1960s that active smoking was a cause of lung cancer (Royal College of Physicians of London, 1962; U.S. Department of Health Education and Welfare, 1964). IARC published its first monograph on tobacco smoking in 1986 (IARC, 1986).

The potential for tobacco smoke inhaled by nonsmokers to cause disease was first considered in the US Surgeon General's report in 1972 (U.S. Department of Health Education and Welfare, 1972). That report reviewed the evidence on components of tobacco smoke in enclosed spaces and commented on the potential for inhaled pollutants from cigarette smoke to cause disease. Beginning in the late 1960s, epidemiological research addressed adverse effects of smoking in the home on the health of children. In 1981, published reports from Japan (Hirayama, 1981) and Greece (Trichopoulos et al., 1981) indicated increased lung cancer risk in nonsmoking women married to cigarette smokers. These reports sparked a wave of additional epidemiological studies on lung cancer, as well as studies on exposure to SHS, using biomarkers and measurement of tobacco smoke components in indoor air.

By 1986, the evidence had mounted, and three reports published in that year concluded that SHS was a cause of lung cancer. In its Monograph 38, IARC concluded that "passive smoking gives rise to some risk of cancer" (IARC, 1986). The IARC Working Group supported this conclusion on the basis of the characteristics of sidestream and mainstream smoke, the absorption of tobacco smoke materials during involuntary smoking, and the nature of dose-response relationships for carcinogenesis. In the same year, a US National Research Council (NRC) committee (National Research Council, 1986) and the US Surgeon General (U.S. Department of Health and Human Services, 1986) also concluded that involuntary smoking increases the incidence of lung cancer in nonsmokers. In reaching this conclusion, the NRC cited the biological plausibility of the ass-

ociation between exposure to SHS and lung cancer and the supporting epidemiological evidence (National Research Council, 1986). Based on a meta-analysis of the epidemiological data adjusted for bias, the report concluded that the best estimate for the excess risk of lung cancer in nonsmokers married to smokers was 25%. The 1986 report of the US Surgeon General also characterised involuntary smoking as a cause of lung cancer in nonsmokers (U.S. Department of Health and Human Services, 1986). This conclusion was based on the extensive information already available on the carcinogenicity of active smoking, on the qualitative similarities between SHS and mainstream smoke, and on the epidemiological data on involuntary smoking.

Subsequently, the many further epidemiological studies on SHS and lung cancer have better characterised the quantitative risk associated with SHS, and refined understanding of the doses of carcinogens received by nonsmokers who inhale it. Many additional agencies have now concluded that SHS causes lung cancer and other diseases; adverse health effects have also been causally associated with SHS (Table 2.1). The last IARC review on the topic of SHS and cancer was in its Monograph 83, Tobacco Smoke and Involuntary Smoking, based on a Working Group that convened in 2002 (IARC, 2004). The list of cancers investigated for association with SHS is now lengthy, with reports covering many of the cancers caused by active smoking, breast cancer, and childhood cancers. The considerations around biological plausibility of a causal association of

SHS exposure with these cancers, reflect either local deposition of tobacco smoke components and metabolites (sinonasal cancer and gastrointestinal cancers) or their systemic distribution (cancers of the breast, bladder, pancreas, brain, liver, and ovary, and leukemias and lymphomas).

These conclusions on SHS and disease risk have had substantial impact, providing a strong rationale for making public and workplaces smoke-free. The significance of this research, and the related conclusions, have motivated widespread efforts by the multinational tobacco companies to discredit the scientific evidence on SHS and disease, particularly the findings of epidemiological studies (Brandt, 2007). These efforts have now been documented through reviews of the industry's internal documents, and these tactics were one element of the successful litigation in the USA against the industry, which was found guilty of fraud and racketeering (Kessler, 2006).

Prior reviews and methods for this review

The evidence on SHS and cancer has been serially reviewed. Reports have been prepared by various agencies including most recently IARC in 2002 (IARC, 2004), the California Environmental Protection Agency in 2005 (California Environmental Protection Agency: Air Resources Board, 2005), and the US Surgeon General in 2006 (U.S. Department of Health and Human Services, 2006). Additionally, reports in peer-reviewed literature have addressed the topic (Johnson, 2005; Taylor et al., 2007). In preparing the evidence tables for this chapter, these reports provided a starting point for identifying those studies that should be considered. Additionally, literature searches were updated using search strategies described below. Quantitative summaries of the evidence were prepared when the data were sufficiently abundant and with adequate homogeneity of methodology and reporting of findings. The method of DerSimonian and Laird was employed for this pooling, using the statistical package Stata (DerSimonian & Laird, 1986).

Three major reports were the starting point for the literature review on cancer: 1) *The Health Consequences of Involuntary Exposure to Tobacco Smoke: A Report of the Surgeon General* (U.S. Department of Health and Human Services, 2006), 2) *Proposed Identification of ETS as a Toxic Air Contaminant* (California Environmental Protection Agency: Air Resources Board, 2005), and 3) *IARC Monograph 83: Tobacco Smoke and Involuntary Smoking* (IARC, 2004). The literature on SHS and cancer contained in these reports was systematically updated. A computerised literature search of the electronic PubMed database was conducted through December 31, 2007, without time or language restrictions. A keyword search was performed on tobacco smoke pollution, secondhand smoking, passive smoking, household smoking, involuntary smoking, and environmental tobacco smoke, in combination with cancer-related keywords. These keywords included cancer, adenocarcinoma, lymphoma, leukemia, childhood, glioma, menin-gioma, brain, head, neck, oral, nasal sinus, nasopharyngeal, esophageal, lung, breast, kidney, stomach, gastrointestinal, liver, pancreas, colon, colorectal, rectal, bladder, ovarian, prostate, and cervical cancer. Identified studies were screened and bibliographies were examined for related articles. Finally, publications of authors focusing on the field of smoking and cancer were searched. The identified articles were abstracted in a uniform fashion. Data from never smokers were presented in preference to data from current or former smokers. When available, adjusted relative risks were abstracted rather than crude results.

Adult cancers

Lung cancer

Overview

In numerous prior reports, including IARC Monograph 83, the conclusion has been reached that SHS causes lung cancer in people who have never actively smoked (Table 2.1). The evidence has been found sufficient to infer causality based on the extensive evidence showing that active smoking causes lung cancer, the biological plausibility of a causal association of SHS with cancer risk, and the consistency of the epidemiological findings. Alternative explanations to causation, particularly confounding and information bias, have been repeatedly scrutinised and rejected.

A causal association of involuntary smoking with lung cancer derives biological plausibility from the presence of carcinogens in SHS and the lack of a documented threshold dose for respiratory carcinogens in active smokers (U.S. Department of Health and Human Services, 1982, 1986, 2004; IARC, 1986). Moreover, genotoxic activity has been demonstrated for many components of SHS (Claxton *et al.*, 1989; Lofroth, 1989; Weiss, 1989; Bennett *et al.*, 1999; DeMarini, 2004). Experimental and real-world exposures of nonsmokers to SHS leads to their excreting 4-(N-methylnitrosamino)-1-(3-pyridyl)-1-butanol (NNAL), a tobacco-specific carcinogen, in their urine (Carmella *et al.*, 2003; Hecht, 2003). Nonsmokers exposed to SHS also have increased concentrations of adducts of tobacco-related carcinogens (Maclure *et al.*, 1989; Crawford *et al.*, 1994). Additionally, using an animal model, researchers found that whole-body exposure in rats to cigarette smoke increases the risk of neoplastic proliferative lung lesions and induces lung cancer (Mauderly *et al.*, 2004).

Time trends of lung cancer mortality in nonsmokers have been examined, with the rationale that temporally increasing exposure to SHS should be paralleled by increasing mortality rates (Enstrom, 1979; Garfinkel, 1981). These data provide only indirect evidence on the lung cancer risk associated with involuntary exposure to tobacco smoke. Epidemiologists have directly tested the association between lung cancer and involuntary smoking utilising conventional designs: case-control and cohort studies. These studies not only provide evidence relevant to causation, but also provide the characterisation of the risk that is needed to quantify the burden of lung cancer associated with SHS.

The epidemiological studies have primarily used self- or surrogate-report of exposure as the key indicator. Marriage to a smoker, particularly for women, has been the most frequently used exposure indicator. Methodological investigations suggest that accurate information can be obtained by interview in an epidemiological study on the smoking habits of a spouse (i.e. never or ever smoker) (Pron *et al.*, 1988; Coultas *et al.*, 1989; Cummings *et al.*, 1989; Lubin, 1999). However, information concerning quantitative aspects of the spouse's smoking is reported with less accuracy. Misclassification of current or former smokers as never smokers may introduce a positive bias, because of the concordance of spouse smoking habits (Lee, 1998). The extent to which this bias explains the numerous reports of association between spousal smoking and lung cancer has been addressed; findings indicate that bias does not account for the observed association (Wald *et al.*, 1986; Lee, 1988; U.S. Environmental Protection Agency, 1992; Wu, 1999; U.S. Department of Health and Human Services, 2006).

In some countries, including the USA, smoking prevalence now varies markedly with indicators of income and education, more recently tending to rise sharply with decreasing level of education and income (U.S. Department of Health and Human Services, 1989, 2004). In general, exposure to SHS follows a similar trend, and critics of the findings on SHS and lung cancer have argued that uncontrolled confounding by lifestyle, occupation, or other factors may explain the association. In fact, data for the USA do indicate a generally

less healthy lifestyle in those with greater SHS exposure (Matanoski *et al.*, 1995). However, other than a few occupational exposures at high levels, as well as indoor radon, risk factors for lung cancer in never smokers that might confound the SHS association cannot be proffered, and the relevance to past studies of these current associations of potential confounders with SHS exposure is uncertain.

Epidemiological evidence

The first major studies on SHS and lung cancer were reported in 1981. Hirayama's early report (Hirayama, 1981) was based on a prospective cohort study of 91 540 nonsmoking women in Japan. Standardised mortality ratios (SMRs) for lung cancer increased significantly with the amount smoked by the husbands. The findings could not be explained by confounding factors and were unchanged when follow-up of the study group was extended (Hirayama, 1984). Based on the same cohort, significantly increased risk was reported for nonsmoking men married to wives smoking 1-19 cigarettes and ≥20 cigarettes daily (Hirayama, 1984). In 1981, increased lung cancer risk in nonsmoking women married to cigarette smokers was reported (Trichopoulos *et al.*, 1981). These investigators conducted a case-control study in Athens, Greece, which included cases with a final diagnosis of lung cancer other than adenocarcinoma or terminal bronchial carcinoma, and controls from the Hospital for Orthopedic Disorders. The positive findings reported in 1981 were unchanged with subsequent expansion of the study population (Trichopoulos et al., 1983).

Subsequently, numerous case-control and cohort studies have addressed SHS and lung cancer. Among the additional studies, a US multicenter study merits specific discussion because of its size (651 cases and 1253 controls), and its methodology, which addressed the extant criticisms at the time of its being conducted (Fontham et al., 1994). The study found a significant increase in overall relative risk for nonsmoking women married to smokers (odds ratio (OR)=1.26; 95% CI=1.04-1.54). Significant risk was also associated with occupational exposure to SHS.

Beginning with the 1986 NRC report, there have been periodic meta-analyses of the evidence on SHS and lung cancer. One of the first comprehensive meta-analyses was carried out by the US Environmental Protection Agency for its 1992 risk assessment (U.S. Environmental Protection Agency, 1992). A meta-analysis of the 31 studies published to that time was central in the Agency's decision to classify SHS as a Group A carcinogen - namely a known human carcinogen. The meta-analysis considered the data from the epidemiologic studies by tiers of study quality and location and used an adjustment method for misclassification of smokers as never smokers. Overall, the analysis found a significantly increased risk of lung cancer in never smoking women married to smoking men; for the studies conducted in the USA, the estimated relative risk was 1.19 (90% CI=1.04-1.35).

In 1997, a comprehensive meta-analysis was carried out which included 37 published studies (Hackshaw et al., 1997). An excess risk of lung cancer was estimated for nonsmokers married to smokers as 24% (95% CI=13-36%). Adjustment for potential bias and confounding by diet did not alter the estimate. This meta-analysis was part of the basis for the conclusion by the UK Scientific Committee on Tobacco and Health that SHS is a cause of lung cancer (Scientific Committee on Tobacco and Health, 1998). A subsequent IARC meta-analysis (IARC, 2004) including 46 studies and 6257 cases, yielded similar results: 24% (95% CI=14-34%). Incorporating the results from a cohort study with null results overall, but only 177 cases (Enstrom & Kabat, 2003), did not change the findings (Hackshaw, 2003).

The most recent summaries from the 2006 Surgeon General's report are provided in Table 2.2. The summary estimates continue to show an excess risk of around 20% (e.g. pooled relative risk estimates around 1.2) for nonsmokers married to smokers. There is not strong evidence for heterogeneity by gender or location. Workplace exposure is also associated with increased risk. The evidence is less convincing for childhood exposure.

Several other recent meta-analyses further quantify the association between SHS and lung cancer. A meta-analysis of 22 studies published through 2003 on workplace SHS exposure and lung cancer was performed (Stayner et al., 2007). The pooled relative risk (RR) was 1.24 (95% CI=1.18-1.29) associated with exposure to workplace SHS. Among highly exposed workers, the RR was 2.01 (95% CI=1.33-2.60). Another meta-analysis was carried out to calculate a pooled estimate of RR of lung cancer associated with exposure to SHS in never smoking women exposed to smoking spouses (Taylor et al., 2007). Using 55 studies (seven cohort, 25 population-based case-control, and 23 non-population-based case-control studies) published through 2006, the authors found a pooled RR for lung cancer associated with SHS from spouses of 1.27 (95% CI=1.17-1.37). For North America the RR was 1.15 (95% CI=1.03-1.28), for Asia, 1.31 (95% CI=1.16-1.48) and for Europe, 1.31 (95% CI=1.24-1.52).

Since the two meta-analyses above and the 2006 Surgeon General's report on SHS, two new case-control studies have been published that confirm the association between SHS and lung cancer. A multicenter, population-based case-control study in Mexico City was conducted. For males and females combined, the OR for lung cancer associated with SHS exposure at home was 1.8 (95% CI=1.3-2.6) after adjusting for age, sex, educational level, and access to social security (Franco-Marina et al., 2006). Among male and female never smokers, the crude OR for lung cancer associated with SHS exposure at home was 1.8 (95% CI=1.1-3.0) (Franco-Marina, 2008). A study in never smoking Chinese women aged 18-70 years, included cases diagnosed with lung cancer from hospitals in Beijing, Shanghai, and Chengdu, and population controls matched for age and sex (Fang et al., 2006). The OR for lung cancer associated with >50 person-years of exposure to SHS from home or work was 1.77 (95% CI=1.07-2.92).

Table 2.2 Quantitative estimate of the risk of lung cancer with differing sources of exposure to secondhand smoke (adapted from U.S. Department of Health and Human Services, 2006)

Study	Data source	Exposure vs. Referent	RR	95% CI
Hackshaw *et al.*, 1997	37 studies	Smoking vs. nonsmoking spouse	1.24	1.13-1.36
IARC, 2004	38 studies	Smoking vs. nonsmoking husband	1.23	1.13-1.34
US Surgeon General, 2006	Case-control (44 studies)	Smoking vs. nonsmoking spouse	1.21	1.13-1.30
Spouse	Cohort (8 studies)	Smoking vs. nonsmoking spouse	1.29	1.12-1.49
54 studies	Men	Smoking vs. nonsmoking wife	1.37	1.05-1.79
	Women	Smoking vs. nonsmoking husband	1.22	1.13-1.31
	USA and Canada	Smoking vs. nonsmoking spouse	1.15	1.04-1.26
	Europe	Smoking vs. nonsmoking spouse	1.16	1.03-1.30
	Asia	Smoking vs. nonsmoking spouse	1.43	1.24-1.66
US Surgeon General, 2006	Nonsmokers (25 studies)	Workplace SHS vs. not	1.22	1.13-1.33
Workplace	Nonsmoking Men (11 studies)	Workplace SHS vs. not	1.12	0.86-1.50
25 studies	Nonsmoking Women (25 studies)	Workplace SHS vs. not	1.22	1.10-1.35
	Nonsmokers USA & Canada (8 studies)	Workplace SHS vs. not	1.24	1.03-1.49
	Nonsmokers Europe (7 studies)	Workplace SHS vs. not	1.13	0.96-1.34
	Nonsmokers Asia (10 studies)	Workplace SHS vs. not	1.32	1.13-1.55
US Surgeon General, 2006	Men and Women	Maternal smoking	1.15	0.86-1.52
Childhood	Men and Women	Paternal smoking	1.10	0.89-1.36
24 studies	Men and Women	Either parent smoking	1.11	0.94-1.31
	Women	Maternal smoking	1.28	0.93-1.78
	Women	Paternal smoking	1.17	0.91-1.50
	USA (8 studies)	Either parent smoking	0.93	0.81-1.07
	Europe (6 studies)	Either parent smoking	0.81	0.71-0.92
	Asia (10 studies)	Either parent smoking	1.59	1.18-2.15

Three prospective cohort studies examining the relationship between SHS in nonsmokers have also been published since the meta-analyses by Taylor *et al.* (2007) and Stayner *et al.* (2007). Most recently, in Japan, a population-based cohort study of 28 414 lifelong nonsmoking women aged 40-69 years was conducted, collecting information on exposures from spousal smoking, workplace exposure, and childhood exposure (Kurahashi *et al.*, 2008). The hazard ratio (HR) for all lung cancer types associated with living with a smoking husband was 1.34 (95% CI=0.81-2.21). The HR for adenocarcinoma associated with living with a smoking husband was significantly elevated at 2.03 (95% CI=1.07-3.86). For all lung cancer types, the HR associated with SHS in the workplace was 1.32 (95% CI=0.85-2.04), while the HR specifically for adenocarcinoma associated with SHS in the workplace was 1.93 (95% CI=0.88-4.23).

A cohort study in 10 European countries in the European Prospective Investigation into Cancer and Nutrition (EPIC) was conducted to examine the relationships of SHS and air pollution with lung cancer (Vineis *et al.*, 2007). It was found that among never smokers, the HR of lung cancer for SHS exposure at home or work was 1.05 (95% CI=0.60-1.82); at home: 0.84 (95% CI=0.38-1.9), at work: 1.28 (95% CI=0.67-2.4) (Vineis, 2008).

Also examined was the association between household exposure to SHS and lung cancer mortality in two cohorts of New Zealand lifelong nonsmokers aged 45-77 years, by linking census records, which included smoking information, to mortality records (Hill

et al., 2007). The age and ethnicity standardised RR for mortality from lung cancer associated with home exposure to SHS was 1.00 (95% CI=0.49-2.01) in the 1981-1984 cohort and 1.16 (95% CI=0.70-1.92) in the 1996-1999 cohort.

For this chapter, the prior meta-analyses were not updated with these new estimates, as the existing estimates are based on an already substantial body of research; they are robust to additional data and IARC has already concluded that passive smoking causes cancer.

The extent of the lung cancer burden associated with involuntary smoking remains subject to some uncertainty, but estimates have been made that are useful indications of the magnitude of the disease risk (U.S. Department of Health and Human Services, 1986; Weiss, 1986; California Environmental Protection Agency : Air Resources Board, 2005). In 1990, researchers reviewed the risk assessments of lung cancer and passive smoking and estimated the numbers of lung cancer cases in US nonsmokers attributable to passive smoking (Repace & Lowrey, 1990). The range of the nine estimates, covering both never smokers and former smokers, was from 58 to 8124 lung cancer deaths for the year 1988, with an overall mean of 4500 or 5000 excluding the lowest estimate of 58. The 1992 estimate of the California EPA, based on the epidemiologic data, was about 3000, including approximately 1500 and 500 deaths in never smoking women and men, respectively, and about 1000 in long-term former smokers of both sexes (U.S. Environmental Protection Agency, 1992). The California EPA

estimated that at least 3423, and perhaps as many as 8866, lung cancer deaths were caused by SHS in the USA (California Environmental Protection Agency: Air Resources Board, 2005). These calculations illustrate that passive smoking must be considered an important cause of lung cancer death from a public health perspective; exposure is involuntary and not subject to control.

Bladder cancer

The US Surgeon General (U.S. Department of Health and Human Services, 2006), California EPA (California Environmental Protection Agency: Air Resources Board, 2005), and IARC (2004) reports did not address cancer of the bladder. The literature search for this chapter identified nine studies with information on the association between exposure to SHS and bladder cancer (Tables 2.3a,b) with cases identified between 1963 and 2004. A meta-analysis of these studies was conducted to obtain a pooled estimate of risk for bladder cancer associated with exposure to SHS. Since several studies presented risk estimates stratified by mutually exclusive exposure categories (Burch *et al.*, 1989; Zeegers *et al.*, 2002; Chen *et al.*, 2005; Samanic *et al.*, 2006), the Working Group pooled these estimates using random effects meta-analysis. Risk estimates were then pooled across studies using random effects meta-analysis (Figure 2.1). The most comprehensive exposure from each study was used in calculating the combined risk estimate of 0.97 (95% CI=0.74-1.28, *p for heterogeneity*=0.153). Neither

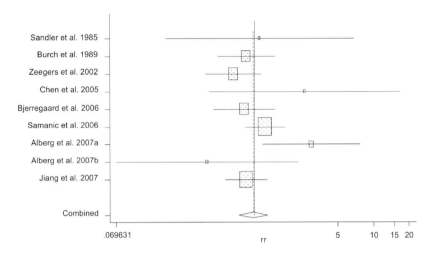

Figure 2.1 **Pooled risk estimates from random effects meta-analysis of exposure to SHS and bladder cancer**

Alberg et al., 2007a and 2007b refer to estimates from the 1963 and 1975 cohorts respectively. All data included in the reference Alberg et al., 2007

Sandler et al., 1985 refers to estimates cited in the reference Sandler et al., 1985a

cases and 202 controls matched on age and sex were examined (Phillips *et al.*, 2005). Among never smokers, exposure to SHS from smoking by a spouse was associated with a significantly increased risk of intracranial meningioma (OR=2.0; 95% CI=1.1-3.5). Risk increased with increasing years of exposure (*p for trend*=0.02). Neither exposure to SHS from another household member nor exposure at work was associated with risk, with ORs of 0.7 (95% CI=0.4-1.1) and 0.7 (95% CI=0.4-1.2), respectively (Tables 2.4a,b).

Breast cancer

In considering whether passive smoking causes breast cancer, the evidence for active smoking needs to be considered in assessing the plausibility of an association of breast cancer risk with SHS in nonsmokers. There is some evidence to suggest that an association between tobacco smoke and breast cancer is biologically plausible. Studies have shown that carcinogens in tobacco smoke reach breast tissue (Petrakis *et al.*, 1978, 1988 ; Li *et al.*, 1996) and are mammary mutagens (Nagao *et al.*, 1994; Dunnick *et al.*, 1995; el-Bayoumy *et al.*, 1995). However, other studies using biomarkers have found an association between smoking and decreased levels of estrogen (MacMahon *et al.*, 1982 ; Michnovicz *et al.*, 1986), which implies that active smoking might decrease the risk of breast cancer.

the Begg's nor Egger's tests indicated publication bias with p-values of 0.602 and 0.654, respectively.

Brain cancer

The California EPA report on SHS in 2005 reviewed the previous literature regarding the association between SHS exposure and brain cancer in adults; four studies were considered. In the first published study, brain tumor mortality in a large scale cohort of nonsmoking married women in Japan was examined (Hirayama, 1984). It was reported that the rate ratio (RR) of death from brain cancer was increased among women with smoking husbands when compared to women who were married to nonsmokers. For

a husband's consumption of 1-14 cigarettes/day the RR was 3.03 (90% CI=1.07-8.58), for 15-19 cigarettes/day the RR was 6.25 (90% CI=2.01-19.43), and the RR was 4.23 (90% CI=1.53-12.19) for 20+ cigarettes/day. However, there were only 34 cases of death from brain cancer. The 2005 California EPA report concluded that the epidemiological evidence for an association between SHS and risk of brain tumors was weak and inadequately researched, the same conclusion reached earlier in the 1997 California EPA report on SHS. Since the 2005 California EPA report, only one new report was identified. Associations between SHS exposure and the risk of intracranial meningioma in a population-based case-control study that included 95

Table 2.3a Exposure to SHS and bladder cancer - Cohort studies

Reference, location, period	Cohort description	Exposure assessment	Exposure categories	Relative risk (95% CI)	Adjustment for potential confounders	Comments
Zeegers et al., 2002 The Netherlands 1986-1992	3346 adults 55-69 years at enrollment (619 microscopically confirmed incident carcinomas of the urinary bladder, ureters, or urethra); 6.3 years of follow-up with no subjects lost	Self-administered questionnaire	Never-smoking partner (adulthood)	1	Age and gender	Results for never smokers
			Ex-smoking partner (adulthood)	0.95 (0.46-2.0)		
			Current-smoking partner (adulthood)	0.74 (0.29-1.9)		
			Parents did not smoke (childhood)	1		
			Parents smoked (childhood)	1.2 (0.56-2.4)		
			Low exposure to SHS at work (adulthood)	1		
			High exposure to SHS at work (adulthood)	1.4 (0.70-2.6)		
			No exposure to SHS at home or at work (adulthood)	1		
			1 to <3 hours per day of exposure to SHS at home or work (adulthood exposure)	0.69 (0.33-1.4)		
			3+ hours per day of exposure to SHS at home or work (adulthood exposure)	0.64 (0.29-1.4)		
Bjerregaard et al., 2006 Denmark, France, Sweden 1991-2004	126 908 adults 25-70 years at enrollment (115 cases of primary bladder cancer in never smokers); average follow-up time was 6.3 years	Self- and interviewer-administered questionnaire	No SHS exposure (at baseline) at home and/or work	1	Fruit and vegetable intake, SHS exposure in childhood	Results for never smokers
			SHS exposure (at baseline) at home and/or work (adulthood exposure)	0.82 (0.46-1.48)		
			No SHS exposure during childhood	1		
			SHS exposure during childhood (from parents or others)	2.02 (0.94-4.35)		

Reference, location, period	Cohort description	Exposure assessment	Exposure categories	Relative risk (95% CI)	Adjustment for potential confounders	Comments
Alberg et al., 2007 Maryland, USA 1963–1978 cohort	24 823 never smoking women, aged ≥ 25 years at enrollment with no prior cancer (23 cases of invasive bladder cancer)	Self-administered questionnaire	Never smokers with noncurrent SHS exposure in the home	1	Age, education, marital status	Results for never smokers
			Current SHS exposure in the home (any source)	2.3 (1.0–5.4)		
			Former SHS exposure in the home (any source)	0.3 (0.1–2.5)		
			Current SHS exposure in the home (any source)	1.8 (0.8–4.5)		
			Exposed to SHS in the home from spouse only	1.1 (0.3–3.8)		
			Exposed to SHS in the home from other (than spouse) household members only	3.0 (1.2–7.9)		
Alberg et al., 2007 Maryland, USA 1975–1994 cohort	26 381 women, aged ≥ 25 years at enrollment with no prior cancer (30 cases of invasive bladder cancer)	Self-administered questionnaire	Never smokers with noncurrent SHS exposure in the home	1	Age, education, marital status	Results for never smokers
			Current SHS exposure in the home (any source)	0.9 (0.4–2.3)		
			Former SHS exposure in the home (any source)	0.8 (0.3–2.0)		
			Current SHS exposure in the home (any source)	0.9 (0.3–2.2)		
			Exposed to SHS in the home from spouse only	1.2 (0.4–3.6)		
			Exposed to SHS in the home from other (than spouse) household members only	0.4 (0.1–3.3)		

Table 2.3b Exposure to SHS and bladder cancer - Case-control studies

Reference, location, period	Characteristics of cases	Characteristics of controls	Exposure assessment	Exposure categories	Relative risk (95% CI)	Adjustment for potential confounders	Comments
Sandler *et al.*, 1985a North Carolina, USA 1979-1981	6 patients 15-59 years with cancer of the urinary tract; 40% response rate	489 friend and community controls individually matched on gender, age, and race; 75% response rate	Self-administered questionnaire	Nonsmoking spouse or never married	1	Age and education	Only married individuals were eligible to be considered "exposed"
				Spouse smoked regularly (at least 1 cig/day for at least 6 months) any time during marriage	1.1 (0.2-7.6)		
Sandler *et al*, 1985b North Carolina, USA 1979-1981	5 patients 15-59 years with cancer of the urinary tract; 70% response rate	438 friend and community controls individually matched on gender, age, and race; control response rate not stated	Self-administered questionnaire	Not exposed to SHS from father during first 10 yrs of life	1		None of the bladder cancer cases were exposed to SHS from the mother
				SHS exposure from father during first 10 yrs of life	0.8 (0.1-5.7)		
Burch *et al.*, 1989 Alberta and Ontario, Canada 1979-1982	826 adults 35-79 years with primary bladder cancer without recurrent malignant neoplasms of the bladder or invasion of the bladder from primary prostatic cancer; 67% response rate	826 population controls individually matched for age, gender, and area of residence; 53% response rate	Interviewer-administered questionnaire	**Among nonsmokers:** No SHS exposure at home	1		
				Males: exposure at home	0.94 (0.45-1.95)		
				Females: exposure at home	0.75 (0.33-1.71)		
				No SHS exposure at work	1		
				Males: exposure at home	0.97 (0.50-1.91)		
				Females: exposure at home	0.93 (0.48-1.79)		
Chen *et al.*, 2005 Taiwan 1996-1999	14 adults ≥50 years with newly diagnosed bladder cancer	202 hospital controls (fracture and cataract patients) ≥50 years	Interviewer-administered questionnaire	**Men:** No SHS exposure	1	Age, BMI, cumulative arsenic, hair dye usage, education	Interaction present for arsenic measured by secondary methylation index Results among nonsmokers presented
				SHS exposure	7.16 (1.87-27.4)		
				Women: No SHS exposure	1		
				SHS exposure	1.09 (0.42-2.80)		

Reference, location, period	Characteristics of cases	Characteristics of controls	Exposure assessment	Exposure categories	Relative risk (95% CI)	Adjustment for potential confounders	Comments
Samanic et al., 2006 Spain 1998-2000	1219 White adults aged 21-80 years with incident bladder cancer without previous cancer of the lower urinary tract, or patients with bladder tumors secondary to other malignancies; 84% response rate	1271 hospital controls (with conditions considered unrelated to smoking), individually matched on age, gender, race, and hospital; 88% response rate	Interviewer-administered questionnaire	**Men:** No childhood SHS	1	Age, hospital region, fruit or vegetable consumption, and high-risk occupation	Sum of the years spent at each childhood residence up to age 18
				<18 yrs SHS exposure	1.2 (0.6-2.3)		
				18 yrs SHS exposure	0.9 (0.3-2.6)		
				No residential adulthood SHS	1	*p for trend*= 0.92	Sum of the years spent at each adult residence times N of smokers per / res.
				>0 to 26 person-yrs of adulthood residential SHS	1.1 (0.5-2.4)		
				>26 to 54 person-yrs of adulthood residential SHS	0.8 (0.3-2.2)		
				>54 person-yrs of residential adulthood SHS	1.3 (0.5-3.2)		
				p for trend	0.74		
				No occupational adulthood SHS	1		Sum of the years spent at each job times N of smokers per job
				>0 to 135 person-yrs of occupational adulthood SHS	0.6 (0.2-1.6)		
				>135 to 240 person-yrs of occupational adulthood SHS	0.2 (0.1-0.7)		
				>240 person-yrs of occpationaladulthood SHS	0.6 (0.2-1.4)		
				p for trend	0.58		
				Women: No childhood SHS	1		
				<18 yrs childhood SHS	0.7 (0.3-1.4)		
				18 yrs childhood SHS	0.6 (0.2-1.7)		
				p for trend	0.24		
				No residential adulthood SHS	1		
				>0 to 26 person-yrs of residential adulthood SHS	2.2 (0.8-6.2)		

Table 2.3b Exposure to SHS and bladder cancer - Case-control studies

Reference, location, period	Characteristics of cases	Characteristics of controls	Exposure assessment	Exposure categories	Relative risk (95% CI)	Adjustment for potential confounders	Comments
Samanic *et al.*, 2006 Spain 1998-2000				>26 to 54 person-yrs of residential adulthood SHS	1.9 (0.7-4.8)		
				>54 person-yrs of residential adulthood SHS	0.8 (0.3-1.9)		
				p for trend	0.27		
				No occupational adulthood SHS	1		
				>0 to 135 occupational person-yrs of adulthood SHS	1.7 (0.7-4.0)		
				>135 to 240 person-yrs of occupational adulthood SHS	1.7 (0.6-4.4)		
				>240 person-yrs of occupational adulthood SHS	3.3 (1.1-9.5)		
				p for trend	0.03		
Jiang *et al.*, 2007 California, USA 1987-1999	148 never smoking Asian adults aged 25-64 years, with histologically-confirmed bladder cancer; 89.7% response rate	292 never smoking population controls, matched for age, gender, race, and area of residence; 96.4% response rate	Interviewer-administered questionnaire	**No SHS exposure during childhood**	1	Age, gender, race, education, adulthood SHS	Confidence intervals not provided
				SHS exposure during childhood	0.91		
				SHS exposure during childhood (1 smoker)	0.88		
				SHS exposure during childhood (>1 smoker)	0.97		
				No SHS exposure during adulthood in a domestic setting	1	Age, gender, education, childhood SHS, adulthood SHS (occupational and social settings)	
				SHS exposure during adulthood (domestic setting)	0.85		
				SHS exposure during adulthood (domestic setting, <10 yrs)	0.88		

Reference, location, period	Characteristics of cases	Characteristics of controls	Exposure assessment	Exposure categories	Relative risk (95% CI)	Adjustment for potential confounders	Comments
Jiang et al., 2007 California, USA 1987-1999				SHS exposure during adulthood (domestic setting, ≥10 yrs)	0.82		
				No SHS exposure during adulthood in an occupational setting	1	Age, gender, education, childhood SHS, adulthood SHS (domestic and social settings)	
				SHS exposure during adulthood (occupational setting)	0.98		
				SHS exposure during adulthood (occupational setting, <10 yrs)	0.93		
				SHS exposure during adulthood (occupational setting, ≥10 yrs)	0.98		
				No SHS exposure during adulthood in a social setting	1	Age, gender, education, childhood SHS, adulthood SHS (domestic and occupational settings)	
				SHS exposure during adulthood (social setting)	1.06		
				SHS exposure during adulthood (social setting, <10 yrs)	1.29		
				SHS exposure during adulthood (social setting, ≥10 yrs)	0.92		
				Low (0) cumulative index of SHS exposure	1	Age, gender, education	
				Intermediate (1-3) cumulative index of SHS exposure	1.61		
				High (4-8) cumulative index of SHS exposure	1.28		

Table 2.4a Exposure to SHS and brain cancer - Cohort studies

Reference, location, period	Cohort description	Exposure assessment	Exposure categories	Relative risk (90% CI)	Adjustment for potential confounders	Comments
Hirayama, 1984 Japan 1966-1981	91 540 nonsmoking, married women ≥40 years (34 deaths due to brain tumors)	Interviewer-administered questionnaire	Nonsmoking husband	1	Husband's age	Same data used in Hirayama, 1985
			Husband smokes 1-14 cig/day	3.03 (1.07-8.58)		
			Husband smokes 15-19 cig/day	6.25 (2.01-19.43)		
			Husband smokes ≥20 cig/day	4.32 (1.53-12.19)		
Hirayama, 1985 Japan 1966-1981	91 540 nonsmoking, married women ≥40 years (34 deaths due to brain tumors)	Interviewer-administered questionnaire	Nonsmoking husband	1	Husband's age	Same data used in Hirayama, 1984
			Husband is ex-smoker or smokes 1-19 cig/day	3.28 (1.21-8.92)		
			Husband smokes ≥20 cig/day	4.92 (1.72-14.11)		

Table 2.4b Exposure to SHS and brain cancer in adults - Case-control studies

Reference, location, period	Characteristics of cases	Characteristics of controls	Exposure assessment	Exposure categories	Relative risk (95% CI)	Adjustment for potential confounders	Comments
Sandler et al., 1985a North Carolina, USA 1979-1981	38 patients 15-59 years with eye, brain, and other nervous system cancers; 66% response rate	489 friend and community controls; 75% response rate	Self-administered questionnaire	Non exposed to SHS	1	Age, sex, active smoking	Smoking wives included
				Spouse smoked regularly (at least 1 cig/day for at least 6 months) any time during marriage	0.7 (0.3-1.5)		
Ryan et al., 1992 Australia 1987-1990	170 adults 25-74 years with newly diagnosed cancer of the brain and meninges (110 glioma cases and 60 meningioma cases); 90.5% response rate	417 community controls, frequency matched on age, gender, and postal code; 63.3% response rate	Interviewer-administered questionnaire		RR (95% CI) for glioma	Age, sex, active smoking	Active smokers included
				Non exposed to SHS	1		
				Ever exposed to SHS	1.24 (0.76-2.00)		
				1-12 yrs SHS exposure	1.33 (0.69-2.56)		
				13-27 yrs SHS exposure	1.17 (0.60-2.27)		
				28+ yrs SHS exposure	1.21 (0.62-2.37)		
				Nonsmokers, ever exposed to SHS	1.30 (0.62-2.7)		

Reference, location, period	Characteristics of cases	Characteristics of controls	Exposure assessment	Exposure categories	Relative risk (95% CI) RR (95% CI) for meningioma	Adjustment for potential confounders	Comments
Ryan et al., 1992 Australia 1987-1990				Non exposed to SHS	1		
				Ever exposed to SHS	1.91 (1.01-3.63)		
				1-12 yrs SHS exposure	1.55 (0.66-3.65)		
				13-27 yrs SHS exposure	2.15 (0.91-6.38)		
				28+ yrs SHS exposure	2.12 (0.98-4.71)		
				Nonsmokers, ever exposed to SHS	2.45 (0.98-6.14)		
Hurley et al., 1996 Australia 1987-1991	416 histologically confirmed gliomas	422 population controls matched by age and sex	Questionnaires and interviews	Spouse does not smoke	1		Results among nonsmokers
				Living with smoker	0.97 (0.61-1.53)		
Phillips et al., 2005 Washington, USA 1995-1998	95 adult patients never smokers/haven't smoked in last 10 years with intracranial meningioma; 84% overall response rate	202 community controls, individually matched on age and sex; 55% response rate from random digit dialing and 67% response rate from Medicare eligibility lists		Spouse does not smoke	1	Conditional regression matched on age and sex and adjustment for education	
				Spouse smokes	2.0 (1.1-3.5)		
				Spouse smoked <13 yrs	1.4 (0.7-3.1)		
				Spouse smoked 13-28 yrs	2.3 (0.9-5.9)		
				Spouse smoked >28 yrs	2.7 (1.0-7.1)		
				p for trend	0.02		
				No SHS exposure at home from other household members	1		
				SHS exposure at home from other household members (not spouse)	0.7 (0.4-1.1)		
				No SHS exposure at work	1		
				SHS exposure at work	0.7 (0.4-1.2)		

The 2001 and 2004 reports of the US Surgeon General reviewed further evidence related to smoking and estrogen, finding that smoking was associated with a decreased risk of endometrial cancer and an earlier age at menopause (U.S. Department of Health and Human Services, 2001, 2004). These anti-estrogenic consequences of active smoking have been construed as implying that breast cancer risk would be reduced for active smokers in comparison with never smokers. The evidence is not consistent, however, and uncertainty remains about the effect of smoking on blood estrogen levels. These possibly opposing biological consequences of active smoking may explain why review of the epidemiologic data has found an overall null effect of active smoking on the risk of breast cancer.

Since the 1960s, there have been more than 50 studies investigating the association between active smoking and breast cancer. In 2002, a pooled analysis of data from 53 studies was conducted and found a relative risk of 0.99 (95% CI=0.92-1.05) for women who were current smokers compared with women who were lifetime nonsmokers (Hamajima et al., 2002). One possible explanation for the null results is that the anti-estrogenic effects of smoking may offset the potentially carcinogenic effects on the risk of breast cancer. Subsequently, the 2004 reports of the US Surgeon General and IARC concluded that the weight of evidence strongly suggests that there is no causal association between active smoking and breast cancer (IARC, 2004). One year later, the California EPA concluded that active smoking

is a cause of breast cancer, although it did not carry out a full, systematic review (California Environmental Protection Agency: Air Resources Board, 2005). Two cohort studies published in 2004 found a significant increase in risk of breast cancer (Al-Delaimy et al., 2004; Reynolds et al., 2004). However, the US Surgeon General concluded that sufficient evidence has not accumulated to suggest a causal association between active smoking and breast cancer (U.S. Department of Health and Human Services, 2006).

More than 20 epidemiologic studies have been published specifically addressing the association between SHS and breast cancer. Several major reports, including the IARC Monograph 83, the 2005 California EPA report, and the 2006 US Surgeon General's report, have reviewed the evidence for an association between SHS exposure and breast cancer (IARC, 2004 ; California Environmental Protection Agency: Air Resources Board, 2005 ; U.S. Department of Health and Human Services, 2006). The California EPA conducted a meta-analysis using six cohort studies and 12 case-control studies that were deemed to provide the "best evidence." They found an increased risk of 25% (95% CI=8-44%) overall, and concluded that there is sufficient evidence for a causal association among premenopausal women (California Environmental Protection Agency: Air Resources Board, 2005). Among post-menopausal women, there was no indication of an association. In 2004, IARC concluded that the evidence is inconsistent, and although some case-control studies found positive

effects, cohort studies overall did not find a causal association (IARC, 2004). Additionally, the lack of a positive dose-response relationship and association with active smoking weigh against the possibility of an increased risk of breast cancer from SHS exposure. Subsequently, the US Surgeon General came to similar conclusions (U.S. Department of Health and Human Services, 2006). Using data from seven prospective cohort studies and 14 case-control studies, a meta-analysis was performed. Sensitivity analyses showed that cohort studies overall found null results and studies that adjusted for potential confounding showed weaker associations (U.S. Department of Health and Human Services, 2006). Furthermore, the possibility of publication bias was evaluated, and found that less precise studies tended to have more positive results. Finally, after reviewing all of the evidence using the criteria for causality, the US Surgeon General's report found that overall the evidence is inconsistent and concluded that the data is suggestive, but not sufficient to infer a causal association between SHS exposure and breast cancer.

Since the 2006 US Surgeon General's report, three new case-control studies examining the association between SHS and breast cancer have been identified. A large population-based case-control study in Poland (2386 cases and 2502 controls) examining the associations between active and passive smoking and risk of breast cancer was conducted (Lissowska et al., 2006). Never smoking women ever exposed to SHS at home or at work did not have a significantly elevated risk of breast

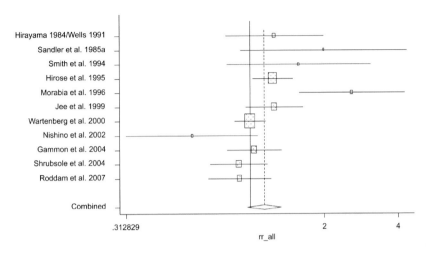

Figure 2.2a Pooled risk estimates from random effects meta-analysis of exposure to SHS from spouse and breast cancer in all women

cancer (OR=1.10; 95% CI=0.84-1.45). In addition, a trend was not observed between increasing hours/day-years of SHS and risk of breast cancer (*p for trend*=0.24) (Lissowska *et al.*, 2007). A population-based case-control study of breast cancer in women aged 36-45 years (639 cases and 640 controls) was conducted. Among never smoking women, there was no significant association between SHS exposure from a partner in the home and risk of breast cancer (RR=0.89; 95% CI=0.64-1.25). Additionally, there was not a trend with increasing duration of SHS exposure (p=0.31) and heterogeneity of the association comparing pre- and postmenopausal women (p=0.35) (Roddam *et al.*, 2007). The association between SHS and risk of breast cancer was evaluated in non-Hispanic white (NHW) and Hispanic/American Indian (HAI) women from the

Southwestern USA (1527 NHW and 798 HAI cases; 1601 NHW and 924 HAI controls) (Slattery *et al.*, 2008). Among never smokers, exposure to SHS only increased the odds of premenopausal breast cancer in HAI women (OR=2.3; 95% CI=1.2-4.5). In addition, HAI premenopausal never smoking women with the rs2069832 IL6 GG genotype exposed to ≥10 hours of SHS per week, compared to those with no SHS exposure, had over four times the odds of breast cancer (OR=4.4; 95% CI=1.5-12.8, *p for interaction*=0.01).

The meta-analysis of SHS exposure and breast cancer risk in the 2006 US Surgeon General's report on involuntary smoking, was updated for this Handbook to include the three new case-control studies identified by literature search. Since many of the studies provided risk estimates that were stratified by mutually exclusive

exposure categories, these estimates were pooled using random effects meta-analysis. Risk estimates were then also pooled across studies using random effects meta-analysis (Table 2.5; Figures 2.2a-c). Pooled estimates were calculated for three population samples: all women in a study (regardless of menopausal status), premenopausal women, and postmenopausal women. Three exposure categories were considered: spouse/partner in adulthood, adulthood work exposure, and childhood parental exposure in the home.

For all women, the updated, combined relative risk from exposure from a spouse or partner was 1.14 (95% CI=0.97-1.34, *p for heterogeneity*=0.002), slightly smaller than the US Surgeon General's report's combined estimate of 1.18 (95% CI=0.99-1.39, *p for heterogeneity*=0.002). The updated, combined estimate used the pooled (random effects) results for duration of exposure to SHS from a partner in never smoking women aged 36-45 years (RR=0.91; 95% CI=0.67-1.22) (Roddam *et al.*, 2007). The combined RR for all women from occupational SHS exposure was 1.10 (95% CI=0.88-1.38, *p for heterogeneity*=0.004), slightly larger than the US Surgeon General's report's combined estimate of 1.06 (95% CI=0.84-1.35, *p for heterogeneity*=0.008). No new data were available for updating estimates for childhood parental SHS exposures since the 2006 US Surgeon General's report. The Begg's and Egger's tests provided evidence for publication bias in studies among all women for occupational SHS exposure during adulthood.

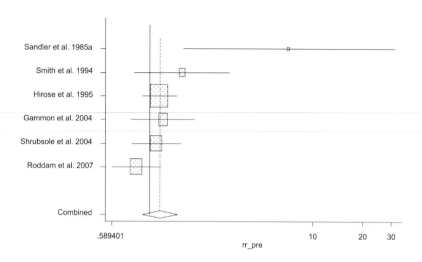

Figure 2.2b Pooled risk estimates from random effects meta-analysis of exposure to SHS from spouse and breast cancer in premenopausal women

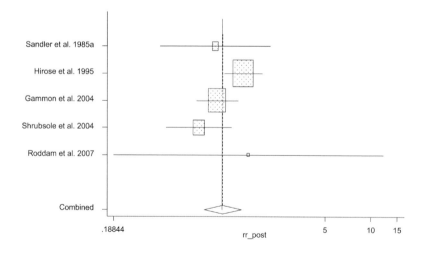

Figure 2.2c Pooled risk estimates from random effects meta-analysis of exposure to SHS from spouse and breast cancer in postmenopausal women

Updated combined estimates from this meta-analysis were also calculated for studies stratified by menopausal status. For premenopausal women, the updated combined relative risk from exposure from a spouse or partner was 1.16 (95% CI=0.91-1.48, *p for heterogeneity*=0.074), slightly smaller than the US Surgeon General's report's combined estimate of 1.25 (95% CI=0.97-1.62, *p for heterogeneity*=0.164). Among postmenopausal women, the updated combined relative risk from exposure from a spouse or partner was 1.02 ((95% CI=0.76-1.36), *p for heterogeneity*=0.143), almost the same as the US Surgeon General's report's combined estimate of 1.00 (95% CI=0.73-1.38, *p for heterogeneity*=0.080). These updated combined estimates include results from Roddam *et al.* (2007). No new data were available, since the 2006 US Surgeon General's report, for updating combined estimates for pre- and postmenopausal women's workplace or childhood SHS exposures. The Begg's and Egger's tests did not provide evidence of publication bias for studies among premenopausal women for SHS exposure from spouse or partner.

The results for the relationship between SHS exposure and breast cancer risk from this meta-analysis diverge from those of the 2005 California EPA report on environmental tobacco smoke. In addition to inclusion of the recently published studies contained in this Handbook, the selection of studies included in the California EPA meta-analyses is a likely explanation for this difference.

Table 2.5 Random effects meta-analysis results of SHS and breast cancer (2006 US Surgeon General's report and updated estimates by Volume 13 Working Group)

Exposure	All women				Premenopausal				Postmenopausal			
	n	SG (2006)	n	Updated	n	SG (2006)	n	Updated	n	SG (2006)	n	Updated
Adult (spousal)	10	1.18 (0.99-1.39) [0.002]	11	1.14 (0.97-1.34) [0.002]	5	1.25 (0.97-1.62) [0.164]	6	1.16 (0.91-1.48) [0.074]	4	1.00 (0.73-1.38) [0.080]	5	1.02 (0.76-1.36) [0.143]
Adult (work)	6	1.06 (0.84-1.35) [0.008]	7	1.10 (0.88-1.38) [0.004]	4	1.21 (0.70-2.09) [0.000]	4	1.21 (0.70-2.09) [0.000]	3	0.83 (0.53-1.29) [0.086]	3	0.83 (0.53-1.29) [0.086]
Child (parental)*	9	1.01 (0.90-1.12) [0.101]	9	1.01 (0.90-1.12) [0.101]	4	1.14 (0.90-1.45) [0.339]	4	1.14 (0.90-1.45) [0.339]	3	1.04 (0.86-1.26) [0.242]	3	1.04 (0.86-1.26) [0.242]

SG: US Surgeon General
*No new studies
n: number of studies included in each analysis
[in brackets]: p-value for test of heterogeneity (null hypothesis is no heterogeneity)

Using six case-control studies judged unlikely to have missed three major sources of lifetime SHS exposure (childhood home, adulthood home, and work), the California EPA report presented a combined relative risk estimate among all women of 1.89 (95% CI=1.52-2.36, *p for heterogeneity*=0.265). The analysis, which included all 17 studies, yielded a combined relative risk among all women of 1.40 (95% CI=1.17-1.68, *p for heterogeneity*=0.0). Among studies which presented results for premenopausal women, the California EPA report presented a combined relative risk estimate from six case-control studies deemed unlikely to have missed major sources of lifetime SHS exposure to be 2.20 (95% CI=1.70-2.85, *p for heterogeneity*=0.361), while using all 11 case-control studies yielded a combined relative risk of 1.99 (95% CI=1.49-2.66).

Cervical cancer

The US Surgeon General (U.S. Department of Health and Human Services, 2006), the California EPA (California Environmental Protection Agency: Air Resources Board, 2005), and the IARC (2004) reports all addressed the relationship between SHS exposure and risk of cervical cancer. A literature search identified a total of 12 studies with 13 study samples (Tables 2.6a,b) that examined the association between exposure to SHS and cervical cancer.

Table 2.6a Exposure to SHS and cervical cancer - Cohort studies

Reference, location, period	Cohort description	Exposure assessment	Exposure categories	Relative risk (95% CI)	Adjustment for potential confounders	Comments
Hirayama, 1981 Tokyo, Japan, 1966-1979	91 540 nonsmoking wives followed for 14 years	Interviewed about risk factors		**RR (90% CI)**		
			Husband nonsmoker	1		
			Husband ex-smoker or 1-19 cig/day	1.15		
			Husband smokes 20+ cig/day	1.14		
			p for trend	0.249		
Hirayama, 1984 Tokyo, Japan 1966-1981	91 540 nonsmoking wives followed for 16 years	Interviewed about risk factors		**RR (90% CI)**	Age by Mantel-Haenszel method	
			Husband nonsmoker	1		
			Husband smokes 1-14 cig/day	1.67 (0.67-4.20)		
			Husband smokes 15-19 cig/day	2.02 (0.64-6.33)		
			Husband smokes 20+ cig/day	2.55 (1.04-6.27)		
			p for trend	0.0248		
Jee et al., 1999 Korea 1994-1997	Korean women aged 40-88 who received health insurance from KMIC	Questionnaires from 1992, 1993, and 1994 conducted in 416 hospitals	Husband's smoking status		Age of wives and husbands, SES, residency, husband's vegetable consumption, husband's occupation	
			Husband never smoker	1.0		
			Husband ever smoked	0.9 (0.6-1.3)		
			Husband current smoker	0.9 (0.6-1.2)		
Nishino et al., 2001 Japan 1984-1993	9675 Japanese lifelong nonsmoking women	Self-administered questionnaire completed in 1984	Husband nonsmoker	1.0		
			Husband smokes	1.1 (0.26-4.5)		
			p value	0.925		

Reference, location, period	Cohort description	Exposure assessment	Exposure categories	Relative risk (95% CI)	Adjustment for potential confounders	Comments
Tay & Tay, 2004 Singapore 1995-2001	623 women attending colposcopy clinic for evaluation between 1995 and 2001			OR (95% CI)	Age, parity, age at first intercourse, birth control pill use, patients smoking	Not restricted to never smokers
			Husband nonsmoker	1		LSIL: Low grade squamous intra-epithelial lesion
			LSIL: Husband smokes 1 more cig/day	1.03 (0.990-1.071)		
			HSIL: Husband smokes 1 more cig/day	1.046 (1.013-1.080)		HSIL: High grade squamous intraepithelial lesion
Trimble et al., 2005 Washington County, MD, 1963-1978	Female residents of Washington County, MD who agreed to participate in original cohorts	Mailed questionnaires and door-to-door interviews	No Passive Smoking (PS)	1.0	Age	Analysis among Never smokers. PS refers to passive smoking
			PS only	2.5 (1.3-3.3)		
			Other household member	2.6 (1.6-4.0)		
			Spouse	2.2 (1.2-4.3)		
			Never smoker, no PS	1.0	Age, education, marital status, religious attendance	
			PS only	2.1 (1.3-3.3)		
			Other household member	2.3 (1.1-4.9)		
			Spouse	2.0 (1.2-3.3)		
Washington County, MD, 1975-1994			No PS	1.0	Age	
			PS only	1.3 (0.7-2.3)		
			Other household member	1.3 (0.7-2.5)		
			Spouse	1.6 (0.7-3.9)		
			Never smoker, no PS	1.0	Age, education, marital status, religious attendance	
			PS only	1.4 (0.8-2.4)		
			Other HH member	1.3 (0.6-3.2)		
			Spouse	1.6 (0.7-3.9)		

Table 2.6b Exposure to SHS and cervical cancer - Case-control studies

Reference, location, period	Characteristics of cases	Characteristics of controls	Exposure assessment	Exposure categories	Relative risk (95% CI)*	Adjustment for potential confounders	Comments
Buckley et al., 1981 England 1974-1979	31 husbands of married women with cervical dysplasia, carcinoma in situ, or invasive cervical cancer	62 husbands of patients without cervical dysplasia, carcinoma in situ, or invasive cervical cancer matched for age and age at first intercourse	Husbands and wives interviewed either at health clinic or at home	**Cervical dysplasia, carcinoma in situ:** husband's smoking status	RR	Matched for age and age at first intercourse	
				Nonsmoker	1		
				Ex-smoker	4.42		
				Current smoker	1.91		
				Chi-square for trend	2.42		
				Invasive carcinoma: husband's smoking status	RR	Matched for age and age at first intercourse	
				Nonsmoker	1		
				Ex-smoker	1.82		
				Current smoker	4.44		
				Chi-square for trend	2.17		
				Invasive cervical cancer: husband's smoking status	RR	Matched for age and age at first intercourse	
				Nonsmoker	1		
				Ex-smoker	2.69		
				Current smoker	3.21		
				Chi-square for trend	4.59		
Brown et al., 1982 Canada 1959-1968	33 patients with invasive or in situ cervical cancer	29 with hysterectomies for non-cancer reasons	Interview using questionnaire	**Invasive cancer:** Husband nonsmoker	1	Matched for age at surgery, parity, social class, and date of surgery	Unmatched crude ORs calculated from table
				Husband smokes <20 cig/day	0.55		
				Husband smokes 20-40 cig/day	1.25		
				Husband smokes >40 cig/day	6.00		

Reference, location, period	Characteristics of cases	Characteristics of controls	Exposure assessment	Exposure categories	Relative risk (95% CI)*	Adjustment for potential confounders	Comments
Brown et al., 1982 Canada 1959-1968				**Total cervical cancer:** Husband nonsmoker	1		
				Husband smokes <20 cig/day	1.36		
				Husband smokes 20-40 cig/day	5.00		
				Husband smokes >40 cig/day	15.00		
Sandler et al., 1985b University of North Carolina 1979-1981	All cancer cases (except basal cell skin) from North Carolina Memorial Hospital tumor registry diagnosed between 1979 and 1981 and alive in 1981; aged 15-59	Friends or acquaintances of case without cancer, of similar age (±5 yrs), sex, and race, or through telephone sampling	Mailed questionnaire and telephone call	Mother nonsmoker	1	None	Results presented among nonsmokers; CIs not presented
				Mother smoked	0.77		
				Father nonsmoker	1		
				Father smoked	1.7		
Sandler et al., 1985a University of North Carolina 1979-1981	All cancer cases (except basal cell skin) from North Carolina Memorial Hospital tumor registry diagnosed between 1979 and 1981 and alive in 1981; aged 15-59	Friends or acquaintances of case without cancer, of similar age (+/- 5 yrs), sex, and race, or through telephone sampling	Mailed questionnaire and telephone call	Spouse did not smoke	1		Results among nonsmokers presented
				Spouse smoked	2.1 (1.2-3.9)		
Hellberg et al., 1986 Falu Hospital, Sweden 1977-1981	140 pregnant women histologically diagnosed with cervical intraepithelial neoplasia using colposcopy	280 pregnant age-matched women (2 for each case) also visiting the maternity clinic on the same occasion with normal smears	Midwife administered questionnaire and mailed it	Male partner nonsmoker	1		Unmatched OR calculated from table
				Male partner smokes	2.01 (1.84-2.21)		
				p value	<0.001		
Slattery et al., 1989 Utah 1984-1987	266 histologically confirmed incident cases of carcinoma in situ or invasive carcinoma identified through rapid reporting system	408 age- and residence-matched controls using random digit dialing sampling without history of hysterectomy before 1984 or missing data	Personal interviews in respondents' homes	No hrs/day of passive smoking (PS)	1	Age, education, church attendance, # sexual partners of woman; age and residence matched	Results among never smokers presented (81 cases and 305 controls). PS refers to passive smoking
				0.1-0.9 hrs/day	1.14 (0.45-2.94)		
				1.0-2.9 hrs/day	1.57 (0.52-4.73)		
				≥3.0 hrs/day of	3.43 (1.23-9.54)		

Table 2.6b Exposure to SHS and cervical cancer - Case-control studies

Reference, location, period	Characteristics of cases	Characteristics of controls	Exposure assessment	Exposure categories	Relative risk (95% CI)*	Adjustment for potential confounders	Comments
Slattery et al., 1989				**No hrs/day of PS in-home**	1		
Utah 1984-1987				0.1-1.5 hrs/day	0.62 (0.25-1.53)		
				>1.5 hrs/day	2.66 (1.15-6.13)		
				No hrs/day of PS away from home	1		
				0.1-1.5 hrs/day	1.33 (0.58-3.07)		
				>1.5 hrs/day	2.3 (0.89-5.95)		
				None in-home PS	1		
				Little in-home PS	1.86 (0.37-9.37)		
				Some in-home PS	1.49 (0.44-5.09)		
				A lot in-home PS	2.93 (1.08-7.94)		
				None away from home PS	1		
				Little away from home PS	1.58 (0.68-3.66)		
				Some away from home PS	1.11 (0.49-2.50)		
				A lot away from home PS	1.59 (0.57-4.45)		
Coker et al., 1992 University of North Carolina 1987-1988	103 cases with CIN grades II and III; aged 18-45 years; Black or White and non-pregnant; response rate 92%	268 normal controls; aged 18-45 years; black or white and non-pregnant; response rate 91.8%	Interviewed by telephone or in person	**No PS at home**	1	Age, race, education, # sex partners, # Paps in last 5 yrs, genital warts	Results for nonsmoking women
				<17 yrs at home	1.5 (0.5-4.9)		
				18+ yrs at home	0.4 (0.1-1.3)		
				No PS at work	1		
				1-4 yrs at work	1.7 (0.5-5.1)		
				5+ yrs at work	0.4 (0.1-2.5)		
				Not exposed	1		
				Parent only	0.4 (0.1-1.2)		

Reference, location, period	Characteristics of cases	Characteristics of controls	Exposure assessment	Exposure categories	Relative risk (95% CI)*	Adjustment for potential confounders	Comments
Coker et al., 1992 University of North Carolina 1987-1988				Husband only	1.5 (0.3-6.2)		
				Parent and husband	0.4 (0.1-1.9)		
				Others only	1.8 (0.4-8.4)		
Hirose et al., 1996 Aichi Cancer Center, Japan 1996	556 women with first diagnosis, histologically confirmed cervical cancer	26 751 first visit outpatients aged ≥20 without ever being diagnosed with cancer	Self-administered questionnaire		AOR (95% CI)	Age, first-visit year, drinking, physical activity	Results for nonsmoking women
				Husband nonsmoker	1		
				Husband smokes	1.3 (1.07-1.59)		
				Husband smokes <20 cig/day	1.0 (0.76-1.33)		
				Husband smokes ≥20 cig/day	1.55 (1.24-1.94)		
Coker et al., 2002 South Carolina Health Department, 1995-1998	High-grade SIL (HSIL) cases, 313 low-grade SIL (LSIL) cases, with mean age near 25 years; response rate 82.1%	427 controls with mean age near 28 years; response rate 72.5%	Interviewed by telephone	HSIL: No passive smoking (PS) by either parent/ sex partner	1	Age, age at first sexual intercourse, race, HR-HPV status, and active smoking	Not restricted to nonsmokers. High grade squamous intraepithelial lesion.
				PS by either parent/ sex partner	2.2 (1.0-4.8)		
				No PS by parent as a child	1		
				PS by parent as a child	1.9 (1.0-3.7)		
				No PS by sex partner	1		
				PS by sex partner	1.0 (0.5-2.1)		
				No PS	1		
				1-9 yrs of PS	0.7 (0.2-2.6)		
				10+ yrs of PS	1.8 (0.9-3.6)		
				LSIL: No PS by either parent or sex partner	1		Low grade squamous intraepithelial lesion
				PS by either parent or sex partner	1.4 (1.0-2.0)		PS refers to passive smoking

Table 2.6b Exposure to SHS and cervical cancer - Case-control studies

Reference, location, period	Characteristics of cases	Characteristics of controls	Exposure assessment	Exposure categories	Relative risk (95% CI)*	Adjustment for potential confounders	Comments
Coker et al., 2002 1995-1998				No PS by parent as a child	1		
				PS by parent as a child	1.2 (0.9-1.7)		
				No PS by sex partner	1		
				PS by sex partner	1.1 (0.8-1.5)		
				Never PS	1		
				1-9 yrs of PS	1.8 (1.1-3.0)		
				10+ yrs of PS	1.4 (0.9-2.0)		
Wu et al., 2003 Taiwan 1999-2000	100 histologically confirmed women (CIN2: 39, CIN3:12, CIS: 46, invasive cancer: 3) aged ≥19	197 women age (±2 yrs) and residence matched with negative Pap smears	Nurse interviewer-administered questionnaire	No childhood, home ETS exposure	1	Age and residence-matched, education, # pregnancies, age at first intercourse, cooking ventilation	Results for nonsmoking women
				Childhood, home ETS exposure	0.99 (0.54-1.83)		ETS refers to environmental tobacco smoke
				No childhood, work ETS exposure	1		ETS refers to environmental tobacco smoke
				Childhood, work ETS exposure	1.03 (0.47-2.26)		
				No adulthood, home ETS exposure	1		
				Adulthood, home ETS exposure	2.73 (1.31-5.67)		
				No adulthood, work ETS exposure	1		
				Adulthood, work ETS exposure	1.56 (0.83-2.92)		
				Lifetime, childhood, home ETS exposure			
				No	1		
				1-10 cig/day	1.35 (0.78-2.35)		
				>10 cig/day	1.02 (0.43-2.40)		

Reference, location, period	Characteristics of cases	Characteristics of controls	Exposure assessment	Exposure categories	Relative risk (95% CI)*	Adjustment for potential confounders	Comments
Wu et al., 2003				Lifetime, childhood, work ETS exposure			
Taiwan 1999–2000				No	1		
				1-10 cig/day	1.25 (0.54-2.90)		
				>10 cig/day	0.79 (0.24-2.55)		
				Lifetime, childhood, home ETS exposure			
				No	1		
				1-10 cig/day	1.11 (0.59-2.09)		
				>10 cig/day	0.82 (0.31-2.19)		
				Lifetime, childhood, work ETS exposure			
				No	1		
				1-10 cig/day	1.34 (0.53-3.36)		
				>10 cig/day	0.79 (0.21-2.97)		
				Lifetime, adulthood, home ETS exposure			
				No	1		
				1-10 cig/day	2.13 (0.96-4.73)		
				>10 cig/day	3.97 (1.65-9.55)		
				Lifetime, adulthood, work ETS exposure			
				No	1		
				1-10 cig/day	1.47 (0.64-3.37)		
				>10 cig/day	1.65 (0.73-3.75)		
				Lifetime, adulthood, all ETS exposure			
				No	1		
				1-10 cig/day	1.90 (0.72-5.03)		
				>10 cig/day	2.99 (1.10-8.09)		

Table 2.6b Exposure to SHS and cervical cancer - Case-control studies

Reference, location, period	Characteristics of cases	Characteristics of controls	Exposure assessment	Exposure categories	Relative risk (95% CI)*	Adjustment for potential confounders	Comments
Sobti et al., 2006 India	103 histologically confirmed cervical cancer patients	103 controls free of any cancer	Interviewer-administered questionnaire	**GSTM1 null:** Never smoker Passive smoker	1 6.95		ORs calculated from table
				GSTM1 present: Never smoker Passive smoker	1 4.32		GSTM1 gene (glutathione S-Transferese mu1)
				GSTT1 null: Never smoker Passive smoker	1 28.57		GSTT1 (glutathione S-transferese theta1)
				GSTM1 present: Never smoker Passive smoker	1 3.72		
				GSTP1 ile/ile: Never smoker Passive smoker	1 4.33		
				GSTP1 ile/val: Never smoker Passive smoker	1 5.53		GSTP1 gene (glutathione S-transferese pi1)
				GSTP1 val/val: Never smoker Passive smoker	1 5.13		
Tsai et al., 2007 Taiwan 2003-2005	Women aged ≥20 screened by PAP smear with CIN I or over for the first time	Randomly selected from women with negative Pap smear findings, matched on residence and agreeing to interview	Interviewer-administered questionnaire	**Inflammation:** Non-smoker	1	Age, education, times of prior Pap smear, # of lifetime sexual partners, age at first intercourse, family history cervical cancer, cooking oil fume exposure, HPV infection	Results for nonsmoking women
				Secondhand smoker	1.3 (0.6-2.7)		
				Nonsmoker	1		
				Lifetime 1-10 pack/yrs	0.9 (0.4-1.9)		
				Lifetime 11-20 pack/yrs	1.7 (0.5-5.6)		
				Lifetime >20 pack/yrs	4.1 (1.3-12.5)		
				CIN1: Nonsmoker	1		CIN (Cervical Intra-epithelial neoplasia grade 1)
				SHS	1.6 (0.8-3.2)		
				Nonsmoker	1		

Reference, location, period	Characteristics of cases	Characteristics of controls	Exposure assessment	Exposure categories	Relative risk (95% CI)	Adjustment for potential confounders	Comments
Tsai et al., 2007 Taiwan 2003-2005				Lifetime 1-10 pack/yrs	1.3 (0.6-2.8)		
				Lifetime 11-20 pack/yrs	2.4 (0.7-7.7)		
				Lifetime >20 pack/yrs	4.0 (1.2-13.8)		CIN2 (Cervical Intra-epithelial neoplasia grade 2)
				≥CIN2: Nonsmoker	1		
				Secondhand smoker	1.8 (0.9-4.1)		
				Nonsmoker	1		
				Lifetime 1-10 pack/yrs	1.3 (0.6-2.9)		
				Lifetime 11-20 pack/yrs	2.1 (0.6-7.9)		
				Lifetime >20 pack/yrs	7.2 (2.5-20.6)		

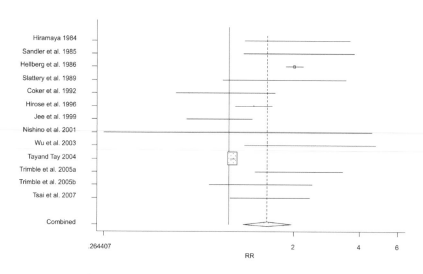

Figure 2.3 Pooled risk estimates from random effects meta-analysis of exposure to SHS and cervical cancer

Trimble et al., 2005a and 2005b refer to estimates from the 1963 and 1975 cohorts respectively. All data included in the reference Trimble et al., 2005

Risk estimates are plotted in Figure 2.3 for the most comprehensive SHS exposure index available. Since several studies presented risk estimates stratified by mutually exclusive exposure categories (Hirayama, 1984; Slattery et al., 1989; Coker et al., 1992; Hirose et al., 1996; Wu et al., 2003; Tay & Tay, 2004; Tsai et al., 2007), these estimates were pooled using random effects meta-analysis. Although a combined random effects estimate is shown, none of these studies adequately accounted for prior human papillomavirus (HPV) infection. Consequently, the evidence is not informative as to whether SHS increases the risk of cervical cancer in HPV-infected women. Overall, increased risk was found in association with SHS exposure (Figure 2.3). However, the increase cannot be separated from increased risk for HPV infection indirectly associated with SHS exposure.

Colorectal cancer

Several recent studies, addressing genetic markers of risk, have examined the relationship between passive smoking and colorectal cancer. It was found that passive smoking was associated with an increased risk for colorectal cancer only among NAT2 fast acetylators (OR=2.6; 95% CI=1.1-5.9) for exposure in childhood and adulthood (Lilla et al., 2006). After adjusting for active smoking, total long-term exposure to passive smoke was found to be associated with increased risk of rectal cancer among men exposed to >10 hours/week compared to none (OR=1.4; 95% CI=1.0-2.1), but no significant associations were found between exposure to SHS and rectal cancer among women (Slattery et al., 2003).

Esophageal cancer

This review identified one published study examining the relationship between SHS exposure and esophageal cancer (Wang et al., 2006). The researchers conducted a population based case-control study in 107 esophageal squamous cell carcinoma cases and 107 controls matched on residency, age, and sex in five townships of Huaian, China. They found that exposure to SHS was associated with an increased risk of esophageal cancer (OR=2.04; 95% CI=1.14-3.70). However, these results were not restricted to nonsmokers.

Liver cancer

The relationship between passive smoking and risk for cancer of the liver has also been investigated. A prospective cohort study conducted in 160 130 Korean women, aged 40-88, found no association between liver cancer and husbands' smoking habit (Jee et al., 1999). There were 83 cases of liver cancer identified in the follow-up period from July, 1994 to December, 1997. Wives with former smoking husbands had RR=0.8 (95% CI=0.5-1.5) and wives of current smoking husbands had RR=0.7 (95% CI=0.4-1.1). Another cohort study conducted in Japanese nonsmoking women, found an elevated, but not significant, age-adjusted risk of liver cancer after nine years of follow-up (OR=1.2; 95% CI=0.45-3.2) (Nishino et al., 2001); however, there were only 20 cases of liver cancer. It was hypothesised that parental smoking during pregnancy might plausibly increase risk for childhood hepatoblastoma by exposing the fetus' liver through the fetal circulation (Pang et al., 2003). Though there were only 10 cases, they found a significantly elevated OR of developing hepatoblastoma associated with smoking by both parents (OR=4.74; 95% CI=1.68-13.35). An increased risk of hepatoblastoma was also reported if both parents smoked relative to neither parent smoking (RR=2.28; 95% CI=1.02-5.09) (Sorahan & Lancashire, 2004).

Lymphoma

Only one study has been published examining the relationship between SHS exposure and cancer of the lymph nodes in adults. A population-based case-control study was conducted examining the association between SHS exposure and Hodgkin lymphoma (HL) among US women aged 19-44 years and those aged 45-79 years (Glaser et al., 2004). Though not limited to never smokers, exposure to SHS during childhood was significantly associated with risk of HL in the 19-44 year age group (OR=1.6; 95% CI=1.03-2.4) after adjusting for age, race, having a single room at 11 years, birth place (USA vs. other), renting a house/dwelling at age eight, being Catholic, and ever breastfeeding. Exposure to SHS during adulthood was not significantly associated with risk of HL (adjusted OR=0.8; 95% CI=0.6-1.2).

Nasal sinus cancer

The 2006 Surgeon General's report on involuntary smoking addressed SHS exposure and risk of nasal sinus cancer. Only three studies were found (Hirayama, 1984; Fukuda & Shibata, 1990; Zheng et al., 1993) with up to a three-fold increase in nasal sinus cancer risk associated with SHS exposure (Tables 2.7a,b). The report concluded that the evidence regarding SHS exposure and nasal sinus cancer was suggestive, but not sufficient to infer a causal relationship, and that more studies by histological type and subsite were needed. New studies were not found.

Nasopharyngeal cancer

The 2006 US Surgeon General's report on involuntary smoking also addressed SHS exposure and the risk of nasopharyngeal cancer. Only three studies were found in the literature (Yu et al., 1990; Cheng et al., 1999; Yuan et al., 2000) showing slightly elevated related relative risks. The US Surgeon General's report concluded that though biologically plausible, the evidence regarding SHS exposure and nasopharyngeal cancer was inadequate to infer a causal relationship. Since this review, no new studies have been published in the literature regarding SHS exposure and risk of nasopharyngeal cancer (Table 2.8).

Oral cancer

Few studies have examined the role of SHS in the etiology of oral cancer. In a case-control study of overall cancer and adult exposure to passive smoking, it was found that exposure to passive smoke was not significantly associated with cancer of the lip, oral cavity, and pharynx after adjusting

for age and education (OR=1.1; 95% CI=0.4-3.0) (Sandler et al., 1985a). Another case-control study found that neither exposure to maternal nor paternal smoking during childhood was associated with an unadjusted risk of cancer of the lip, oral cavity, and pharynx (maternal smoking OR=0.8; 95% CI=0.2-3.5, paternal smoking OR=1.3; 95% CI=0.4-3.8) (Sandler et al., 1985b). Neither of these studies was limited to never smokers.

Ovarian cancer

A cohort study conducted in Japanese nonsmoking women, found an elevated, but not significant, increased risk of ovarian cancer associated with husbands smoking status after adjusting for age (OR=1.7; 95% CI=0.58-5.2) (Nishino et al., 2001). However, there were only 15 cases of ovarian cancer reported during nine years of follow-up for 9675 women. A population-based case-control study in the USA, examined the hypothesis that active and passive tobacco smoking are associated with the risk of epithelial ovarian cancer (558 women with epithelial ovarian cancer and 607 population controls) (Goodman & Tung, 2003). Significant associations were not found among never smokers with exposure to passive smoke from either parent for gestational or childhood exposure. In a study among never smokers (434 cases and 868 age and region matched hospital controls), a decreased risk of ovarian cancer was found to be associated with daily exposure to passive smoke (OR=0.68; 95% CI=0.46-0.99) (Baker et al., 2006).

Table 2.7a Exposure to SHS and nasal sinus cancer - Cohort study

Reference, location, period	Cohort description	Exposure assessment	Exposure categories	Relative risk (95% CI)	Adjustment for potential confounders
Hirayama et al., 1984 Japan 1966-1981	91 540 nonsmoking, married women, aged ≥40 years (28 deaths due to nasal sinus cancer)	Interviewer-administered questionnaire	Husband's smoking: None 1-14 cig/day 15-19 cig/day ≥ 20 cig/day	RR (90% CI) 1 1.67 (0.67-4.20) 2.02 (0.64-6.33) 2.55 (1.04-6.27)	Husband's age

Table 2.7b Exposure to SHS and nasal sinus cancer - Case-control study

Reference, location, period	Characteristics of cases	Characteristics of controls	Exposure assessment	Exposure categories	Relative risk (95% CI) or odds ratio	Adjustment for potential confounders
Fukuda & Shibata, 1990 Japan 1982-1986	46 women 40-79 years with incident neoplasms of the maxillary sinuses; 96.6% response rate	88 population controls, individually matched on age, gender, and health-center region; 93.4% response rate	Self-administered questionnaire	**Among nonsmokers:** No smokers in household 1 smoker in household >1 smoker in household	1 1.40 (0.57-3.49) 5.73 (1.58-20.73)	none
Zheng et al., 1993 USA 1986	147 deaths from nasal sinus cancer in White males aged ≥45 years who participated in the 1986 US National Mortality Followback Survey	449 White controls aged ≥45 years who died from other causes	Questionnaire sent to next of kin	Nonsmoker in household Smoking spouse Smoking spouse, maxillary sinus cancers	1 3.0 (1.0-8.9) 4.8 (0.9-24.7)	age, alcohol age, alcohol

Table 2.8 Exposure to SHS and nasopharyngeal cancer - Case-control studies

Reference, location, period	Characteristics of cases	Characteristics of controls	Exposure assessment	Exposure categories	Relative risk (95% CI)	Adjustment for potential confounders
Yu et al., 1990 China 1983-1985	306 patients <50 years old with incident nasopharyngeal carcinoma; 100% response rate	306 population controls, individually matched on age, gender, and neighborhood; response rate not stated	Interviewer-administered questionnaire	**Among nonsmokers:**		Age and gender
				Never exposed to SHS at home	1	
				Father smoked when subject was age 10	0.6 (0.3-1.2)	
				Mother smoked when subject was age 10	0.7 (0.3-1.5)	
				Other household members smoked when subject was age 10	1.0 (0.5-2.2)	
				Lived with any smoker at age 10	0.7 (0.4-1.3)	
				Spouse smoked	0.8 (0.4-1.9)	
				Ever exposed to SHS at home	0.7 (0.4-1.4)	
Cheng et al., 1999 Taiwan 1991-1994	375 histologically confirmed incident nasopharyngeal cancers (NPC), ≤75 years old, no previous NPC, residence in Taipei last 6 months; 99% response rate	327 healthy community controls individually matched to cases on sex, age and residence; 88% response rate	Questionnaire	**Nonsmokers:**		Age, sex, education, family history of NPC
				No childhood SHS	1	
				Childhood SHS	0.6 (0.4-1.0)	
				No adulthood SHS	1	
				Adulthood SHS	0.7 (0.5-1.2)	
Yuan et al., 2000 China 1987-1991	935 histologically confirmed nasopharyngeal cancers; 84% response rate	1032 persons from the community frequency matched by age (± 5 yrs) and sex	In-person interview by 4 trained interviewers employing a structured questionnaire	**Male and female nonsmokers:**		Age, sex, education, preserved foods, citrics, cooking smoke, occupational exposure to chemical fumes, history of chronic ear, nose condition, family history of NPC

Table 2.8 Exposure to SHS and nasopharyngeal cancer - Case-control studies

Reference, location, period	Characteristics of cases	Characteristics of controls	Exposure assessment	Exposure categories	Relative risk (95% CI)	Adjustment for potential confounders
Yuan et al., 2000				Never exposed over lifetime	1	
China 1987-1991				Mother smoked	2.30 (1.23-4.28)	
				Mother smoked <20 cig/day	1.65 (0.83-3.29)	
				Mother smoked ≥20 cig/day	4.24 (1.84-9.77)	
				Father smoked	1.99 (1.18-3.35)	
				Father smoked <20 cig/day	1.73 (0.99-3.02)	
				Father smoked ≥20 cig/day	2.28 (1.31-3.99)	
				Non-parental household member smoked	2.37 (1.20-4.71)	
				Any household member smoked	2.05 (1.22-3.44)	
				Total household <20 pack-yrs	1.78 (1.02-3.13)	
				Total household 20-39 pack-yrs	2.23 (1.28-3.89)	
				Total household 40+ pack-yrs	2.51 (1.18-5.34)	
				Spouse smoked	2.48 (1.42-4.31)	
				Spouse smoked <20 yrs	2.37 (1.28-4.41)	
				Spouse smoked 20+ yrs	2.59 (1.38-4.84)	
				Spouse smoked <20 cig/day	2.44 (1.35-4.42)	
				Spouse smoked 20+ cig/day	2.52 (1.36-4.65)	
				Spouse <20 pack-yrs	2.47 (1.37-4.45)	

Reference, location, period	Characteristics of cases	Characteristics of controls	Exposure assessment	Exposure categories	Relative risk (95% CI)	Adjustment for potential confounders
Yuan et al., 2000				Spouse 20-39 pack-yrs	2.12 (1.07-4.19)	
China 1987-1991				Spouse 40+ pack-yrs	4.69 (1.60-13.70)	
				Non-spousal household member smoked	1.86 (1.09-3.18)	
				Any household member smoked	1.88 (1.12-3.16)	
				Total household smoked <20 cig/day	1.81 (1.03-3.19)	
				Total household smoked 20-39 cig/day	1.70 (0.97-2.98)	
				Total household 40+ cig/day	2.72 (1.39-5.31)	
				Co-worker smoked	1.99 (1.19-3.32)	
				Co-worker smoked <3 hrs	1.76 (1.03-3.02)	
				Co-worker smoked 3+ hrs	2.28 (1.32-3.93)	

The authors hypothesised that immunosuppression by nicotine or upregulation of enzymes that metabolise carcinogens may be responsible for the protective effects observed.

Pancreatic cancer

For pancreatic cancer, the literature review identified both cohort and case-control studies (Tables 2.9a,b). The three cohort studies provided no evidence for increased risk of pancreatic cancer associated with the exposure indicators (Nishino *et al.*, 2001; Gallicchio *et al.*, 2006). The case-control studies also provided little evidence for increased risk, except for one study carried out in Egypt (Lo *et al.*, 2007). This hospital-based case-control study used two institutions to identify the cases and drew controls from the otolaryngology and ophthalmology inpatient services; most cases did not have histological confirmation and there is concern about the comparability of cases and controls, given the methods of recruitment. The pooled estimate calculated by the Working Group for exposure at home as an adult was OR=1.35 (95% CI=0.88-2.07) (Figure 2.4).

Stomach cancer

The relationship between exposure to SHS and cancer of the stomach has been investigated in five study populations (Tables 2.10a,b). In a cohort of 91 540 nonsmoking Japanese women ≥40 years, followed from 1966 to 1981, there were 854 cases of stomach cancer (Hirayama, 1984). Husband's smoking was not

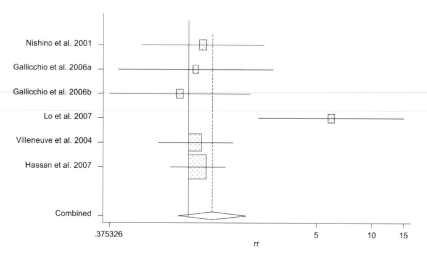

Figures 2.4 Pooled risk estimates from random effects meta-analysis of exposure to SHS and pancreatic cancer

Gallicchio et al., 2006a and 2006b refer to estimates from the 1963 and 1975 cohorts respectively.
All data included in the reference Gallicchio et al., 2006

significantly associated with risk of stomach cancer; the ORs associated with husband being an ex-smoker or of smoking 1-19 cigarettes/day was 1.03 (90% CI=0.89-1.18) and for 20+ cigarettes/day, OR=1.05 (90% CI=0.89-1.24). Another prospective cohort study conducted in Korean women aged 40-88 years, examined the association between SHS exposure from the husband's smoking and risk of stomach cancer (Jee *et al.*, 1999). It was found that neither husband's former smoking (OR=1.0; 95% CI=0.7-1.5) nor current smoking (OR=0.9; 95% CI=0.6-1.2) were associated with risk of stomach cancer in their wives. Also examined was the association between SHS and stomach cancer in a population-based prospective study among Japanese women aged 40 years and older during nine years

of follow-up (Nishino *et al.*, 2001). The age-adjusted RR for stomach cancer associated with husband's smoking was 0.95 (95% CI=0.58-1.6).

Two case-control studies examined the relationship between SHS exposure and risk of stomach cancer. Using information on 65 incident stomach cancer cases and 343 population controls, identified between 1994 and 1997 in Canada, it was found that among male never smokers there was a strongly increased risk associated with residential and occupational exposure to SHS among subjects with cardial stomach cancer (Mao *et al.*, 2002). For men with cardial cancer, the ORs ranged from 2.5 (95% CI=0.5-13.1) for 1-55 lifetime person-years of exposure, to OR=4.5 (95% CI=0.9-21.8) for 56-125 lifetime

Table 2.9a Exposure to SHS and pancreatic cancer - Cohort studies

Reference, location, period	Cohort description	Exposure assessment	Exposure categories	Relative risk (95% CI)	Adjustment for potential confounders	Comments
Nishino et al., 2001 Japan 1984-1992	9675 never smoking married women ≥40 years at enrollment (19 pancreatic cancer cases) with no previous diagnosis of cancer	Self-administered questionnaire	Husband does not smoke Husband smokes	1 1.2 (0.45-3.2)	Age	
Gallicchio et al., 2006 Maryland, USA 1963-1978	18 839 never smoking adults ≥25 years at enrollment (22 pancreatic cancer cases) with no prior cancer diagnosis	Self-administered questionnaire	No household members smoke Any household member smokes	1 1.1 (0.4-2.8)	Age, education, marital status	Two separate cohort studies described in this article; men excluded from SHS exposure analyses
Maryland, USA 1975-1994	20 181 never smoking adults ≥25 years at enrollment (34 pancreatic cancer cases) with no prior cancer diagnosis	Self-administered questionnaire	No household members smoke Any household member smokes	1 0.9 (0.4-2.3)	Age, education, marital status	Two separate cohort studies described in this article; men excluded from SHS exposure analyses

person-years of exposure to SHS, after controlling for 10 year age group; province; education; social class; and meat, fruit, vegetable, and juice consumption. Among never smoking men, the adjusted ORs were lower for the distal subsite of stomach cancer than cardia. In a case-control study based in the USA, it was found that the unadjusted RR for digestive cancer associated with father's smoking was 1.7 (95% CI=0.8-3.9), and for maternal smoking, RR=0.6 (95% CI=0.2-2.1) (Sandler et al., 1985b). In the same study population, the researchers found the RR for digestive cancer associated with spousal smoking to be 1.0 (95% CI=0.5-2.2) after adjusting for age and education (Sandler et al., 1985a).

Childhood cancers

Childhood leukemia

The 2006 US Surgeon General's report on SHS summarised the evidence on childhood leukemia and SHS exposure. The report concluded that the evidence was suggestive, but not sufficient to infer a causal relationship between prenatal and postnatal exposure to SHS and childhood leukemia. Since this report, three new studies have been published on SHS and risk of childhood leukemia. The relationship between parental smoking and childhood leukemia in the Northern California Childhood Leukemia Study was investigated (Chang et al., 2006).

Table 2.9b Exposure to SHS and pancreatic cancer - Case-control studies

Reference, location, period	Characteristics of cases	Characteristics of controls	Exposure assessment	Exposure categories	Relative risk(95% CI)	Adjustment for potential confounders	Comments
Villeneuve et al., 2004 Canada 1994-1997	105 never-smoking adults ≥30 years with pancreatic cancer; female response rate: 56%; male response rate: 55%	1145 adult population controls, matched on province and frequency matched on age and gender; female response rate: 71%; male response rate: 65%	Self-administered questionnaire	Never exposed to SHS	1	Age, BMI, income, province, sex	
				SHS exposure at home or work up to age 19	1.37 (0.46-4.07)		
				SHS exposure at home or work during adulthood	1.01 (0.41-2.50)		
				SHS exposure at home or work in lifetime	1.21 (0.60-2.44)		
				1-20 yrs SHS exposure at home	0.97 (0.42-2.26)		
				21-34 yrs SHS exposure at home	0.90 (0.39-2.11)		
				35+ yrs SHS exposure at home	1.43 (0.66-3.11)		
				All: 1-9 yrs SHS exposure at work	1.55 (0.68-3.56)		
				10-21 yrs SHS exposure at work	1.16 (0.49-2.74)		
				22+ yrs SHS exposure at work	1.20 (0.54-2.67)		
				SHS exposure only at home	0.97 (0.43-2.18)		
				SHS exposure only at work	1.43 (0.61-3.36)		
				1-35 yrs SHS exposure at home or work	1.33 (0.60-2.93)		
				36-56 yrs SHS exposure at home or work	1.09 (0.49-2.41)		
				57+ yrs SHS exposure at home or work	1.15 (0.54-2.47)		

Reference, location, period	Characteristics of cases	Characteristics of controls	Exposure assessment	Exposure categories	Relative risk(95% CI)	Adjustment for potential confounders	Comments
Hassan *et al.*, 2007 Texas, USA 2000-2006	735 patients with newly diagnosed, histologically-confirmed pancreatic adenocarcinoma who were English speaking US citizens	805 visitors who accompanied cancer patients (usually spouses), frequency matched on age, race, and sex	Interviewer-administered questionnaire	**Nonsmokers:** Never exposed to SHS	1	Age, sex, race, diabetes, alcohol consumption, education, state of residence, marital status	294 nonsmoking cases and 412 nonsmoking controls
				Ever exposed to SHS (childhood or adulthood)	1.1 (0.8-1.6)		
				Occasional SHS exposure during childhood	0.9 (0.5-1.6)		
				Regular SHS exposure during childhood	1.1 (0.7-1.6)		
				Occasional SHS exposure at home during adulthood	1.4 (0.7-2.5)		
				Regular SHS exposure at home during adulthood	1.03 (0.7-1.6)		
				Occasional SHS exposure at work during adulthood	0.8 (0.5-1.3)		
				Regular SHS exposure at work during adulthood	1.2 (0.7-1.9)		
				SHS exposure only during childhood	1.2 (0.7-1.9)		
				SHS exposure only during adulthood	1.3 (0.8-2.2)		
				SHS exposure during both childhood and adulthood	1.0 (0.6-1.5)		
				1-5 yrs SHS exposure during childhood	0.6 (0.2-1.7)		
				6-10 yrs SHS exposure during childhood	0.6 (0.2-1.5)		
				>10 yrs SHS exposure during childhood	1.1 (0.7-1.6)		

Table 2.9b Exposure to SHS and pancreatic cancer - Case-control studies

Reference, location, period	Characteristics of cases	Characteristics of controls	Exposure assessment	Exposure categories	Relative risk (95% CI)	Adjustment for potential confounders	Comments
Hassan et al., 2007 Texas, USA 2000-2006				1-10 yrs SHS exposure during adulthood	1 (0.5-1.7)		
				11-20 yrs SHS exposure during adulthood	1.1 (0.6-2.01)		
				>20 yrs SHS exposure during adulthood	1.2 (0.8-1.9)		
				1-10 yrs SHS exposure during lifetime	0.8 (0.4-1.6)		
				11-20 yrs SHS exposure during lifetime	1.1 (0.7-1.7)		
				>20 yrs SHS exposure during lifetime	1.2 (0.8-1.8)		
Lo et al., 2007 Egypt 2001-2004	194 adults 19-90 years with newly diagnosed pancreatic cancer	194 hospital controls from the ear/nose/throat, ophthalmology units frequency-matched on age and sex	Interviewer-administered questionnaire	**Nonsmokers:** Never lived with a smoker	1	Age, sex, rural/urban residence	41 nonsmoking cases and 97 nonsmoking controls
				Ever lived with a smoker, <30 yrs	6.0 (2.4-14.8)		

This case-control study included 327 acute childhood leukemia cases (281 acute lymphoblastic leukemia (ALL) and 46 acute myeloid leukemia (AML)) and 416 controls matched on age, sex, maternal race, and Hispanic ethnicity. The investigators found that maternal smoking was not associated with an increased risk of either ALL (OR=1.12; 95% CI=0.79-1.59) or AML (OR=1.00; 95% CI=0.41-2.44). The OR for AML associated with paternal preconception smoking was 3.84 (95% CI=1.04-14.17). The corresponding OR for ALL associated with paternal preconception smoking was 1.32 (95% CI=0.86-2.04).

The role of maternal alcohol and coffee consumption and parental smoking on the risk of childhood acute leukemia was investigated in a multicenter, hospital-based, case-control study in France with 280 incident cases and 288 hospitalised controls, frequency matched with the cases by age, gender, and center (Menegaux et al., 2005). Significant associations of maternal smoking with ALL (OR=1.1; 95% CI=0.7-1.6) and acute non-lymphocytic leukemia (ANLL) (OR=1.0; 95% CI=0.5-2.1) were not found. Paternal smoking was also not significantly associated with risk of ALL (OR=1.1; 95% CI=0.7-1.5) or ANLL (OR=1.3; 95% CI=0.6-2.7). Another case-control study was conducted in France of coffee, alcohol, SHS, and risk of acute leukemia (Menegaux et al., 2007). The researchers identified 472 cases of childhood acute leukemia (407 ALL and 62 with AML) and frequency-matched 567 population controls by age, sex, and region of residence. Only the risk of ALL associated with maternal smoking during pregnancy was significantly elevated (OR=1.4; 95% CI=1.0, 1.9), after adjusting for age, gender, region, socio-professional category, and birth order. Paternal smoking before, during, or after pregnancy was not significantly associated with risk of either ALL or AML. These new studies provide more evidence suggesting a causal relationship between prenatal and postnatal exposure to SHS and childhood leukemia.

Childhood brain cancer

The US Surgeon General (U.S. Department of Health and Human Services, 2006), the California EPA (California Environmental Protection Agency: Air Resources Board, 2005), and the IARC (2004) publications have reviewed the evidence relating the risk of childhood brain tumors (CBTs) to SHS exposure. In addition to the studies presented in these reports, the effect of parental smoking on the risk of CBT was examined in a small hospital-based case-control study in China (Hu et al., 2000). Parents of 82 children with newly diagnosed primary malignant brain tumors were individually matched to 246 hospital controls from 1991 to 1996. There was little evidence to support an association between parents' smoking before or during pregnancy and risk of CBT. More recently, the association between CBTs (all histological types combined) and exposure of parents and children to cigarette smoke was evaluated in a comprehensive, large, international case-control study (Filippini et al., 2002).

Table 2.10a Exposure to SHS and stomach cancer - Cohort studies

Reference, location, period	Cohort description	Exposure assessment	Exposure categories	Relative risk (95% CI)	Adjustment for potential confounders
Hirayama, 1981 Japan 1966-1979	91 540 nonsmoking, married women ≥40 years (716 deaths due to stomach cancer)	Interviewer-administered questionnaire	Nonsmoking husband	1	Husband's age and occupation. Confidence intervals not provided
			Husband is ex-smoker or smokes 1-19 cig/day	1.02	
			Husband smokes ≥20 cig/day	0.99	
Hirayama, 1984 Japan 1966-1981	91 540 nonsmoking, married women ≥40 years (854 deaths due to stomach cancer)	Interviewer-administered questionnaire	Nonsmoking husband	RR (90% CI) 1	Husband's age
			Husband is ex-smoker	1.15 (0.93-1.43)	
			Husband smokes 1-14 cig/day	1.00 (0.86-1.17)	
			Husband smokes 15-19 cig/day	1.00 (0.81-1.22)	
			Husband smokes ≥20 cig/day	1.01 (0.86-1.19)	
			Nonsmoking husband	1	Husband's age and occupation
			Husband is ex-smoker or smokes 1-19 cig/day	1.03 (0.89-1.18)	
			Husband smokes ≥20 cig/day	1.05 (0.89-1.24)	

Table 2.10a Exposure to SHS and stomach cancer - Cohort studies

Reference, location, period	Cohort description	Exposure assessment	Exposure categories	Relative risk (95% CI)	Adjustment for potential confounders
Jee et al., 1999 South Korea 1994-1997	157 436 nonsmoking, married women ≥40 years (197 stomach cancer cases)	Self-administered questionnaire	Husband never smoked	1	Age, husband's age, SES, residence, husband's vegetable consumption, husband's occupation
			Husband is ex-smoker	1.0 (0.7-1.5)	
			Husband is current smoker	0.9 (0.6-1.2)	
Nishino et al., 2001 Japan 1984-1992	9675 nonsmoking women ≥40 years (83 stomach cancer cases)	Self-administered questionnaire	Nonsmoking husband	1	Age
			Husband smokes	0.95 (0.58-1.6)	
			Neither husband nor other household members smoke	1	
			Other household members smoke (and husband does not smoke)	0.90 (0.52-1.5)	
			Husband smokes (and other household members do not smoke)	0.91 (0.48-1.7)	
			Husband and other household members smoke	0.90 (0.45-1.8)	
			Nonsmoking husband	1	Age, study area, alcohol consumption, vegetable intake, fruit intake, miso soup intake, pickled vegetable intake
			Husband smokes	0.98 (0.59-1.6)	
			No other household member smoke	1	
			Other household members smoke	0.87 (0.54-1.4)	

Table 2.10b Exposure to SHS and stomach cancer - Case-control studies

Reference, location, period	Characteristics of cases	Characteristics of controls	Exposure assessment	Exposure categories	Relative risk (95% CI)	Adjustment for potential confounders	Comments
Sandler et al., 1985a North Carolina, USA 1979-1981	518 cancer patients 15-59 years; 72% response rate	518 friend and community controls individually matched on gender, age and race; 75% response rate	Self-administered questionnaire	Nonsmoking spouse or never married Spouse smoked regularly (at least 1 cig/day for at least 6 months) any time during marriage	1 1.0 (0.5-2.2)	Age and education	Only 39 patients 15-59 years with cancer of the digestive system and 489 controls used
Sandler et al., 1985b North Carolina, USA 1979-1981	470 cancer cases (any site); 70% overall response rate	438 controls, individually matched on gender, age and race	Self-administered questionnaire	Not exposed to SHS from mother during first 10 yrs of life SHS exposure from mother during first 10 yrs of life Not exposed to SHS from father during first 10 yrs of life SHS exposure from father during first 10 yrs of life	1 0.7 1 1.3	None	31 digestive cancer cases were used in the SHS analysis and all of the controls; results for nonsmokers presented; no CIs provided
Mao et al., 2002 Canada 1994-1997	1171 cases of newly diagnosed, histologically confirmed cardial or distal stomach cancers; 63.2% overall response rate	207 population controls; 62.6% overall response rate	Self-administered questionnaire	**Cardial stomach cancer:** Never exposed to SHS at work or home 1-22 yrs SHS exposure at home or work 23-42 yrs SHS exposure at home or work 43+ yrs SHS exposure at home or work 1-55 smoker-yrs of SHS exposure at home or work	1 3.5 (0.7-17.3) 2.8 (0.5-14.2) 5.8 (1.2-27.5) 2.5 (0.5-13.1)	Age, province, education, social class, meat, vegetable, fruit and juice consumption	Only never smoking men were used for the SHS exposure analysis

Table 2.10b Exposure to SHS and stomach cancer - Case-control studies

Reference, location, period	Characteristics of cases	Characteristics of controls	Exposure assessment	Exposure categories	Relative risk (95% CI)	Adjustment for potential confounders	Comments
Mao et al., 2002 Canada 1994-1997				56-125 smoker-yrs of SHS exposure at home or work	4.5 (0.9-21.8)		
				126+ smoker-yrs of SHS exposure at home or work	3.4 (0.7-17.0)		
				Distal stomach cancer: Never exposed to SHS at work or at home	1		
				1-22 yrs SHS exposure at home or work	0.5 (0.2-1.1)		
				23-42 yrs exposure at home or work	0.9 (0.5-1.7)		
				43+ yrs exposure at home or work	1.0 (0.5-2.0)		
				1-55 smoker-yrs of exposure at home or work	0.6 (0.3-1.3)		
				56-125 smoker-yrs of exposure at home or work	0.7 (0.3-1.4)		
				126+ smoker-yrs of exposure	1.1 (0.6-2.0)		

The study sample consisted of 1218 cases <20 years old and newly diagnosed with CBT and 2223 population-based controls. There was no association between the risk of CBT and mothers' smoking (OR=0.9; 95% CI=0.8-1.0) or paternal smoking (OR=1.1; 95% CI=0.9-1.2) prior to pregnancy, mother smoking during pregnancy (home or work) (OR=0.9; 95% CI=0.8-1.1), or SHS exposure of the child during the first year of life (OR=1.0; 95% CI=0.8-1.1). The findings did not change after adjusting for the child's age, histological type, or location. There was some variation across histological type. For example, risk of the primitive neuroectodermal tumors was significantly elevated in children who were regularly exposed during gestation through their mothers being involuntarily exposed to SHS at work (OR=1.3; 95% CI=1.0-1.8) or to all sources of SHS combined (OR=1.3; 95% CI=1.0-1.7). However, risk of other histological types was reduced in persons whose mother smoked until pregnancy (OR=0.7; 95% CI=0.5-1.0) and who were exposed during the first year of life (OR=0.7; 95% CI=0.5-1.0). However, these findings should be considered in the context of the large number of exposure groups and histological types and the related risk for type I error.

Is there a safe level of exposure to SHS?

Studies of the relation between level of exposure to SHS and risk of disease have not shown evidence of a level below which the excess risk is zero. That is, there are no empirical data to support the concept of a safe (harm-free) level of exposure to SHS. This is not the same, of course, as demonstrating that there is no threshold (other than zero exposure). However, the epidemiological findings need to be considered alongside what is known about the toxicology of SHS and the likely biologic mechanisms of action, which are referred to earlier in this chapter. It was on this basis that the 2006 US Surgeon General's report concluded "the scientific evidence indicates that there is no risk-free level of exposure to secondhand smoke" (U.S. Department of Health and Human Services, 2006). The Working Group agrees with this assessment.

Burden of disease

Because of widespread exposure to SHS and the numerous adverse consequences of exposure, the impact on the health of children and adults is substantial. The burden of disease attributable to SHS has

been estimated for a number of populations. Making such estimations requires assumptions about exposure patterns and the risks of SHS-related diseases applicable to particular populations. While consequently subject to uncertainty, the available estimates document that SHS has substantial, while avoidable, public health impact. For example, estimates made by the State of California for both the state and for the entire USA (see Table ES-2 from the California EPA report), document thousands of premature deaths from cancer and ischemic heart disease, as well as over 400 deaths attributable to SIDS each year in the USA (Table 2.11). The morbidity burden for children is high (Table 2.11).

Estimates made for Europe with a similar approach led to the same conclusion on the public health significance of SHS exposure (Smoke Free Partnership, 2006). The report, *Lifting the Smokescreen: 10 Reasons for a Smokefree Europe*, provides estimates of the numbers of deaths attributable to SHS

among nonsmokers in 25 European countries in 2002. The estimates are made with the assumptions of causal associations of SHS exposure with stroke and chronic respiratory disease, in addition to lung cancer and ischemic heart disease. The total burden is over 19 000 premature deaths annually.

Methods for estimating the burden of disease attributable to SHS (and other environmental exposures) at national and local levels have been reviewed recently by WHO (Prüss-Üstün & Corvalán, 2006). The burden of disease associated with SHS exposure varies from population-to-population with the profile of exposure and the underlying rates of disease. For adults, the burden of attributable disease is strongly dependent on the rate of coronary heart disease, which is a major contributor to mortality in many countries, not just in the wealthiest parts of the world.

Table 2.11 Contribution of SHS to the burden of disease in the United States - examples of health outcomes attributable to SHS

Outcome	Annual excess number due to SHS
Children born weighing <2500 g	24 500
Pre-term deliveries	71 900
Episodes of childhood asthma	202 300
Doctor visits for childhood otitis media	790 000
Deaths due to Sudden Infant Death Syndrome	430
Deaths due to Ischemic Heart Disease	46 000 (22 700 – 69 500)
Lung cancer deaths	3400

Adapted from California Environmental Protection Agency: Air Resources Board (2005)

Summary

This chapter describes the findings of review groups that have conducted comprehensive assessments of the health effects of exposure to SHS. Over the four decades that research findings on SHS and health have been reported, stronger conclusions of reviewing groups have progressively motivated the development of protective policies. The rationale for such policies is solidly grounded in the conclusions of a number of authoritative groups: that SHS exposure contributes to the causation of cancer, cardiovascular disease, and respiratory conditions.

The Working Group found a high degree of convergence of the research findings. In fact, since 1986, an increasing number of reports have added to an ever growing list of causal effects of SHS exposure. These reports have given exhaustive consideration to the epidemiological findings and the wide range of research supporting the plausibility of causal associations. They have also considered and rejected explanations other than causation for the associations observed in the epidemiological studies. Particular attention has been given to confounding by other risk factors and to exposure misclassification, both of active smoking status and of exposure to SHS.

Chapter 3
The evolution of smoke-free policies

Introduction

The previous chapter summarised the evidence that led to the conclusion that exposure to secondhand smoke (SHS) is harmful to the health. Once the public health community accepted this evidence in the 1980s, avoiding exposure to SHS became a high priority for public health policy and practice. The first time that protection of nonsmokers was included as a major goal for a tobacco control programme was 1993 in the US state of California (Pierce *et al.*, 1994). Over time, jurisdictions have tried many approaches to protect the nonsmoker, providing an evidence base on which to judge the effectiveness of the different approaches.

This chapter will present the current consensus guidelines, developed by the Conference of the Parties of the WHO Framework Convention on Tobacco Control (FCTC), for implementing effective smoke-free public health policy and then retrace the evolution of concern about exposure to SHS over time and the resulting policies for protection against it in different parts of the world. This history highlights the political nature of this topic. Even as governments became aware of the mortality and morbidity attributed to SHS exposure in the 1980s and 1990s, many were reluctant to act promptly and decisively. In many

cases, governments preferred voluntary agreements that were acceptable to, and even promoted by, the tobacco industry (Saloojee & Dagli, 2000; Dearlove *et al.*, 2002; Sebrie & Glantz, 2007). It took time for evaluations to demonstrate that these agreements were clearly insufficient to achieve the public health goal, as exposure to SHS was not eliminated and at best reduced (Siegel, 2002). The political power of the tobacco industry within most jurisdictions was, and still is, considerable, and many governments were extremely cautious to avoid political problems for regulating where to allow smoking and where not to (Bornhauser *et al.*, 2006).

Following this chronology, we present a series of examples of jurisdictions that have implemented policies that, by and large, adhere to the WHO FCTC recommended guidelines and others that partially do. Some of these examples contributed to the evidence that is summarised in later chapters in this Handbook. A number of these jurisdictions have ongoing evaluations in place of the impact of the policies implemented, which will further their evidence base in the future. These examples can serve as a guide for the many jurisdictions considering protection of their non-smoking residents.

Finally, we note the work in progress in jurisdictions that have made considerable progress towards smoke-free legislation, although, as yet, they have not reached the goals outlined in the WHO FCTC guidelines (WHO, 2005).

WHO FCTC guidelines on protection from exposure to tobacco smoke

In response to the pervasive health consequences of tobacco use around the world, and the complex economic and political issues involved in implementing effective policies for tobacco control, the WHO adopted an evidence-based international treaty, the WHO FCTC (WHO, 2005). This Treaty acknowledges and addresses a series of difficult, and sometimes unappreciated, issues in tobacco control including cross-border effects, trade liberalisation, foreign investments, global marketing, transnational tobacco advertising, promotion and sponsorship, as well as contraband and counterfeit cigarettes (WHO, 2005). The provisions of the WHO FCTC focus on the multi-faceted interventions that are needed for tobacco control. These include the following: tax and price measures to reduce the demand for tobacco; protection from exposure to tobacco smoke; regulation and disclosure of tobacco products and its contents, including packaging and labeling; education and public awareness campaigns; policies regarding tobacco advertising, promotion and sponsorship; and provisions for treating tobacco dependence. In addition, the WHO FCTC has provisions regarding illegal tobacco sales, purchase by and distribution to minors, and assistance with economically viable alternatives to tobacco. The Treaty went into effect on February 27, 2005 and 162 parties (governments) were signatories as of January 28, 2008.

On July 3, 2007, the 2nd Conference of the Parties to the WHO FCTC approved unanimously the guidelines to assist Parties in meeting their obligations under Article 8 of the Convention: "in a manner consistent with the scientific evidence regarding exposure to secondhand tobacco smoke and the best practice worldwide in the implementation of smoke-free measures." The Conference of the Parties encourages its members, as well as all other WHO Member States, to refer also to the WHO policy recommendations on protection from exposure to SHS in the development and implementation of smoke-free legislation (WHO, 2007b).

Article 8 states that the Parties to the Treaty shall adopt and implement effective legislation "providing for protection from exposure to tobacco smoke in indoor workplaces, public transport, indoor public places and, as appropriate, other public places" given that "scientific evidence has unequivocally established that exposure to tobacco smoke causes death, disease and disability" (WHO, 2005). The guidelines for Article 8 also identify the key elements of legislation necessary to effectively protect people from exposure to tobacco smoke, as required by Article 8. According to these guidelines, the approval and implementation of smoke-free legislation should be based on the following principles (WHO, 2007a):

1. *100% Smoke-free environments, not smoking rooms* - The guidelines indicate that there is no safe level of exposure to SHS, and, therefore, the only way to protect the population is to create 100% smoke-free environments. The creation of 100% smoke-free environments requires that there are no separately designated areas for smoking. The guidelines state that "ventilation, air filtration systems, and the use of designated smoking areas (whether with separate ventilation systems or not), have repeatedly been shown to be ineffective and there is conclusive evidence, scientific and otherwise, that engineering approaches do not protect against exposure to secondhand smoke."

2. *Universal protection by law* - The guidelines indicate that Article 8 creates an *obligation to provide universal protection, i.e. to all people,* by ensuring that all (1) indoor workplaces, (2) indoor public places, (3) public transport, and (4) as appropriate, other public places, are completely free of SHS. It notes that no exemptions are justified on the basis of arguments related to either health or law. Considerations of exemptions, based on any other arguments, should be considered carefully and cautiously so as to not undermine the public health protection of citizens. In addition, Article 8 carries the governmental duty to protect all people from exposure to SHS by law and not by means of voluntary agreements.

3. *Public education to reduce secondhand smoke exposure* - The guidelines emphasise that it is equally important to educate the population regarding the law to ensure awareness and compliance.

4. *Implementation and adequate enforcement of the policy* - The guidelines outline that experience has proven the importance of simple, clear, and enforceable legislation to provide protection under Article 8. The guidelines recommend designating one or more groups as inspectors who are well-trained and supported, particularly during the first weeks and months after the law goes into effect.

Evolution of protection from SHS

Period 1: pre World War I

While tobacco had been used in society for centuries, cigarettes were not widely used anywhere in the world before the end of the XIXth century. Following the development of the Bonsack machine for making cigarettes in the USA in 1888, the cigarette market started to grow significantly (Kluger, 1996). This machine was critical for mass production of cigarettes at very low prices, which made them affordable. Aggressive marketing was used to consolidate the industry and build demand. As smoking became more prevalent and socially acceptable, exposure to SHS also became a nuisance to many. In 1910, the Non-Smokers Protective League in the USA was formed to lobby for increased bans on smoking in public places. A letter to the editor of the *New York Times* in 1913 stated "Smoking is now general in restaurants and a nonsmoker can seldom take a meal without the sickening fumes of tobacco puffed by a man who has a profound disregard for the rights and comforts of others" (Brandt, 2007). By 1913, smoking activists in the USA lobbied against the ban on smoking on railways, claiming the need for public space that allowed smoking, such as designated smoking cars (Brandt, 2007).

Period 2: 1914-1949

At the start of this period, smoking rooms were set aside in wealthy residencies and social norms proscribed lighting up in front of women in most western societies (Tyrrell, 1999).

While the cigarette market was growing rapidly before World War I, it accelerated enormously during the war. Leaders of the armed forces exhorted the public on the value of the product (Brandt, 2007). Without an effective opposition, there was fairly rapid public acceptance that cigarettes were needed for members of the armed forces in order to "soothe the nerves somewhat, and deaden the loneliness" (Sobel, 1978). The Red Cross, and other organisations,

raised money to dispatch free chewing gum, toothpaste, and cigarettes to American servicemen (Kennett, 1987). The cigarette industry was generous in supplying cigarettes to the Armed Services and, as a result, there was a rapid growth in cigarette smoking among young men with no social limitations on where to pollute the air with tobacco smoke (Kluger, 1996).

In the early 1920s, John H. Kellogg, an American surgeon, Seventh-day Adventist, the inventor of corn flakes breakfast cereal, and partner in the W.K. Kellogg Company, noted that smoking restrictions were possible when smokers were clearly a minority. However, with the rapid growth in dependent smokers who returned from the war, these smoking restrictions were increasingly hard to maintain even in respected society (Kellogg, 1922). The prospect of voluntary restrictions to protect women in households became increasing less likely, as the tobacco industry effectively targeted women themselves to become smokers.

Until the early 1920s, social norms restricted advertisers from explicitly targeting women, although women frequently appeared in cigarette advertisements in poses epitomised by the "blow some my way" advertising campaign for Chesterfields (Pierce & Gilpin, 1995; Brandt, 2007). The first campaign targeted directly at women smoking was the 1926 Lucky Strike "Reach for a Lucky instead of a sweet" campaign. This campaign has been associated with the launching of cigarette smoking among women (Kluger, 1996); and their level of initiation has increased every year

until the 1970s in the USA (Pierce & Gilpin, 1995).

During the decades following World War I, two factors lowered the social norms denouncing SHS exposure. First, the number of smokers increased dramatically, so that by the end of the Second World War more than 70% of men had become smokers and the proportion of women smoking had grown to well over a quarter of the population (Burns *et al.*, 1996). Further, cigarette smoking was a more frequent behaviour than cigar smoking, and smokers "invaded all indoor public and private spaces" with their smoke. By 1933, Thomas H. Roach, of the Non-Smokers League of Australia, noted the aggressive behaviour of smokers in the nonsmoking sections of trains and train stations, and a major magazine in the country noted in 1935 that the rules against smoking in food preparation areas were largely ignored (Tyrrell, 1999).

Period 3: 1950-1962

Although concerns about increasing lung cancer rates were published in the scientific literature in the late 1920s (Lombard & Doering, 1980), and, in Germany, a rudimentary case-control study in the late 1930s suggested that smoking caused lung cancer (Muller, 1939; Brandt, 2007), the first solid evidence that smoking was a primary cause of lung cancer came with five case-control studies published in 1950 (Doll & Hill, 1950; Levin *et al.*, 1950; Mills & Porter, 1950; Schrek *et al.*, 1950; Wynder & Graham, 1950). Throughout the 1950s, new evidence that smoking caused lung cancer and other health problems continued to accumulate. Studies reported on the induction of cancer by cigarette components in animal models (Wynder *et al.*, 1953), the results from large prospective cohort studies on disease rates among smokers and nonsmokers were presented (Doll & Hill, 1954; Hammond & Horn, 1954), and histopathological differences in smokers and nonsmokers in humans were observed (Auerbach *et al.*, 1956, 1957). A public health consensus review panel was convened by the US Surgeon General and the results published in the journal *Science* (Study Group on Smoking and Health, 1957). The Royal College of Physicians in the UK also published their first report on the likelihood that smoking caused cancer (Medical Research Council, 1957).

However, this public health consensus did not flow over to the US medical community, as was apparent in 1961 when the *New England Journal of Medicine* solicited articles from the leading scientific advocate for the public health viewpoint, Ernst Wynder, and from Pete Little, a respected cancer researcher who headed the Tobacco Institute, the public relations voice of the tobacco industry (Little, 1961; Wynder, 1961). The accompanying editorial advised the medical audience that they should weigh the evidence for each side and make up their own minds about which to believe (Author Unknown, 1961). This equivocation was not evident in the medical community in the UK. The Royal College of Physicians began its own review of the scientific evidence in the late 1950s (Medical Research

Council, 1957), and presented a very influential report in 1962 concluding a causal association between smoking and lung cancer (Royal College of Physicians, 1962). This evidence of a medical consensus in the UK was sufficient to initiate a presidential inquiry in the USA (Kluger, 1996), which resulted in the first US Surgeon General's Report on Smoking and Health (U.S. Department of Health, Education and Welfare, 1964). This report is widely recognised as the first definitive review of the data in the USA, and the beginning of the public health agencies' campaign against smoking in that country (U.S. Department of Health and Human Services, 1989).

The strong evidence of serious health effects caused by "active" smoking generated during this period, gave credence to the suspicion that there were similar dangers from "passive" smoking. These concerns were strengthened by scientific evidence of physiopathological changes in the oxygen-carrying function of the blood of nonsmokers exposed to SHS, as well as by the general annoyance smoking provoked in many nonsmokers.

Period 4: 1963-1979

In 1963, in a prescient editorial of the *South African Medical Journal*, members of the medical association advocated not only for public education, increasing taxation on tobacco products, prohibiting of cigarette advertising, but also for prohibiting smoking in public buildings and on public transport, because "the discomfort and disease of the non-smoker must be

considered before the convenience of the smoker" (Mackenzie & Campbell, 1963). The first sign of high level political concern about the detrimental effects of SHS was the 1969 Commission for the Investigation of Health Hazards of Chemical Compounds in the Work Area (MAK Commission) of the German Research Foundation. Although not an official agency, its recommendations were usually followed by the German government. The MAK Commission discussed the existing evidence on smoking and examined the potential dangers of SHS within an occupational health framework. In 1973 and 1975, the lower house of the West German parliament (Bundestag) passed a resolution calling on the federal government to prepare a comprehensive programme for "protecting the health concerns of nonsmokers in the different settings of life." However, under pressure from the tobacco industry, the parliamentary and governmental initiatives were not implemented (Bornhauser *et al.*, 2006).

In 1969, Bulgaria passed legislation to ban smoking in workplaces where nonsmokers worked, unless the nonsmokers agreed otherwise. In cases of expectant or nursing mothers working in the premises, the ban was not subject to permission by nonsmokers (WHO, 1975).

In 1970, Singapore banned smoking in cinemas, theatres, public lifts, and specific buildings (Tan *et al.*, 2000). That same year, the World Health Assembly (WHA), the conclave of all health ministers of the world, passed a resolution to ban smoking in their meeting rooms[1] (WHO, 1970).

In 1971, US Surgeon General Jesse L. Steinfeld declared to the Interagency Committee on Smoking and Health "Nonsmokers have as much right to clean indoor air... as smokers have to their so-called right to smoke. It is high time to ban smoking from all confined public spaces such as restaurants, theaters, airplanes, trains and buses. It is time that we interpret the Bill of Rights for the nonsmokers as well as the smoker" (Brandt, 2007).

In 1973, after a plane crashed from a fire that started in an airplane bathroom waste bin, the US Federal Aviation Administration banned smoking in aircraft bathrooms (Holm & Davis, 2004). This same year, following years of passengers and cabin crew complaints about poor air quality in aircraft cabins caused by SHS, the US Civil Aeronautics Board established nonsmoking sections in passenger aircraft cabins; many international airlines followed suit (Brandt, 2007).

In 1975, the first WHO expert committee report on smoking and its effects on health pointed out that although the main concern was with health effects in the smoker, the nonsmoker exposed to SHS may be exposed to harmful concentrations of smoke *in ill-ventilated small places* (emphasis added) (WHO, 1975). The effects of inhaling carbon monoxide were highlighted. This report recommended that "Public information programs should emphasise the rights of the nonsmokers, especially children and pregnant women, to be

protected from involuntary exposure to secondhand smoke." Legislative advice was also offered, but preceded by recommendations of moderation because "legislation that is too far out of tune with public opinion may provoke unfavorable reactions" or prevent its enforcement. In the same year, the Australian National Health and Medical Research Council issued a report with very similar recommendations (Noonan, 1976). By 1975, WHO reported that smoking was banned in hospitals and schools in a number of countries. However, many countries emphasised designating nonsmoking areas with or without physical separation from smoking areas.

In 1976, a resolution of the WHA urged Member States to seriously consider the following legislative recommendation: to create or extend nonsmoking areas in hospitals, health care institutions, public transportation, working environments, and other public places. The emphasis was on nonsmoking areas - on gaining spaces for nonsmokers. In 1978, another resolution of the WHA urged Member States "to protect the rights of nonsmokers to enjoy an atmosphere unpolluted by secondhand smoke," because the smoke had harmful effects on those who are involuntarily exposed to it.

In 1973, Norway restricted smoking on public transport, meeting rooms, work premises, and institutions (Ministry of Health & Care Services, 1973). In the same year, the US state of Arizona also restricted smoking to designated areas in libraries, theaters, concert halls, and buses. This was

followed by a US state of Connecticut law restricting smoking in restaurants, and a 1975 US state of Minnesota law that included restrictions on smoking in private workplaces, in addition to restaurants, meeting rooms, and public places (U.S. Department of Health and Human Services, 1989).

Period 5: 1980-1991

Prior to the early 1980s, the most frequently recommended measure for the public's protection from SHS exposure was the segregation of smoking into separate areas, usually without consideration of physical separation or ventilation issues. There were significant concerns regarding the potential political and economic consequences of advancing 100% smoke-free proposals in any location.

However, in 1980, the damage to small-airways in the lungs as a result of workplace exposure to tobacco smoke among nonsmokers, was documented (White & Froeb, 1980), and another study concluded that "We showed, both experimentally and theoretically, that under the practical range of ventilation and building occupation densities, the RSP levels generated by smokers overwhelm the effect of ventilation and inflict significant air pollution burdens on the public" (Repace & Lowrey, 1980). In 1981, Dr. Takeshi Hirayama, a Japanese epidemiologist published the seminal study in the field of SHS (Hirayama, 1981). It reported that nonsmoking women living with smoking husbands had double the risk of lung cancer, compared to wives living with nonsmoking husbands.

---

[1] Resolution WHA23.32 (1970). Considering that smoking of tobacco during meetings may constitute a nuisance to nonsmokers; RESOLVES that all those present at meetings of the Assembly and its committees be requested to refrain from smoking in the rooms where such meetings are held.

By 1986, 13 studies had linked SHS to lung cancer, and the evidence was strong and consistent enough for the US Surgeon General to issue the first report dealing entirely with the effects of passive smoking, which concluded that "involuntary smoking causes disease, including lung cancer, in healthy nonsmokers" (U.S. Department of Health and Human Services, 1986). The US National Academy of Sciences released a report with the same conclusion shortly afterwards (National Research Council, 1986). That same year a report by IARC concluded that there was sufficient evidence that tobacco smoke is carcinogenic to humans and that "passive smoking gives rise to some risk of cancer" (IARC, 1986).

In 1986 and 1990, the WHA passed general resolutions urging Member States to ensure that non-smokers received effective protection from exposure to SHS (WHO, 1986, 1990). In 1991, the WHA recommended banning smoking in relation to public conveyances, adding the caveat "where protection against involuntary exposure to secondhand smoke cannot be ensured."

Following a lawsuit by an employee who contracted lung cancer and claimed that SHS exposure on airlines caused the disease, the US National Research Council's Committee on Airliner Cabin Air Quality, in 1986, unanimously and forcefully proposed prohibiting smoking on all commercial flights of short duration within the USA. This recommendation was endorsed by the Association of Flight Attendants, the American Medical Association, and the American Lung Association.

In 1987, Air Canada instituted highly successful nonsmoking flights on three busy corridors, and a law was implemented in the USA that banned smoking on flights of two hours or less. In 1990, the US Congress expanded this law to include all domestic flights of six hours or less.

In 1988, Norway extended its legislation to require smoke-free air in all enclosed public places and means of transportation; however, this did not include restaurants and bars.

By 1989, 45 US states had laws restricting smoking in public places and 17 states included some restrictions in private sector workplaces.

In 1990, the New Zealand legislature passed a Smoke-free Environments Act (Ministry of Health, 1990). The provisions of this act included some smoke-free areas (e.g. public facilities, including retail areas, and most shared offices), as well as many partial restrictions (more than half of the area nonsmoking) for work cafeterias, restaurants, and meal serving areas of pubs and other licensed venues. However, smoking restrictions were not implemented for non-meal serving areas of pubs, members' clubs, nightclubs, casinos, or in many non-office workplaces.

In 1990, the US Environmental Protection Agency (EPA) issued a draft report identifying SHS as a known human carcinogen. During the same year, using a population survey of California, it was estimated that, compared to workers in a smoke-free worksite, those with only a work area ban were almost three times more likely to be exposed to SHS, and those without any policy were eight times more likely to be exposed (Borland et al., 1992).

In 1991, a class action law suit sought damages from the tobacco industry for diseases and deaths caused to flight attendants by exposure to SHS in airline cabins. This suit was successfully settled and established a not-for-profit medical research foundation (Flight Attendants Medical Research Institute) with $300 million funding from the tobacco industry (Flight Attendants Medical Research Institute, 1991). At the same time, flight attendant unions in many different countries joined forces with non-government organisations to start a broad-scale lobbying campaign for smoke-free skies. As a result of this pressure, the International Civil Aviation Organization approved a resolution in 1992 to eliminate smoking on international commercial flights by July 1, 1996. Though not legally binding, the resolution soon became an accepted standard for airlines, and national airlines began banning smoking on commercial flights as well.

Period 6: 1992-2003

In 1992, the US EPA issued a report classifying SHS as a major human carcinogen. In California, local and city governments have the power of passing local clean air laws, and tobacco control advocates were active from the late 1980s in getting such ordinances passed. By 1994, 195 municipalities had implemented such ordinances. In 1994, the California Legislature approved the California Smoke-Free Workplace Law, which required indoor workplaces in the state to be smoke-free. This law became effective January 1, 1995 in all workplaces, except bars and taverns where it was delayed until January 1, 1998. Not only was this the first comprehensive law, but for many years it was the only comprehensive law worldwide.

In 1998 in India, a woman filed a petition[2] seeking to have the High Court of Kerala require the government to adopt measures to protect her from exposure to SHS on public transport. In 1999, the Court found in her favor noting that public smoking of tobacco violated her constitutional rights. Smoking in public places was declared punishable as a public nuisance and SHS was declared to be air pollution that was subject to India's environmental protection laws. The Court ordered the government of Kerala to educate and legislate in order to eliminate exposure to SHS in public places.

In 2001, the Supreme Court of India settled litigation by directing the central and state governments of the Indian Union to take effective steps to prohibit smoking in health and educational institutions, public offices, court buildings, auditoriums, libraries, and public conveyances, including railways. In response, a law was passed in 2003 and the government implementation rules in 2004 required hotels of more than 30 rooms and restaurants of more than 30 seats to have physically segregated smoking areas.

Following the Indian example, in 2001, environment lawyers in Uganda, with assistance from Environmental Law Alliance World-wide, a non-profit network of lawyers, filed suit against the Attorney General and the environment authority stating that SHS violates nonsmokers' constitutional right to life and the right to a clean and healthy environment. The High Court found that smoking in public places was a violation of the constitutional right to life of non-smokers and the right to a clean and healthy environment guaranteed in both the Ugandan Constitution and the National Environment Statute of 1995. In 2004, the National Environment Management Authority complied with the court order and regulated smoking in public places.

In 2002, Delaware was the second US state to adopt a comprehensive smoke-free workplace law.

Period 7: post 2003

In 2003, WHO adopted the FCTC, as outlined earlier in this chapter. This was the start of considerable governmental action to enact smoke-free workplace laws as part of a comprehensive set of tobacco control interventions. Countries that have enacted smoke-free legislation covering all types of places and institutions according to WHO MPOWER (2008) are presented in Table 3.1; governmental jurisdictions at the sub-national level that have enacted smoke-free legislation are presented in Table 3.2.

In 2003, New York became the third US state to adopt a comprehensive smoke-free work-place law.

Table 3.1 Countries* by WHO region with smoke-free legislation covering all types of places and institutions assessed as reported in MPOWER (WHO, 2008)
Country
Africa
Botswana
Guinea
Niger
Uganda
The Americas
Uruguay
Eastern Mediterranean
Iran
Europe
Estonia
France
Ireland
Italy
Malta
Norway
Sweden
UK
South-East Asia
Bhutan
Western Pacific
New Zealand

*Degree of enforcement varies across countries listed

[2] The Indian judiciary allows individuals and organisations to approach the court seeking its interventions in matters of public interest even if plaintiffs are not directly affected. A letter to the High Court is enough to seek its involvement. The same applies to Ugandan courts.

Table 3.2 Countries with sub-national legislation banning smoking inside enclosed restaurants and bars (with smoking rooms/areas completely prohibited)

BY CONTINENT AND NATIONAL JURISDICTIONS

EUROPE

Province, state, region, county	Date
Switzerland	
Canton of Ticino	01.07.08
United Kingdom	
Scotland	26.03.06
Wales	02.04.07
Northern Ireland	30.04.07
England	01.07.07

NORTH AMERICA

Province, state, region, county	Date
Canada	
Northwest Territories	01.05.04
Nunavut Territories	01.05.04
New Brunswick	01.10.04
Manitoba	01.10.04
Saskatchewan	01.01.05
Newfoundland & Labrador	01.07.05
Ontario	31.05.06
Quebec	31.05.06
Nova Scotia	01.12.06
Alberta	01.01.08
British Columbia	31.03.08
Yukon Territory	15.05.08
Mexico	
Mexico City	07.04.08
Tabasco	09.08.08
United States	
California	01.01.98
Delaware	27.11.02

PACIFIC

Province, state, region, county	Date
Australia	
Tasmania	01.01.06
Queensland	01.07.06
Western Australia	31.07.06
Australian Capital Territory	01.12.06
Victoria	01.07.07
New South Wales	02.07.07
South Australia	31.10.07

SOUTH AMERICA

Province, state, region, county	Date
Argentina	
Santa Fe	21.03.06
Tucuman	29.06.06
Neuquen	15.11.07
Mendoza	12.02.08

OTHER

Province, state, region, county	Date
Bermuda	01.04.06
Guernse	02.07.06
Jersey	02.01.07
Puerto Rico	02.03.07
British Virgin Islands	31.05.07
Isle of Man	30.03.08
Hong Kong	01.07.09

State	Date
New York	24.07.03
Maine	01.01.04
Connecticut	01.01.04
Massachusetts	05.07.04
Rhode Island	31.03.05
Vermont	01.09.05
Washington	08.12.05
New Jersey	15.04.06
Colorado	01.07.06
Hawaii	16.11.06
Ohio	07.12.06
District of Columbia	02.01.07
Arizona	01.05.07
New Mexico	15.06.07
New Hampshire	17.09.07
Minnesota	01.10.07
Illinois	01.01.08
Maryland	01.01.08
Iowa	01.07.08
Utah	01.01.09
Oregon	01.01.09
Nebraska	01.06.09
Montana	01.10.09

Date indicates effective law implementation
Source: As reported by Rob Cunningham and Michael DeRosenroll, Canadian Cancer Society, on September 8, 2008 in Globalink (http://www.globalink.org)

In 2004, Ireland became the first country to enact a comprehensive smoke-free workplace law nationwide. Norway and New Zealand also enacted legislation in 2004. During the same year, three more US states (Maine, Connecticut, and Massachusetts) also adopted such a law, as well as three Canadian provinces and two Canadian territories.

In 2005, two more Canadian provinces and three US states (total of nine states) adopted this law.

In 2006, Uruguay became the first South American country, and the fourth overall, to adopt smoke-free workplace laws. Scotland also implemented its smoke-free law, as well as two Argentinian provinces, two more Canadian provinces (total of five provinces), four more US states, and three Australian states.

In 2007, Lithuania and Iceland joined the countries with smoke-free workplace laws. Three more Australian states enacted legislation, making this country essentially smoke-free. The remainder of the UK, five more US states (total of 18), and an additional Argentinian province also adopted this legislation.

Examples of implementation of smoke-free legislation

WHO reports that 16 countries, comprising only 5% of the world's population, have a comprehensive national smoke-free law, with high compliance in many of these countries (WHO, 2008). State and provincial initial efforts in Australia, Canada, and the USA set the pace for others to follow. A few examples are presented.

The 1994 California legislation: the precursor

California is the most populous US state, with a resident population that grew from 30 to 34 million between the 1990 and 2000 censuses. Beginning in the early 1980s, tobacco control advocates in California were active in trying to protect nonsmokers from SHS (Glanz & Balbach, 2000) and had started a successful strategy of targeting local and city governments to implement their power of passing local clean air ordinances. In 1992, two things occurred that led to the rapid diffusion of these local ordinances. First, the US EPA report (followed quickly by the California EPA publication) listed SHS as a human carcinogen. Second, the results of the first California Tobacco Survey were reported in a major medical journal indicating that Californians in a smoke-free workplace were 3-8 times less exposed to SHS than other workers (Borland *et al.*, 1992). By 1994, 195 municipalities had implemented smoke-free workplace ordinances.

As state law could preempt these proliferating ordinances, both industry and health groups lobbied the California Legislature. In January 2004, the state law requiring smoke-free public buildings was extended to ban smoking within 20 feet of main entrances, exits, and operable windows. Later that year, the California legislature enacted the California smoke-free workplace law, which became effective January 1, 1995, in all workplaces except bars and taverns, where implementation was delayed until January 1, 1998. However, this law did contain a number of important exemptions, included long-term patient care facilities and businesses with fewer than five employees (provided a number of provisions were met). This law did not contain a preemption clause sought by the tobacco industry interest groups, although the language was not completely clear. Immediately, the tobacco industry organised a resident petition to have a proposition (#188) that would overturn this law put on the ballot in the scheduled November election[3]. However, Proposition 188 was defeated with a resounding 71% "no" vote on Election Day.

In 2005, California banned smoking throughout its large prison system (over 170 000 adult inmates). The law requires workers, as well as inmates, to abide by the prohibition when inside the walls, although staff housing on prison grounds are exempt when inmates are not present. However, as of January 2009, there are 31 US states with tighter restrictions on prisons than California (America for Nonsmokers' Rights, 2009).

---

[3] Citizens in California may put a referendum on the statewide ballot that will: a) amend their constitution, b) adopt a new state statute, c) overturn legislation passed by the state legislature, or d) recall politicians. Before such initiatives are put on the ballot, they need to have been endorsed by 5-8% of the number of residents who voted in the previous gubernatorial election. The number of signatures needed in 2008 was 433 952 for a statute and 694 323 for a constitutional amendment. (http://ballotpedia.org/wiki/index.php/California-Initiative-and-Referendum-Law)

Local ordinances versus state law

The city of San Jose, in California, had enacted a clean indoor air ordinance that included long-term care facilities. In 1995, a nursing home resident complained about exposure to SHS in the common areas of the nursing home. The City advised the facility that it was in violation of the local law. The State Department of Health sued claiming that the state law preempted the local law. However the courts did not support the state's position. The 1998 Court of Appeal judged that the local law was not preempted by any state or federal law and that the Department's rules and regulations did not have the authority and force of statutory law. This led to the rapid passage of a network of local ordinances across the state to cover the exemptions in the California state law, so that all state workplaces were smoke-free. Thus, the combination of state and local laws meant that California was the first large population to be fully protected as later envisaged by Article 8 of WHO's FCTC.

Enforcement provisions

The California law did not contain a separate appropriation for enforcement. Local and city governments were given the responsibility of choosing which of a series of potential agencies should have enforcement responsibilities for the law. The law established a graded and not-too-punitive fine structure ($100 first offence, increasing to $500 for 3rd offence within a year), prior to requiring that the company be referred to the California Occupational Safety

and Health Administration, which could (and did in at least one instance) impose fines as high as $50 000.

Without enforcement power, the California Tobacco Control Program (TCP) embarked on a campaign to build a social norm that would ensure voluntary compliance. Educational approaches included paid mass media messages about the dangers of SHS, so that by 2007, over 90% of California smokers surveyed agreed with the statement that any exposure to SHS could harm the health of babies and children, and 76% agreed that inhaling smoke from someone else's cigarette can cause lung cancer (California Department of Public Health, 2007).

Further, the California TCP supported direct mail and outreach campaigns to businesses, including free distribution of signage for walls and tables, as well as bar napkins with smoke-free messages. Educational articles were placed in trade publications, such as the Chamber of Commerce and Business Association newsletters. Local activists conducted volunteer observational surveys, with follow-up letters of congratulations for those in compliance or letters notifying businesses of the observed smoking, which were copied to the law enforcement agencies; and training and collaboration with law enforcement agencies to designate processes for addressing complaints and conducting enforcement operations.

An example of the effectiveness of this approach was provided by the city of San Francisco (population 1 million), California. In 2001, the local health department for the city identified 30 non-compliant

bar owners and implemented an intervention, which included an informational letter informing them that smoking had been observed in their establishment and that there were potential legal liabilities for non-compliance with the law (Moore & Hrushow, 2004). This was followed by a series of three large, colorful postcards sent over a two year period with the message "Bar Owners Alert: Citations on the Rise." Observed compliance rose from 0% in 2002 to 70% in 2004. Observational surveys of a random sample of 300 San Francisco bars, from 2001 to 2003, identified that overall compliance was high and increasing over time (91% to 95%).

Statewide surveys of enforcement agencies were conducted in 1998, 2000, 2004, and 2007; the response rate was approximately 65%. The survey topics included actions taken in response to inquiries and/or complaints, as well as the conduct of agency-scheduled compliance checks. Actions included educational activities, as well as the issuance of warnings or citations. In 2007, 69% of agencies reported undertaking agency-scheduled compliance checks, and over 50% reported initiating a compliance check in response to either an inquiry or complaint. The majority of the actions taken involved education of bar owners and others; 42% of the agencies issued at least one official warning, and 23% reported issuing at least one citation in response to a detected violation. Reported enforcement action (including inquiries and complaints) was significantly lower in 2007 than in earlier years (Rogers *et al.*, 2008). This is in line with the reduction in SHS exposure reported in Chapter 6.

Summary

The 1994 California state law does not comply with the Article 8 guidelines described at the start of this chapter, and therefore cannot be considered a model law. However, local ordinances were enacted quickly to remove the exemptions in the state law. As a result, by 1998 the 34 million residents of California were effectively covered by smoke-free policies in the manner envisaged by Article 8 guidelines, making it the first large jurisdiction to be smoke-free.

The 2004 Irish legislation: the first country

Enactment

In 2002, the Irish legislature gave the power to create smoke-free workplaces to the Minister for Health and Children. Two separate agencies (the Office of Tobacco Control and the Health and Safety Authority) commissioned independent scientists to review and report on the evidence on SHS and health. This report included a recommendation that employees needed to be protected from it in the workplace by legislative measures. At the press release following this report, in January 2003, the Minister for Health and Children announced that he would issue the necessary regulations to make all enclosed workplaces, including bars, smoke-free on January 1, 2004 (Howell, 2004). Extensive lobbying by the hospitality sector to have bars and restaurants exempted was unsuccessful, and on March 29, 2004, Ireland became the first nation to implement legislation creating smoke-free enclosed workplaces, including bars and restaurants. This legislation does not allow designated smoking rooms; however, prisons, hotel rooms, and psychiatric hospitals are exempt.

Enforcement

The performance reports from local health boards was compiled by the Office of Tobacco Control for the first nine months following enactment of the law (Office of Tobacco Control, 2005). A total of 34 957 inspections/compliance checks by environmental health offices were reported in this period; 94% of premises inspected were assessed as smoke-free (no evidence of smoking), and 86% had the required "No smoking" signage. A smoke-free compliance telephone line received 3121 calls over this period, including 1881 complaints (the majority in the first month). At the end of the nine months, complaint calls had stabilised at 40-50 per month.

In its annual report for 2007, the Office of Tobacco Control included details on inspections and compliance with the smoke-free law (Office of Tobacco Control, 2007): there were 7033 inspections of licensed premises with an 87% compliance with the law; 6401 inspections of restaurants (98% compliance); 1162 inspections of hotels (93% compliance); and 14 386 inspections of other workplaces (98% compliance). Combining all these inspections, compliance with the law was assessed to be 95%. A total of 676 complaints were received by the smoke-free compliance telephone line. During the year, there were a total of 49 convictions for infractions of the law with the majority of these relating to licensed premises.

The Irish legislation is widely considered to be a model of smoke-free policy, complying with the requirements of the Article 8 guidelines outlined at the start of this chapter.

The 2004 New Zealand legislation: the first country in the southern hemisphere

New Zealand was an early adopter of policies restricting smoking. In 1987, the New Zealand Department of Health implemented a smoke-free policy in its buildings, and, a year later, domestic airlines went smoke-free. However, early adoption of this partial legislation appeared to be enough to reduce the political pressure for more comprehensive protection of nonsmokers for 13 years and the passage of the Smoke-free Environments Amendment Act 2003, a comprehensive smoke-free law.

The act introduced a range of tobacco control measures, including that all schools and early childhood centers must be smoke-free by January 1, 2004, and nearly all other indoor workplaces by December 10, 2004, including bars, casinos, members' clubs, and restaurants. Smoking was allowed in outdoor "open" areas, including those semi-enclosed, provided they did not meet the Ministry of Health's definition of an enclosed "internal" workplace.

The exact definition of an internal and open area was complex (see http://www.moh.govt.nz/smokefreelaw) (Edwards *et al.*, 2008).

Nevertheless, several partial exemptions were allowed, notably prisons, hotel and motel rooms, and residential establishments, such as long-term care institutions and rest homes. Since then, a number of local governments have implemented smoke-free park policies.

The 2004 Scottish legislation: more European countries join the smoke-free club

Scotland is part of the UK, and, in 1999, became a devolved jurisdiction with legislative and administrative control of issues including health, education, criminal law, home affairs, local government, economic development, the environment, agriculture, sports, and the arts. Other areas, such as the constitution, defense, fiscal and economic systems, employment, safety, social security, and transport, remained under control of the UK Government (The Scotland Office, 1999).

In early 2004, the Scottish Executive, the administrative arm of the Scottish government, launched the first Scottish tobacco control action plan called "A Breath of Fresh Air for Scotland" (Scottish Executive, 2004). This plan included proposals for a Scottish debate on SHS and a separate Parliamentary Members Bill, entitled *Prohibition of Smoking in Regulated areas (Scotland) Bill*, was introduced for legislative debate (Scottish Parliament, 2004). There was a large response to the ensuing Executive's formal public

consultation, with the vast majority supporting a law creating smoke-free enclosed public places, with few exemptions (Scottish Parliament, 2006).

The Smoking, Health and Social Care (Scotland) Bill was introduced to Parliament on December 17, 2004, and was enacted on March 26, 2006 (National Health Service, 2006). The legislation makes it an offence to smoke or to allow smoking in virtually all enclosed public and workplaces, including pubs and restaurants, with only a few exemptions (Scottish Parliament, 2006). Exempted premises include private residential accommodations and private cars; designated rooms in workplaces that are also communal living establishments, such as adult care homes, hospices, and off-shore installations; designated places where people are detained against their will, e.g. psychiatric units, prison cells, and police interview rooms. Designated hotel bedrooms are also exempt, but no minimum number of smoke-free rooms is required.

Local health authorities have the responsibility for enforcement and Environmental Health Officers (EHOs) are authorised to enter no-smoking premises to determine whether the law is being upheld. Inspections are usually incorporated within other health and safety or food hygiene inspections (Scottish Government, 2005); however, independent pro-active (to confirm compliance) or re-active (in response to a complaint) inspections are also undertaken. In the three months following implementation of the law, EHOs carried out 32 000 inspections across Scotland. In this period,

compliance with the legislation was high; inspections recorded 97% compliance with smoking regulations and 80% with signage regulations.

Over time, the number of quarterly inspections decreased to around 8000 a quarter, as observed compliance with smoking regulations remained high at between 95 and 97%. Compliance with display signage increased to 97% for the period April-June 2008 (Scottish Government, 2008). Explicit in the enforcement guidance was the expressed intention to adopt a non-confrontational approach (Scottish Government, 2005). This is reflected in the small number of fixed penalty notices issued, which on average were nine against premises and 232 against individuals per three month reporting period. Thus, for most areas, it would appear that the legislation has become largely self-enforcing. However, within the pub and bar sector, the possibility of prosecution is used by staff as a rationale for strongly enforcing the smoke-free law (Eadie *et al.*, 2008).

The 2005 Italian legislation: approaching the spirit of the FCTC

In January 2005, an Italian law was enacted to regulate smoking in enclosed public places (Gasparrini *et al.*, 2006). This law does not meet the criteria for being fully smoke-free, as designated smoking rooms are still allowed in the hospitality sector (although the conditions for such rooms are very strict and expensive to implement, and only implemented by a small number of establishments). The smoking rooms must be: a) physically separated by four walls from floor to ceiling, less than half of the size of the whole premises; b) enclosed by automatic sliding doors regularly kept in the closed position; and c) with a negative pressure of at least 5 pascal provided by forced ventilation with a flow rate of at least 30 L per second per person, considering a crowding rate of 0.7 persons per m^2. The regulation also states that the designated smoking area should not be a pass way for nonsmokers, but it is not clear if this includes workers and therefore service to these areas. While this law does not meet the criteria for model legislation, it approaches its spirit. Most businesses have decided not to create smoking rooms due to the high cost of implementing the strict standards on air quality. A survey conducted in 2005, estimated that less than 1% of businesses, including bars, restaurants, and pizzerias have built smoking areas for their premises (http://www.ministerosalute.it/resources/static/primopiano/255/conferenzaFumo.pdf)

The Italian legislation was the culmination of a series of public policy changes over the previous decade. In 1996, a constitutional court opened up the possibility of considering SHS as a health hazard under the law, and, in 1999, a bank lost a lawsuit for not protecting a worker from SHS. The Health Minister built a wide public coalition and parliament passed the law protecting citizens from SHS in December 2002. However, this law was challenged in the courts by bar and restaurant owner associations and was not enacted until 2005.

The government focused on enforcement and carried out thousands of inspections in the first 10 months of the enactment of the law. Compliance appeared high; less than 2% of businesses were charged. Spot checks of environmental nicotine concentrations decreased in the hospitality sector, and surveys of Italians suggest that businesses are generally compliant with the law. Although not model legislation, it has achieved the desired goals, and several European countries have chosen this Italian law as the one that most fits their needs.

The 2006 Uruguay legislation: the first middle income developing country

Uruguay was the first developing country in the world to pass and enforce 100% smoke-free legislation for all workplaces, including bars and restaurants, with no exceptions whatsoever. The origin of this success dates back to 2000, when WHO initiated the negotiation of the FCTC. At that time, the Uruguayan Medical Association created a section devoted to tobacco control and the Director General of Health Services of the Ministry of Health, a member of the coalition government of the two traditional right wing parties, promoted the creation of an umbrella organisation, the National Alliance for Tobacco Control (NATC). For the first time governmental and quasi-governmental health agencies, health professionals associations, and academic institutions interested in tobacco control worked together.

In 2003, the Pan American Health Organization (PAHO) and WHO convened a workshop for countries of the southern cone of South America to discuss possible national tobacco control projects. Leaders of the Uruguayan Alliance attended and proposed to make all facilities of the local government of the city of Montevideo (Intendencia) smoke-free. The following year, the Smoke-free Intendencia project started with a small grant from PAHO/WHO. Leaders of the project were health professionals working for the city government and members of NATC. They involved and got the support of the mayor of Montevideo, and other city officials, part of the center-left ruling coalition at that time in opposition to the national government. In 2003, the city of Montevideo enforced 100% smoke-free environments in all its government offices and health services to the public.

Also in 2003, the Global Youth Tobacco Survey reported on exposure levels to SHS among 13- to 15-year-olds in Uruguay, and another international study reported high concentrations of vapor-phase nicotine in indoor workplaces. These results convinced the national government to declare all health settings 100% smoke-free. The government ratified the WHO FCTC in July 2004.

In 2005, the centre-left Broad Front Coalition (Frente Amplio in Spanish) won the parliamentary elections and Tabaré Vazquez, the former Mayor of Montevideo and an oncologist and radiotherapist, became President of the Republic. The Ministry of Health immediately created the national tobacco control programme with three persons. Under the President's leadership, the government raised tobacco taxes, banned tobacco sponsorship of sport events, implemented pictorial health warnings occupying 50% of the principal areas of cigarette packages, and created smoke-free environments in public and workplaces.

In 2006, all public and workplaces, including bars and restaurants, went 100% smoke-free. In six years Uruguay went from not having any significant tobacco control legislation to being highly advanced with regards to smoke-free restrictions, according to the WHO MPOWER report (WHO, 2008).

Summary

The guidelines for the implementation of Article 8 of the WHO's FCTC represent "best practices" and provide public health officials and policymakers with a clear description of the elements of an effective smoke-free policy. Such a policy needs to create 100% smoke-free spaces, by law, in all indoor public and workplaces and public transportation. The policy should emphasise that protection from exposure to SHS is a basic human right, and that protection should be universal. The focus needs to be on ensuring 100% smoke-free environments, as opposed to protecting only targeted populations or permitting smoking in restricted areas. It would appear that an organised strategy for public education and enforcement is critical for successful implementation.

In the early 20th century, cigarette smoking was not a common behaviour and it was proscribed in certain settings. Although advocacy groups tried to maintain this status quo, the rapid dissemination of smoking led to it quickly pervading

every setting. It was not until some 40 years later that advocacy for smoke-free environments began again. The first jurisdiction with legislation that adhered to the FCTC guidelines was the US state of California in 1998, and its experience has been studied and reported widely. However, the critical trigger that diffused this legislation widely was the adoption of the WHO FCTC starting in 2003. The first countrywide legislation was enacted in Ireland in 2004.

Since then, the number of countries that have enacted legislation (at the national and sub-national levels) has increased with each year and is expected to continue to increase in the future. There are now many examples of legislation that completely adhere to the FCTC guidelines and the implementation experiences of some of these are discussed in the chapter. However, a number of countries have implemented legislation that does not meet the guidelines. Some of these, such as Italy, have requirements for smoking rooms that are so stringent and cost prohibitive that establishments voluntarily go smoke-free. Others, however, have implemented legislation with looser standards. While this legislation may have resulted in a reduction in SHS exposure, it is not clear how these countries will be able to amend the legislation so that they adhere to the WHO FCTC guidelines.

Conclusions

The first jurisdiction to go smoke-free did so in 1998, and this experience led to the development of the WHO FCTC "best practice" guidelines in 2003.

Countries ratified the WHO FCTC, agreeing to introduce legislation that adhered to these guidelines. This, in addition to the availability of technical support from WHO, resulted in the rapid diffusion of smoke-free legislation around the world, which appears to be still gathering momentum. The global experience in tobacco control has produced valuable exemplars that can be used to further advance efforts to reduce exposure to SHS. Based on the review of smoke-free policies, the following recommendations should be considered:

1. The guidelines for implementation of WHO FCTC Article 8 should be followed wherever possible, as these are evidence-based from different approaches to tobacco control and have been shown to have all the necessary detail to minimise exposure of the citizenry to SHS and its harmful consequences.

2. Passing a policy is only one part of the process of protecting a population from exposure to SHS; both public education and enforcement efforts are necessary when the smoke-free policy is implemented.

3. The need for enforcement efforts usually decreases after the policy becomes established, when it typically becomes self-enforcing.

Chapter 4
Impact of smoke-free policies on businesses, the hospitality sector, and other incidental outcomes

Introduction

The widespread implementation of smoke-free policies in many countries has been slowed by fears that restrictions on smoking may have an adverse impact on businesses. It is clear, however, that allowing smoking in the workplace adds considerable costs for businesses. Lost productivity results from disease and premature death caused by smoking and exposure to tobacco smoke in the workplace. Establishments which allow smoking face higher health and hazard insurance premiums, and cleaning and maintenance costs. Those that restrict smoking to designated areas assume the costs of building and maintaining them.

Particularly prominent in the debate over smoke-free policies have been concerns about the economic impact on restaurants, bars, and other hospitality sector establishments. Some restaurant and bar owners, for example, express concerns that smoke-free policies will drive their smoking patrons to other venues where smoking is allowed (particularly those in nearby jurisdictions without smoke-free policies), or lead them to cut their visit short or even stay home, reducing their establishments' business. Others argue that decisions

to go smoke-free should be left to the businesses themselves and that if these policies are good for their establishment, owners will voluntarily adopt them. The tobacco industry has supported these arguments with claims that smoke-free policies result in lost revenue for restaurants, bars, and other hospitality establishments; fewer jobs in the hospitality sector; and business closings (KPMG, 1998; Deloitte & Touche LLP, 2003; U.S.Departement of Health and Human Services, 2006). This strategy, of making claims about the harmful economic effects of tobacco control policies, is not unique to the industry's attack on smoke-free policies. It has also been used in opposition to other policies, including higher tobacco taxes and comprehensive bans on tobacco product advertising and promotion (Jha & Chaloupka, 1999; Chaloupka & Warner, 2000).

This chapter reviews the evidence on the costs to businesses of allowing smoking in the workplace, and of the potential costs and benefits to businesses that restrict or ban workplace smoking. The extensive and growing literature on the economic impact of smoke-free policies on the hospitality sector is reviewed

in more detail, after a discussion of the strengths and limitations of the methods used in these studies. This is followed by a brief review of the limited evidence on other incidental and/or unanticipated effects of smoke-free policies not covered in other chapters of this Handbook.

Potential costs and benefits to businesses of smoke-free policies

Cigarette smoking among employees and customers imposes a variety of costs on businesses, ranging from lost productivity among employees to higher insurance, cleaning, and other costs (Hallamore, 2006; Javitz et al., 2006). Businesses can incur costs, however, from policies limiting or banning smoking in the workplace. For instance, there are the costs of creating and maintaining smoking areas, potential lost productivity due to increased smoking breaks for smoking employees, and the loss of business from customers who smoke. Policy implementation and enforcement costs will be shared by businesses and governments. Nonetheless, these policies can significantly reduce the expenses to businesses that more than offset any costs that result from their implementation. The potential costs and benefits for businesses of smoke-free policies are summarised in Table 4.1. This section briefly reviews the limited evidence on these costs and benefits; those related to gains and losses to businesses in the hospitality sector, that result from changes in patronage by smoking and nonsmoking customers, are described in more detail in the following section.

Costs of smoking to businesses

A growing body of research clearly illustrates the costs to businesses that allow smoking by employees and customers. These costs include: increased absenteeism and reduced productivity on the job, resulting from the diseases caused by smoking and exposure to tobacco smoke; time spent on smoking breaks by smoking employees; increased health and life insurance costs for employees; increased fire and hazard insurance costs; higher cleaning and maintenance costs; and the potential for significant legal costs resulting from claims filed by employees seeking compensation for damages caused by exposure to tobacco smoke in the workplace, or by customers seeking protection from tobacco smoke. The relative magnitude of costs will vary by type of businesses that have many smoking patrons (e.g. bars, restaurants), com-pared to those where the costs are primarily from a limited number of smoking employees (e.g. white collar offices).

While the subject of considerable discussion, limited empirical evidence exists on the magnitude of these costs to businesses, particularly those in developing countries. Briefly, existing evidence includes:

- *Lost productivity from health consequences of smoking:* In a recent study from Sweden, using nationally representative data from 1988 through 1991, the Swedish Survey of Living Conditions was linked to register-based data on the number of days missed from work due to sickness, from the National Board of Social Insurance (Lundborg, 2007). It was estimated that smokers were absent between 7.7 and 10.7 days more each year than were nonsmokers. Based on a

Table 4.1 Potential costs and benefits to businesses of smoke-free policies

Costs	Benefits
Lost business due to smokers visiting less frequently or cutting visits short	Increased business from nonsmokers visiting more frequently or staying longer
Costs of establishing and maintaining smoking lounges for smoking employees	Reduced cleaning and maintenance costs
Implementation and enforcement costs	Reduced fire, accident, and life insurance premiums
Lost productivity due to increased or longer smoking breaks for smoking employees	Increased productivity as smoking employees quit or cut back and require fewer smoking breaks
Costs of establishing and maintaining smoking areas for patrons	Increased productivity due to reduced absenteeism and improved health among smoking employees
	Increased productivity due to reduced absenteeism and improved health among nonsmoking employees
	Reduced health care costs from reductions in smoking among smoking employees
	Reduced health care costs from reductions in exposure to secondhand smoke among nonsmoking employees
	Avoidance of potential litigation costs from nonsmoking and smoking employees and/or customers

telephone survey of 200 randomly selected Scottish businesses with 50 or more employees, linked to evidence on the costs of smoking drawn from a review of the literature, it was estimated that absenteeism among Scottish smokers reduced productivity by £40 million, while productivity losses due to the premature death caused by smoking totaled approximately £450 million in 1997 (Parrott *et al.*, 2000). More comprehensive estimates of the lost productivity costs resulting from premature deaths caused by smoking, based on well developed methods for estimating economic expenditures, have been produced for many other developed countries, including Australia (Collins & Lapsley, 1996, 2002, 2008), Canada (Kaiserman, 1997), Ireland (Madden, 2003), the USA (Centers for Disease Control and Prevention, 2005a), and a growing number of others.

• *Lost productivity from smoking breaks:* Based on a comprehensive review of existing literature on the costs to employers resulting from smoking in the workplace, it was estimated that smoking employees take an additional four to thirty minutes in break time each day for on-the-job smoking (Javitz *et al.*, 2006). Using similar estimates, the Conference Board of Canada (Hallamore, 2006) estimated that unsanctioned smoking breaks cost Canadian employers an average of CA$3053 per year in 2005.

• *Lost productivity from exposure to secondhand smoke:* As described in Chapter 2, there is strong evidence that exposure to secondhand tobacco smoke (SHS) causes a variety of health consequences in nonsmokers. Among nonsmoking workers, the death and disease caused by this exposure in the workplace leads to additional lost productivity and increased health care costs for businesses. To date, only one study has estimated these costs. In 2005, using the same well developed methods used to estimate the lost productivity costs resulting from premature death caused by smoking, the Society of Actuaries (Behan *et al.*, 2005) estimated that SHS exposure increased health care costs in the USA by nearly US$5 billion, and led to an additional almost US$5 billion in lost productivity, due to lost wages, fringe benefits, and value of services. This clearly underestimates lost productivity costs to businesses, as it does not account for the lost productivity due to work days missed from diseases caused by smoking.

• *Higher insurance premiums:* Similarly, studies have documented the higher costs of insurance coverage for smoking employees and/or workplaces that allow smoking. For example, in the USA, using data on paid health care claims for a large group indemnity plan, it was estimated that average health care insurance premiums for smoking employees were about 50% higher than those for nonsmokers (Penner &

Penner, 1990). A thorough review estimated that fire insurance costs were US$11-21 higher per smoker in the USA (Javitz *et al.*, 2006), while fire insurance costs attributable to smoking for Scottish workplaces were estimated to be approximately £4 million annually (Parrott *et al.*, 2000). Similarly, smoking increased life insurance premiums by CA$75 per smoking employee (Conference Board of Canada, 1997), while the cost to a business of providing US$ 75 000 in life insurance was an approximately additional US$90 per year for a smoking employee (Javitz *et al.*, 2006).

• *Increased cleaning and maintenance costs:* The US Environmental Protection Agency (Mudarri, 1994) estimated that the adoption of a comprehensive smoke-free policy in 1994 would have reduced building operation and maintenance costs for US businesses by US$4.8 billion per year, based on detailed estimates of the costs of cleaning and maintaining different types of workspaces (office, assembly, and warehouse/industrial space). These figures, updated to account for inflation, estimated that in 2005 the additional smoking-related costs per 1000 square feet of workspace ranged from US$305 for warehouse space to US$728 for office space (Javitz *et al.*, 2006).

• *Potential litigation costs:* There are a variety of potential legal challenges businesses may face as a result of allowing smoking in the workplace (Sweda, 2004).These range from claims for workers compensation and disability benefits, resulting from exposure to smoking in the workplace, to lawsuits from customers arguing that persons sensitive to smoke are being discriminated against by being denied the ability to enjoy a smoke-free environment. In the USA, hundreds of legal challenges document key successes in litigation brought on by those exposed to SHS. Anecdotal evidence indicates that similar legal disputes have been successful in a variety of other countries. While the award amounts in these cases vary widely, it is clear that the potential costs of unsuccessfully defending against these litigations can be significant.

In summary, cigarette smoking imposes significant costs on businesses, which can be considerably reduced if policies that restrict or ban smoking in the workplace are enacted. Some costs can be entirely avoided by complete bans on smoking in the workplace, but only somewhat reduced by more limited restrictions (i.e. the need would still exist for cleaning and maintenance due to smoking). Other costs will be reduced (e.g. lost productivity and higher insurance costs), as employee smoking declines (as discussed in Chapter 7) and nonsmoking workers' exposure to tobacco smoke in the workplace falls (as discussed in Chapter 6) in response to smoke-free policies.

Costs of smoke-free policies to businesses and governments

While allowing smoking in the workplace results in potentially significant expenses to businesses, policies that limit or ban workplace smoking are not without cost. This is particularly true for policies that allow for smoking in restricted or designated areas. These costs include:

• *Costs for smoking areas:* As described in Chapter 3, smoke-free policies vary in how restrictive or permissive they are with respect to allowing for smoking areas. Some workplace policies permit the creation of designated smoking rooms for smoking employees, while others completely ban smoking in all enclosed areas, but allow smoking in non-enclosed areas; others designate smoking and nonsmoking sections for their customers. If employers opt to provide a smoking area for their employees and/or patrons, there will be expenses associated with building and maintaining these areas. Costs will vary considerably depending on the size of the area, whether or not it is enclosed, how it is ventilated, local construction costs, and other factors. The Ontario Campaign for Action on Smoking (Wong, 2002), estimates that the cost of establishing a designated smoking room for use by employees who smoke can range from about CA$55 000 to over CA$268 000, with monthly maintenance fees adding CA$200-600, based on the size of the room and the number

of persons using it. The costs of establishing seven smoking rooms for employees, patients, and visitors in a new building being constructed by the Royal Victoria Hospital in Belfast, were estimated to be approximately £500 000 (McKee *et al.*, 2003). Similarly, it was reported that the cost of creating seven smoking rooms for employees and travelers in St. Louis' Lambert Airport in 1997 was US$450 000 (Manor, 1997). In response to comprehensive smoke-free policies, some businesses have turned to building "smoking huts" or "smoking shacks" (partially enclosed shelters to accommodate their smoking employees and patrons). These can range in cost from less than US$2000 for small, no-frills shelters, to tens of thousands of dollars for larger shelters with more amenities (Ford, 2008).

• *Implementation and enforcement costs:* In general, within a few months of implementation, compliance with smoke-free policies is high, and the policies become self-enforcing in most places that have adopted them (see Chapter 5 for a thorough discussion of support for and compliance with smoke-free policies). Nearly all of the costs of implementation and enforcement will be taken on by governments rather than by businesses. In addition to the costs associated with creating and maintaining designated smoking areas, as described above, expenses to businesses are largely limited to signage and minimal enforcement costs.

• *Lost productivity:* Some suggest that smoke-free policies will result in lost productivity, as employees who smoke will take more smoking breaks in response to the policies. Others argue that employees who smoke may be less able to concentrate and less productive if their opportunities to smoke during working hours are limited. To date, there is no good empirical evidence to support either issue. These policies could raise the costs of smoking breaks to businesses, by forcing smokers outdoors, and thus, increasing their time away from work. However, this increase in costs is likely to be offset by the reductions in time lost for smoking breaks by some smokers who quit or cut back in response to the policy (as described in Chapter 7). Similarly, reductions in productivity among smoking employees, when they are denied the opportunity to smoke while working, are liable to be offset by the productivity gains that accrue from reductions in absenteeism and premature deaths caused by smoking.

Costs to governments of implementing and enforcing smoke-free policies

The relatively quick compliance with smoke-free policies in most countries suggests that the implementation and enforcement costs to governments will likely be short-term. Little empirical evidence is available on the costs or cost-effectiveness of efforts to enforce smoke-free policies. Anecdotal evidence suggests that "reactive" enforcement efforts (those that respond to complaints from non-smokers) are relatively less costly, while more "proactive" enforcement efforts (those involving active compliance checks) will be more expensive. Greater proactive enforcement efforts, however, seem likely to raise compliance more quickly, suggesting that they will be needed for a shorter period, making it unclear which approach is more cost-effective in the intermediate to long-term. For example, WHO recommends proactive enforcement efforts in the first weeks and months after the implementation of a smoke-free policy (WHO, 2007b).

Limited data from hospitality sector employees in Norway indicate that greater enforcement may be needed for smoke-free policies that restrict, rather than comprehensively ban, smoking given greater non-compliance with the partial policies (Hetland & Aarø, 2005).

As discussed in Chapter 5, some evidence suggests that compliance with smoke-free policies is enhanced by investments in media advocacy and public education campaigns that strengthen social norms against smoking, before and/or during the implementation of these policies (Ross, 2006; U.S. Department of Health and Human Services, 2006). This implies that more active enforcement of these policies, and/or greater investments in mass media campaigns, may be needed in some developing countries where anti-smoking norms are weaker (Ross, 2006).

Summary

Cigarette smoking in the workplace imposes a variety of costs on businesses, including the lost productivity resulting from smoking breaks, absenteeism, and premature deaths; higher health care and other insurance costs; increased maintenance and cleaning costs; and potential costs of litigation. Smoke-free policies will reduce the costs to businesses associated with work-place smoking.

To date, little solid evidence exists about the costs of smoke-free policies to businesses and/or governments. While there is much speculation about these costs, most appear minimal, short-term, and/or likely to be offset by reductions in related costs. It does appear, how-ever, that the costs of a complete ban on smoking will be lower than the costs of policies that allow for smoking in designated areas, given the costs of maintaining these areas, the remaining exposure that results, and the greater need for enforcement of these partial restrictions. More research is needed to fully under-stand the costs to businesses and governments of adopting, implementing, and enforcing smoke-free policies.

Impact of smoke-free policies on the hospitality sector

The most vigorous debate over the economic impact of smoke-free policies has been with respect to the business activities of restaurants, bars, gaming establishments, and other firms in the hospitality sector. The debates center on the potential for lost revenues resulting from smokers visiting these establishments less frequently (or forgoing visits altogether), cutting their visits shorter and spending less money than they would have if smoking were permitted, and/or taking their business to establishments in jurisdictions that do not have similar policies. Many of these arguments have been voiced by the tobacco industry or various groups supported by the industry (e.g. smokers' rights associations, local restaurant and/or bar associations) (U.S.Departement of Health and Human Services, 2006).

In nearly all countries, however, the number of nonsmokers in the population exceeds the number of smokers. This raises the likelihood that any revenues lost from changes in smokers' patronage will be offset by greater revenues from nonsmokers increasing their patronage of businesses who enact smoke-free policies. As described in Chapter 3, smoke-free policies have been widely adopted in recent years, generating a series of natural experiments that allow researchers to assess the impact of smoke-free policies on business activity, attitudes towards these policies (as described in Chapter 5), on exposure to SHS (as described in Chapter 6), and on smoking behaviour (as described in Chapter 7). With respect to business activity, over 160 studies have examined these issues, applying diverse analytic methods to a variety of data from hospitality sector businesses in numerous jurisdictions, and they have been compiled (Scollo & Lal, 2008) in an update of the previous comprehensive review on the impact of smoke-free policies

in this sector (Scollo *et al.*, 2003; Scollo & Lal, 2005, 2008).

Studies of the impact of smoke-free policies on the hospitality sector vary considerably in their methodological quality, with the best of these studies sharing most or all of the following characteristics:

• Use of valid, reliable measures of business activity (e.g. official reports of sales tax or business revenues, employment, and/or the number of licensed establishments; population level, representative survey data) that can be used to detect the real impact of a change resulting from the adoption of a smoke-free policy;

• Use of data for several years covering the period before and after the implementation of a smoke-free policy, in order to separate out the impact of the policy from underlying trends in business activity, and to allow sufficient time for businesses, smokers, and nonsmokers to adapt their behaviour to the policy;

• Use of appropriate statistical methods that include controls for underlying trends in the data, and other factors that lead to fluctuations in business activity (most notably, overall economic conditions), and that apply appropriate tests for the statistical significance of the relationship between the policy and measure of business activity;

• Inclusion of data from comparable jurisdictions where no policy changes occurred that can act as controls for the jurisdiction(s) where the policy change(s) being assessed took place.

While many of the studies to date share these characteristics, others do not. The findings from studies that use less reliable data, fail to control for overall economic activity, or otherwise deviate from these guidelines, are mixed in their conclusions about the economic impact of smoke-free policies. In contrast, as described below, the findings from studies with these characteristics consistently find that smoke-free policies have no negative economic impact on restaurants, bars, and other segments of the hospitality industry, with the possible exception of gaming establishments. Indeed, many studies provide evidence of a small positive effect of smoke-free policies on business activity.

Studies based on official reports of business activity

Studies based on sales data – restaurants and bars

A large and rapidly expanding literature uses measures of taxable sales, sales tax revenues, or other official reports of sales data, to assess the economic impact of smoke-free policies on restaurants and bars. Many of these studies include appropriate controls for underlying economic conditions and/or other jurisdictions where no policy changes occurred, and most apply appropriate statistical methods to data for several years before and after the policy change of interest.

The first of these studies examined the impact of local smoke-free restaurant policies adopted in 15 California and Colorado communities between 1985 and 1992 (Glantz & Smith, 1994). Fifteen nearby communities without a smoke-free restaurant policy were included as controls, with selection of the control communities matched to communities where policy changes occurred based on population, urbanicity, median household income, and smoking prevalence. Using linear regression methods applied to a measure of taxable restaurant sales revenues as a share of total revenues before and after the implementation of the local policies, the authors concluded that businesses were not adversely affected in the communities that adopted and implemented policies banning smoking in restaurants.

A few years later, the 1994 analysis was extended to include three additional years of data for the 30 communities originally analysed, and to add five cities and two counties that had adopted smoke-free bar policies between 1990 and 1994, with comparable control communities/counties for all but one of these (Glantz & Smith, 1997). A few minor errors in the coding for the implementation dates of the policies included in the earlier study were corrected. Using similar outcome measures, linear and non-linear regression methods were applied to both the matched data and pooled data, confirming an earlier finding that the smoke-free restaurant policies did not adversely affect restaurants in the communities

that adopted them. Similarly it was concluded that smoke-free bar policies had no economic impact on bars.

Comparable studies, based on sales data from restaurants and/or bars, have been done for different jurisdictions in the USA. These studies reflect the diversity of the USA geographically, demographically, socioeconomically, and with respect to the strength and history of tobacco control efforts, from North Carolina counties in the heart of the US tobacco growing region (Goldstein & Sobel, 1998), to large cities or states like New York City (Hyland *et al.*, 1999) and New York State (Engelen *et al.*, 2006). Likewise, a growing number of studies have used bar and/or restaurant sales data from developed countries, including Australia (Wakefield *et al.*, 2002; Lal *et al.*, 2003, 2004), Canada (Luk *et al.*, 2006), Norway (Lund *et al.*, 2005; Lund, 2006; Lund & Lund, 2006), and New Zealand (New Zealand Ministry of Health, 2005; Thomson & Wilson, 2006; Edwards *et al.*, 2008). Nearly all of these studies reached the same general conclusion: that smoke-free policies do not adversely affect the business activity of restaurants and bars, with several providing evidence of a small positive impact of the policy on sales.

In contrast, given the slower diffusion of these policies to developing countries described in Chapter 3, almost no studies exist on the economic impact of smoke-free policies in these countries. The one exception is an analysis of the impact of the 1999 amendments to South Africa's tobacco control policies that introduced restrictions on smoking in restaurants beginning in 2001

(Blecher, 2006). Specifically, under the new policy, restaurateurs were given the option of going entirely smoke-free or creating separately ventilated smoking (in up to 25% of the restaurant) and nonsmoking sections. Using annual provincial value-added tax (VAT) revenues for restaurants from 1995 through 2003, alternative models were estimated that controlled for overall economic conditions, and, in one, the efficiency of VAT tax collection. It was concluded that "the restrictions placed on smoking in restaurants in 2001 have had at worst no significant effect on restaurant revenues, and at best a positive effect on revenues."

Studies based on employment data – restaurants and bars

Several studies use measures of employment to assess the economic impact of smoke-free policies on restaurants and bars. These measures include direct counts of employed persons, and more indirect measures, such as official reports of unemployment, insurance claims, and payroll tax collections. As with the studies that use measures of sales, the best of these studies will control for underlying economic conditions, include several years of pre- and post-policy change data, include similar control jurisdictions where no policy changes occurred, and employ appropriate statistical methods.

To date, all studies using employment-based outcomes have been conducted for jurisdictions in developed countries. Given the relatively early diffusion of smoke-free policies at the local level in the

USA, the majority of the studies have focused on this locale. Findings from studies that meet the standards described above are quite consistent with the results from studies based on measures of sales. They generally conclude that smoke-free policies have had either no significant impact or a small positive impact on employment.

For example, the impact of the comprehensive smoke-free policy implemented in April 2004 by Lexington-Fayette County Kentucky, in the middle of one of the largest tobacco growing and manufacturing states in the USA, was studied (Pyles et al., 2007). It was concluded that restaurant employment rose after the policy was put in place, while bar employment was unchanged. In addition, restaurant and bar employment in neighboring counties was unaffected, a finding inconsistent with opponents' arguments that smokers would take their business to nearby jurisdictions that allowed smoking following the Lexington-Fayette County smoking ban.

Though relatively few non-US studies have looked at the impact of smoke-free policies on employment outcomes, the methodologically sound studies have come to the same basic conclusions reached by the ones from the USA. For example, analysis of Ottawa, Canada's August 2001 ban on smoking in restaurants, bars, and pubs found that employment in affected businesses rose in the period immediately following the ban, while unemployment insurance claims fell, despite an overall decline in employment (Bourns & Malcomson, 2001). Similarly, it was concluded that employment in cafes

and restaurants rose by 9%, and by 24% in drinking establishments, while employment in clubs fell by 8% following the implementation of New Zealand's comprehensive smoke-free policy in late 2004 (Thomson & Wilson, 2006).

Studies based on the number of businesses – restaurants and bars

Other studies of the economic impact of smoke-free policies have used various measures of the numbers of restaurants and bars, such as counts of businesses, business openings and closings, and the number of bankruptcies, with the findings from studies that meet the criteria described above consistent with those based on measures of sales and employment. For example, in the study of the impact of the Lexington-Fayette County Kentucky smoke-free policy, it was concluded that there was no significant impact of the policy on business openings and closings, both for those that served alcoholic beverages and for those that did not (Pyles et al., 2007). Similarly, in a study of the Ottawa smoke-free policy, bankruptcy and insolvency indicators were found to be lower in the period immediately after the ban was implemented than in the two years prior to the ban (Bourns & Malcomson, 2001).

Studies based on business value – restaurants and bars

Two innovative studies looked at the impact of smoke-free policies on the value of restaurants (Alamar & Glantz, 2004) and bars (Alamar & Glantz, 2007) using a measure of

value based on the sales price of establishments that were sold during the periods examined. For the 608 restaurants sampled, 118 were in smoke-free jurisdictions, and sold between 1991 and 2002; for the 197 bars sampled, 17 were in smoke-free jurisdictions, and sold between 1993 and 2005. Controlling for underlying economic conditions (using measures of gross state product and state level unemployment rates for the state in which each establishment was located), type of establishment (e.g. fast food versus full-service restaurant), and general trends, it was concluded that the value of restaurants was 16% higher in smoke-free jurisdictions than in those that allowed smoking, while the value of bars was unaffected by policies banning smoking.

Studies based on revenue data - gaming establishments

In contrast to the relatively large literature using objective measures to assess the economic impact of smoke-free policies on restaurants and bars, there are relatively few studies that have examined the impact on gaming establishments. This is largely the result of the exclusion of these establishments from the venues covered by most smoke-free policies, as described in Chapter 3. Nevertheless, there are a few studies that have looked at the impact of smoke-free policies on various gaming activities.

The first study to examine the impact on gaming venues, investigated the effects of local smoke-free policies in Massachusetts that limited smoking in bingo halls and at gambling events sponsored by local charities (Glantz

& Wilson-Loots, 2003). It was found that increases in other gambling opportunities led to reductions in bingo and charitable gambling event profits, but that the magnitude of the drop was not related to the presence or absence of a smoke-free policy. More recently, a similar approach was used to examine the impact of Massachusetts' state-wide smoking ban implemented in mid-2004 on Keno sales. This report concluded that there was no impact of the ban on this type of gaming (Connolly et al., 2005).

Two recent studies considered the effects of Delaware's comprehensive smoke-free policy that covered three horse racing tracks that allowed video lottery gambling ("racinos"). The first of these studies (Mandel et al., 2005) concluded that the state smoking ban had no impact on either total revenues from the video lottery machines, or on the average revenues per machine; a subsequent re-analysis that corrected for a data entry error and for heteroskedasticity (unequal variance in the error term) in the data (Glantz & Alamar, 2005) confirmed the findings from the original analysis. In contrast, the same data was used and reached the opposite finding: that the Delaware smoking ban reduced gaming revenues by nearly 13% in the year following the implementation of the ban (Pakko, 2006). The differences in findings are accounted for by alternative approaches to modeling the seasonality in the data (Mandel et al. included an indicator for winter months only, while Pakko included indicators for winter, spring, and summer), and by differences in the statistical methods employed

(Mandel et al. used relatively simple weighted regression methods based on the number of video lottery machines, while Pakko used a more general approach to accounting for the heteroskedasticity that also corrected for the serial correlation in the data). The approach used by Pakko appears more appropriate than that used by Mandel and colleagues, and is robust to other specifications including those that replace the quarterly indicators for seasonality with monthly indicators, and that drop 1996 (the year the three racinos opened, which appears to account for the heteroskedasticity in the data).

Most recently, the effects of Victoria, Australia's policy banning smoking in most gaming venues, implemented in September 2002, was studied (Lal & Siahpush, 2008). Interrupted time series methods were applied to monthly expenditures on electronic gaming machines (EGM), from July 1998 through December 2005, for both Victoria and South Australia (their control jurisdiction). It was concluded that the Victoria policy led to "an abrupt, long-term decrease in EGM expenditures" of about 14%, comparable to the 13% decline estimated for the Delaware racinos (Pakko, 2006). The report goes on to note that the decline in EGM expenditures was much larger than observed at Victoria's casino, which was also covered by the smoking ban, but subject to a number of exemptions that allowed the proprietor to cater to high-spending patrons in private rooms. Also, employment in Victoria's gaming sector was at historically high levels three years after the ban. In addition to curbing exposure

to SHS, it was found that Victoria's smoke-free policy was effective in reducing problem gambling, and that the money gamblers did not spend gambling would likely be spent in other sectors of the economy.

Clearly, more research is needed to sort out the economic impact of smoke-free policies on gaming establishments, both on the gaming sector directly, as well as the broader economic impact. As described in Chapter 3, the spread of increasingly comprehensive smoke-free policies that ban smoking in casinos and in other gaming establishments will provide new, natural experiments allowing researchers to assess the economic impact of these policies on the gaming sector.

Studies based on revenue and/or employment data – other hospitality sector establishments

Finally, several studies have used measures of economic activity in other parts of the hospitality sector to evaluate the financial impact of smoke-free policies. These studies have generally focused on the impact of the policies on tourism, using measures of revenues generated by hotels and motels and/or employment in these establishments. The most methodologically sound of these studies share the characteristics of the best studies described above, and are consistent in their conclusions that smoke-free policies do not have an adverse economic impact on these segments of the hospitality industry.

A good example of research on the tourism sector is a study which looked at measures of hotel revenues (both absolute revenues and revenues as a share of total retail sales revenues) and number of tourists (Glantz & Charlesworth, 1999). Data were examined before and after the adoption of comprehensive smoke-free policies in three states (California, Utah and Vermont) and six cities (Boulder, Colorado; Flagstaff and Mesa, Arizona; Los Angeles and San Francisco, California; and New York City). It was found that hotel revenues grew faster following the adoption of the smoke-free policy in four of these jurisdictions, the rate of growth was unchanged in four others, and that revenues grew more slowly (but did not fall) in the last. In these analyses, which pooled the data from the communities, no significant impact of the policy adoption on either measure of revenue was detected. Finally, in analyses that used measures of the number of international tourists visiting the three states studied, there was either no impact of the policy or the number of visitors increased following the implementation of the policy. Given these findings, the re-searchers concluded that "smoke-free ordinances do not appear to adversely affect, and may increase, tourist business."

Studies based on survey data

A second set of studies has relied on measures drawn from survey data to assess the economic impact of smoke-free policies on hospitality sector businesses. These studies include data from surveys of patrons or more representative, population level consumer surveys, and surveys of owners/managers of businesses affected by the smoke-free policy.

A number of patron or consumer surveys collected information on actual dining/drinking out behaviour before and after a policy change, while some pre-implementation surveys inquired about anticipated changes in behaviour in response to the policy. In some post-implementation surveys, individuals were asked about actual changes in behaviour resulting from the policy change, while others gathered information on respondent's preferences for smoke-free dining/drinking areas, and other related attitudes and perceptions. Similarly, surveys of business owners or managers collected self-reported information on business revenues that, in general, were not validated, as well as owner/manager perceptions of the impact of the policy on their business (either anticipated or realised), in addition to their attitudes about the policies.

In addition to meeting the other criteria described above, the best of the studies based on survey data used appropriate sampling and sur-vey methods to collect validated measures of relevant outcomes. For example, a convenience survey of bar patrons, prior to the implementation of a ban on smoking in bars, that asks about their anticipated response to the policy, is much more likely to provide biased estimates of the impact of the policy than would randomly selected consumer surveys, representative of the local population, that collect actual data on bar patronage conducted before and after the policy implementation. The vociferous debate over potentially adverse economic effects of smoke-free policies can create a "negative placebo effect" that leads some

business owners/managers to either fear that the ban will have a negative impact on their business, or to attribute any declines in business after the policy implementation to the policy change, rather than to other factors that may account for the decline (Glantz, 2007). Similarly, researchers observed that "it seems likely that owners of businesses that are faring poorly in a highly volatile market may be more likely to blame external forces (such as the adoption of a smoke-free policy) rather than their own business decisions for their problems" (Eriksen & Chaloupka, 2007).

Given the potential for biased responses, particularly in surveys of business owners or managers, it is not surprising that these studies are much more likely to conclude that the economic impact of smoke-free policies is negative. In a comprehensive review of studies published through August 2002 (Scollo *et al.*, 2003), it was noted that studies based on this type of survey data are four times more likely to conclude that these policies have a negative economic impact, than are studies based on official reports of sales, employment, and related data. Despite the potential for bias, the majority of studies based on survey data, particularly those based on patron/consumer survey data, conclude that there is either no impact or a small, positive economic impact from smoke-free policies.

Studies that employ survey data come from a wider variety of countries than the studies based on sales, employment, and other related data described above, including Australia, Canada, Hong Kong, Ireland, Italy, New Zealand, Norway, Scotland,

South Africa, Spain, the UK, and the USA. However, as seen by this list, these studies add relatively little information on the economic impact of smoke-free policies in developing countries, as few of these countries have adopted such policies. Given the potential misuse of studies based on flawed survey data, this section reviews methodologically sound studies and highlights the potential biases that result from the use of unrepresentative survey data and/or unreliable measures.

Studies based on consumer/patron surveys

Analyses of survey data from Norway, collected before and after the June 1, 2004 implementation of the country's ban on smoking in bars and restaurants, helps explain the consistent finding from studies based on sales and employment data that smoke-free policies do not have an adverse economic impact (Lund *et al.*, 2005; Lund, 2006; Lund & Lund, 2006). Annual representative surveys of Norwegian adults showed no significant changes in the frequency of pub/bar and restaurant visits following the implementation of the ban. Responses to the post-ban survey question "has the ban on smoking in hospitality venues changed your patronage habits?" illustrate the differences in the impact of the ban on patronage by smokers and nonsmokers. Nonsmokers were significantly more likely to report that the ban increased their frequency of visiting hospitality venues, with 18% of nonsmokers reporting an increase, as compared to 1% of daily smokers and 3% of non-daily smokers. In contrast,

smokers were much more likely to report a decrease in their frequency of visiting affected establishments, with 42% of daily smokers and 10% of occasional smokers reporting reduced frequency, as compared to 2% of nonsmokers. Given the much greater prevalence of nonsmokers among Norwegian adults, 12% of the overall sample reported an increase in their frequency of visiting hospitality venues, while 12% reported a decrease. The majority of the population (76%) reported no changes in their patronage in response to the smoke-free policy.

These findings are consistent with those from other studies that use population-based consumer surveys to assess the economic impact of smoke-free policies in a variety of other jurisdictions. In general, these studies find that the implementation of the policy has no significant impact on dining/drinking out practices, and that any reductions in the frequency of such practices among smokers are made up for (often more than made up for) by increases in the frequency of dining/drinking among nonsmokers.

These studies also illustrate the bias that results from convenience samples of hospitality sector customers prior to a change in policies. For example, a survey of current patrons' anticipated responses to a proposed ban on smoking in Hong Kong restaurants, bars, and cafes was administered, and concluded that the ban would reduce revenues for these businesses by more than 10% (KPMG, 2001). In general, these types of convenience surveys of current patrons do not include the nonsmokers deterred from

visiting by the smoky environment, and, as a result, do not pick up the increases in their patronage after policy implementation that offsets any anticipated reductions in patronage among existing customers. Moreover, the anticipated reduction in patronage that smokers describe may not end up happening after the implementation of a smoking ban, as opportunities for smokers to go to alternative venues are limited, resulting in few smokers actually altering their establishment patronage in response to the ban (in contrast to nonsmokers who are increasingly attracted to now smoke-free venues) (Cowling & Bond, 2005).

Studies based on owner/manager surveys

The studies most likely to conclude that smoke-free policies have a negative economic impact on the businesses targeted by the policies are those based on surveys of business owners and managers. Many of these studies are based on proprietor expectations, rather than on the actual impact on business after the smoke-free policy has been implemented. Studies based on pre-implementation surveys of business owners/managers appear most likely to be subject to the "negative placebo affect" (Glantz, 2007). In contrast, well-designed, post-implementation surveys of business owners/managers, which collected more valid measures of business activity, often concluded that their businesses were not negatively affected by the policy. The differences between the perceived and actual business impact of smoke-free policies is clearly illustrated by analysis of the Québec policy limiting smoking in restaurants (Crémieux & Ouellette, 2001). Based on a survey of restaurateurs, that included both those in compliance and those not in compliance with the policy, the researchers concluded that "impacts on… restaurant patronage were widely anticipated but not observed."

The most methodologically sound studies in this group are those based on representative surveys of business owners/managers conducted long enough after the implementation of the policy for its impact on their business activity to be clear. Ideally, such studies would also include similar surveys in comparable jurisdictions where no policy changes occurred, and/or other approaches to control for general trends and underlying economic conditions, in order to isolate the effects of the policy from those of other factors. Few of these studies, however, used this approach.

Analysis of the economic impact of New York City's 1995 smoke-free policy is one of the small numbers of studies that uses a representative sample of restaurants and includes appropriate controls (Hyland & Cummings, 1999). Since this policy only applied to restaurants with more than 35 seats, and did not cover establishments that generated at least 40% of their revenues from the sale of alcoholic beverages, small restaurants and restaurants with bars were included as control groups for the larger restaurants that were affected by the policy, as all of these would have been subject to the same underlying economic conditions. The researchers found that 35% of the restaurants subject to the policy

reported a decrease in business following its implementation; however, illustrating the importance of including appropriate controls, they also found that 34% of small restaurants and 36% of restaurants with significant income from alcoholic beverage sales also reported a decline in business. Given this, they concluded that "there is no evidence to suggest that the smoke-free law has had a detrimental effect on the city's restaurant business."

As with the studies based on sales, employment, or related data, the only evidence from developing countries based on survey data comes from South Africa's experiences following its 1999 Tobacco Products Control Amendment Act that limited smoking in restaurants and other public places. Between November 2004 and January 2005, a survey was conducted of 1431 restaurant owners/managers (1011 surveys were successfully completed) identified by searching online, publicly accessible databases (van Walbeek et al., 2007). This survey gathered data both on the costs of complying with the policy and on restaurant revenues. Based on the retrospective reports of restaurant owners/managers, it was found that revenues in most restaurants (59%) were unchanged following the policy, while 22% of restaurants reported an increase in revenues and 19% reported a decrease. Some differences were observed across restaurants, with franchised restaurants more likely to report an increase in revenues and independent restaurants more likely to report a drop. Given this, it was concluded that there was no net negative impact of South Africa's smoking restrictions on restaurant business.

Industry-sponsored studies

The tobacco industry, and groups that support it, have been vocal opponents of smoke-free policies, arguing among other things that these policies will adversely affect the businesses covered by the policies (U.S.Departement of Health and Human Services, 2006). Many of the studies researchers reviewed (Scollo & Lal, 2008) have been funded by the tobacco industry (e.g. through the Accommodation Grant Program) or by groups supported by the tobacco industry (e.g. various bar and/or restaurant associations that received funding from the industry).

In a comprehensive review of the existing literature through August 2002, an assessment was made of the association between funding source and study findings (Scollo et al., 2003). It was concluded that all studies that found smoke-free policies to have a negative economic impact had been funded by the tobacco industry, an organisation that had received tobacco industry funding, or an industry ally. In addition, the vast majority (94%) of the industry-supported studies concluded that smoke-free policies had a negative economic impact.

An updated review available through January 2008, includes more recent non-industry funded studies that find that there is a negative economic impact of smoke-free policies (most notably for gaming establishments), but there continues to be a strong association between industry funding (either direct or through affiliated organisations) and the conclusion that the policies negatively affect the businesses they cover (Scollo & Lal, 2008).

Summary of research on the economic impact of smoke-free policies on the hospitality sector

As of January 2008, 165 studies were identified which examined the economic impact of smoke-free policies on the hospitality sector (Scollo & Lal, 2008). Eighty-six of these studies employed official reports of sales, employment, or other related measures in their analyses, while 79 of them were based on survey data. Other characteristics of these studies including whether or not they were peer reviewed and their findings are summarised in Table 4.2.

Forty-nine of the identified studies based on official reports of business activity met the criteria described above for a methodologically sound evaluation of the economic impact of smoke-free policies; specifically, these studies used data covering a period including several years before and after policy implementation, controlled for underlying economic conditions and other relevant factors, and used appropriate statistical methods. These studies use data on an assortment of economic indicators, including: taxable sales, sales tax revenues, or other sales data; employment; the number of establishments; measures of bankruptcy; and the value of businesses. Several of the studies examine more than one outcome. Of the 49 identified studies, 47 concluded that smoke-free policies have either no economic impact or a positive economic impact on the businesses affected by them.

In addition, 37 other studies met some, but not all, of these criteria; most often they failed to control for underlying economic conditions. These studies were more mixed in their findings, with 18 concluding that the policies had either no economic impact or a small positive effect, and 19 concluding that they had a negative impact. Given their limitations, it is not surprising that only three of these 37 studies were published in peer-reviewed outlets.

Seventy-nine of the studies used survey data to assess the economic impact of smoke-free policies, with 34 of these based on consumer/patron surveys and the remaining 45 based on owner/manager surveys. Given the limitations of these surveys described above (particularly those based on convenience samples and/or that collected information on anticipated rather than realised impact), only about one in five of these studies were published in a peer-reviewed outlet. Nearly all of the peer-reviewed studies (17 of 19) concluded that there are no negative economic effects of smoke-free policies. The majority of studies based on consumer/patron surveys that are published in other outlets also found that there is no negative economic impact of these policies. Of the studies based on survey data, those that relied on owner/manager survey data and that are not published in peer-reviewed outlets (the most methodologically flawed studies) are the only group more likely to conclude that there is a negative economic impact of smoke-free policies.

Other incidental effects of smoke-free policies

In addition to their economic effects (or lack thereof), smoke-free policies can impact a variety of other behaviours and related outcomes. Some of these are covered in other chapters, including the impact of the policies on attitudes towards tobacco and related social norms (Chapter 5), on exposure to tobacco smoke and its health consequences (Chapter 6), and on smoking behaviour (Chapter 7). This section reviews the evidence, often anecdotal, about other incidental and/or unanticipated effects of smoke-free policies. These include effects on other problem behaviours (e.g. drinking, gambling, and violence), litter, and street noise. Finally, the overall, broader economic impact of smoke-free policies and tobacco control efforts is briefly discussed. This section is not a comprehensive review of all possible incidental/unanticipated effects, but rather a short discussion of those that have received some attention and a selected review of the existing evidence on each.

Smoke-free policies and other problem behaviours

Drinking and its consequences

Concerns about the potential economic impact of smoke-free policies on bars are often driven by the observation that smoking and drinking are frequently done together. Given this observation, it is plausible that by reducing smoking, smoke-free policies might also reduce drinking among smokers. Several studies by economists have explored the potential relationships between smoking and drinking by examining the impact of tax or price changes for cigarettes on drinking behaviour and/ or vice-versa (Dee, 1999; Cameron &

Table 4.2 Summary of studies on the economic impact of smoke-free policies on the hospitality sector+ (through 31 January 2008)

Type of data	Methodological quality*	Peer reviewed	Reported a negative impact (Number of studies)		Total
			No	Yes	
Official reports of sales, employment or related measures (n=86)	Meet criteria for methodologically sound studies (n=49)	Yes (n=21)	20	1	49
		No (n=28)	27	1	
		Total for studies meeting all four criteria (n=49)	47	2	
	Met some of but not all criteria for methodologically sound studies (n=37)	Yes (n=3)	3	0	37
		No (n=34)	15	19	
		Total for studies meeting some of criteria (n=37)	18	19	
		Subtotal	65	21	86
Survey data (n=79)	Patron/Consumer surveys (n=34)	Yes (n=9)	8	1	34
		No (n=25)	19	6	
		Total Consumer	27	7	
	Owner/Manager surveys(n=45)	Yes (n=10)	9	1	45
		No (n=35)	10	25	
		Total Owner/Manager (n=45)	19	26	
		Subtotal	46	33	79
		Total	111	54	165

+ In preparation for this chapter, Scollo and Lal (2008) updated their previous, comprehensive review of the literature on the impact of smoke-free policies on the hospitality sector to include studies available through January 2008. These studies were identified by searching a number of citation indices, including Medline, the Science Citation Index, the Social Science Citation Index, Current Contents Search, PsycINFO, and Ovid HealthSTAR. The following search terms were used: "smok" and restaurants," "bars," "hospitality," "economic," "regulation," and "law." Unpublished studies, and those not found through these searches, were identified through other approaches, such as soliciting relevant studies from the members of the International Union Against Cancer's International Tobacco Control Network (GLOBALink), and by searching hospitality industry and tobacco company websites based in major English-speaking countries. Internet searches were conducted with Google, using the search terms "smok" bans" and "restaurants" or "bars," limited by the terms "economic impact" or "study." Finally, additional studies were identified through the monitoring of media reports and various tobacco-related publications.

For their reviews, each identified study was assessed by both Scollo and Lal and the following details were tabulated: author; year published; publisher name and type; whether or not the study was peer reviewed; and the source, if any, of funding for the study. Where the funding source was unclear, Scollo and Lal searched industry document archives to determine if funding was provided by tobacco companies, or associated organisations. In addition, the approach and findings of each study was determined, including date and location of policy implementation, nature of the policy implemented, type of outcome measure employed, analytic method used, whether or not economic conditions were controlled for, and a brief description of the key findings (including whether or not the author(s) concluded that the actual or potential economic impact of the policy at issue on the outcome(s) being analysed was negative). The detailed review is available online at: http://www.vctc.org.au/tc-res/Hospitalitysummary.pdf.

*These studies used data covering a period including several years before and after policy implementation, controlled for underlying economic conditions and other relevant factors, and used appropriate statistical methods.

Williams, 2001), generally concluding that there is some complementarity between these behaviours; that is, increases in the price for one leads to reductions in the consumption of both. A few of these studies have considered similar relationships between smoking and illicit drug use, reaching similar conclusions (Chaloupka et al., 1999; Cameron & Williams, 2001; Farrelly et al., 2001).

Few studies, however, have considered the impact of smoke-free policies on other substance use, with those that have focused on drinking and its consequences. For example, the first six waves of the US Health and Retirement Survey, a longitudinal survey of adults aged 51 to 61 at baseline conducted from 1992 through 2002, were used to examine the impact of smoking restrictions and other factors on self-reported drinking (Picone et al., 2004). It was concluded that more comprehensive restrictions on smoking (those that cover more venues, including bars) significantly reduce drinking among women, but have little impact on drinking among men.

More recently, state level data were used on beverage-specific alcohol consumption in the USA to look at the impact of state smoke-free policies on drinking (Gallet & Eastman, 2007). Relatively crude indicators of the policies were used: an indicator for any smoking ban and an indicator for a ban on smoking in restaurants and/or bars. Estimates indicated that the policies resulted in reductions in consumption of beer and spirits, but an increase in wine consumption. The researchers concluded that "the benefits from reducing tobacco consumption by enacting smoking

bans may crossover to reductions in social maladies tied to excessive drinking."

A different conclusion was reached in the assessment of the impact of selected smoke-free policies on drinking and driving between 2000 and 2005, based on the use of US county level data on fatal motor vehicle accidents attributable to alcohol (Adams & Cotti, 2008). Jurisdictions selected for analyses are large US cities and counties and counties in states that adopted smoke-free bar policies between 2002 and 2005. The researchers found that alcohol-related traffic fatalities rose in counties covered by smoke-free bar policies, but did not change in counties without such policies, attributing this to an increase in driving by smokers who seek out bars where smoking is allowed (either in other jurisdictions not covered by a smoke-free bar policy, or those that are covered but do not comply with the policy) that more than offsets any reductions in drinking caused by the policy. This seems to be a short-term, transitional effect that will eventually disappear as these policies diffuse throughout the USA and as compliance increases.

Clearly, more research is needed to fully understand the impact of smoke-free policies on drinking, other substance use, and their related consequences.

Problem gambling

As described above, the evidence is mixed on the impact of smoke-free policies on business activity in gaming establishments. To the extent that such policies do result in a decline in gambling revenues,

this is likely to be accompanied by a reduction in problem gambling (Lal & Siahpush, 2008). Indeed, it was noted that "Gambling control advocates expected the legislation would be useful in curbing excessive gambling among EGM users in that enforcing a break in play would prompt many gamblers to reconsider their gambling," and suggests that problem gamblers deterred by smoke-free policies may pay off existing debts, save more, spend more on housing, and increase spending in retail establishments. Given the mixed evidence, however, more research is needed to better understand the impact on problem gambling of smoke-free policies that cover gaming establishments.

Domestic violence

Reductions in drinking that might result from smoke-free policies could reduce domestic violence, given the established relationship between alcohol consumption and violence (Markowitz, 2000). For example, it was found that Irish smokers reported less drinking following the implementation of the comprehensive smoke-free policy in Ireland, than did smokers in Scotland and the rest of the United Kingdom, when comparable policies were not in effect (Hyland et al., 2008b). To date, there is no substantive evidence that smoke-free policies have increased domestic violence, but some evidence suggests that they are likely to reduce such violence.

Noise

Anecdotal reports suggest that smoke-free policies, particularly those that cover bars and clubs, increase noise outside of these establishments and result in greater complaints from neighbors. There are, however, very limited, solid data to support this. Data from repeated cross-sectional surveys of pub/bar and restaurant employees in Norway, following the implementation of the country's comprehensive smoke-free policy, indicate that almost half of bar employees and one-third of restaurant employees 'agree completely' that there is more noise outside of the premises, with about one in five bar employees and one in ten restaurant employees reporting an increase in complaints from neighbors (Lund, 2006). To the extent that there are real concerns about increased noise, adoption or enforcement of existing anti-noise policies is appropriate.

Litter

Anecdotal reports also suggest that there may be an increase in litter following the implementation of smoke-free policies, as smokers are forced outside to smoke and drop their cigarette butts on sidewalks and streets. This is supported by the findings from the Norwegian bar/restaurant employee survey described above, with the majority of employees indicating an increase in cigarette litter following the country's smoke-free policy (Lund, 2006). Some have suggested that supplying smokers with portable ashtrays would be an effective approach to reducing potential litter, while others recommend better enforcement of existing litter laws. There is no reliable evidence, however, on the extent to which litter increases following

the implementation of a smoke-free policy, or on the effectiveness of different approaches to reduce it.

Summary

Little reliable evidence exists on the impact of smoke-free policies on other problem behaviours, including other substance use and its consequences, problem gambling, domestic violence, noise, and litter. While concerns about the potential for increased problem behaviours (with the exception of gambling) have been raised, there are almost no data to support these concerns.

Smoke-free policies and the macroeconomy

As noted above, opponents of tobacco control efforts often raise concerns about the broader, macroeconomic effects of tobacco control policies. With respect to smoke-free policies, these concerns are most relevant to the impact on tax revenues and employment. These issues are brief-ly discussed in this section (see Jha & Chaloupka, 1999; Prabhat & Chaloupka, 2000 for more complete discussions of these issues).

To the extent that smoke-free policies reduce cigarette smoking, as described in Chapter 7, the implementation of these policies will reduce revenues generated by cigarette excise and other taxes. However, these reductions in revenues are likely to be offset by increases in other tax revenues, as the money that smokers once spent on cigarettes is now being spent on other goods and services which are subject to VAT and other taxes.

If the loss of cigarette tax revenues is of particular concern, adoption of smoke-free policies as part of a comprehensive approach to reducing tobacco use that includes increases in cigarette and other tobacco tax revenues, is an effective means of both preserving the revenue stream generated by these taxes, for the short- to medium-term, and reducing tobacco use.

Those opposed to tobacco control policies and programmes also raise concerns about the impact of these efforts on employment, arguing that the resulting reductions in tobacco use will lead to job losses in tobacco-related farming, manufacturing, and distribution, as well as in other sectors of the economy. Again, any reductions in tobacco-related employment that result from smoke-free policies, or other tobacco control activities, will be offset by increased employment in other sectors as the money once spent on cigarettes is spent on other goods and services. This is particularly true in many developing countries where smoking is increasing, and where the short-term impact of the policies is more likely to be slowing the growth in tobacco use rather than significantly reducing it.

Summary and conclusions

Smoke-free policies impact bus-inesses in numerous ways, from improving the health and productivity of their employees to reducing their insurance, cleaning, maintenance, and potential litigation costs. Experience to date suggests that there are minimal short-term costs to businesses of implementing comprehensive smoke-free policies. Existing evidence from developed countries indicates that smoke-free workplace policies have a net positive effect on businesses; the same is likely to be the case in developing countries. Establishing and maintaining designated indoor or outdoor smoking areas is more costly to implement than a completely smoke-free policy. There are minimal costs to governments related to enforcement and education.

Much of the debate over the economic impact of smoke-free policies, and as a result, much of the research, has focused on the hospitality sector. Methodologically sound research studies from developed countries consistently conclude that smoke-free policies do not have an adverse economic impact on the business activity of restaurants, bars, or establishments catering to tourists, with many studies finding a small positive effect of these policies. These studies include outcomes such as official reports of sales, employment, and the number of businesses. Very limited evidence from South Africa, an upper middle-resource country, is consistent with these findings. It is likely that the same would be true in other developing countries; nevertheless, research confirming this would be useful as smoke-free policies are adopted in a growing number of these countries. Few studies exist on the impact of smoke-free policies on gaming establishments, and their results are mixed; more research is needed on these venues.

There is insufficient evidence about the effects of smoke-free policies on various problem behaviours, such as other substance use and its consequences, problem gambling, domestic violence, noise, and litter. No credible evidence exists to support claims that smoke-free policies will negatively affect the overall economy.

Chapter 5
Public attitudes towards smoke-free policies – including compliance with policies

Introduction

This Chapter reviews what is known about public attitudes towards both legal and voluntary restrictions on tobacco use to protect against secondhand smoke (SHS) exposure. Attitudinal data was considered in this Handbook, as it is an important moderator in the process of adoption and compliance with smoke-free policies (see the conceptual framework in IARC's Handbook volume 12 (IARC, 2008)). More specifically public attitudes are important for the following reasons:

• In democratic nations, supportive public attitudes are often necessary for facilitating the process of passing smoke-free legislation or regulations by local or national governments.

• Once such legislation or regulations exist, public attitudes are likely to impact how well such laws are complied with and enforced; hence, how well these laws achieve health protection goals of reducing SHS exposure (see Chapter 6). If such laws are successful, there may be other benefits in terms of reduced tobacco consumption, quitting

behaviour, and possibly reduced visible role-modelling of smoking in the presence of children (see Chapter 7).

• The attitudes of the public are likely to be important in terms of the extent to which voluntary control measures (e.g. smoke-free homes and, in most jurisdictions, also cars) are adopted and complied with by individuals and families. There is evidence for this social diffusion model for the adoption of smoke-free homes from a study of smokers in four countries (Borland *et al.*, 2006a).

• Public attitudes concerning SHS may conceivably impact the extent to which governments make progress on other aspects of tobacco control that benefit from public support (e.g. high tobacco taxes, funding of mass media campaigns, and restrictions on tobacco marketing). Similarly, public attitudes can help guide appropriate policy in areas which are controversial among tobacco control experts (e.g. smoking restrictions in some outdoor settings) (Chapman, 2007). Appropriate care with such

policymaking could minimise the risk of a public backlash with regard to tobacco control interventions in general.

Nevertheless, "attitudes" are a complex construct and can involve a number of dimensions. There are inadequate data on which to disentangle attitudes towards smoke-free policies that are attributable to concerns about involuntary exposure to SHS and health hazards, general concerns for protecting infants and children, protection against nuisance impacts, and respect for the law or voluntary policies (once a smoke-free policy is in place). There is also insufficient clarification in the literature about how smoke-free attitudes relate to emotional reactions to smoking and to the imposition of laws that are not supported by some smokers. Attitudes around smoking may also be linked in complex ways with satisfaction of particular experiences (e.g. socialising in restaurants and bars). There is some further consideration of the issue of knowledge and beliefs in the Discussion, but this Chapter has not been able to tease out the different dimensions of what comprise attitudes to smoke-free policies.

In summary, the quality of these studies varies widely from high quality prospective cohort studies to telephone surveys in just a city jurisdiction.

This Chapter has involved systematic review of the peer-reviewed literature published since January 1990 (up to 31 December 2007) with additional specific Medline searches conducted up to 31 March 2008. The major focus was on identifying Medline-indexed articles. More specifically, the stages of the literature search were as follows:

• Identification of country level and any multi-country studies on public attitudes and compliance in developed countries. Particularly rigorous searches were focused on identifying attitudinal changes associated with countries that have introduced comprehensive smoke-free laws (see Chapter 3). The voluminous number of attitudinal studies on SHS at the sub-national level prevented a comprehensive view of these, though this is unlikely to substantively impact the patterns found (see the Discussion section of this Chapter). While focused on "public attitudes," this Chapter also describes, where appropriate, some attitudinal data of specific occupational groups (e.g. school staff, hospital employees, and hospitality workers).

• Where major categories of public settings in developed countries were not covered by such country level studies, searches were then conducted for published sub-national level studies (such as at

the level of US/Australian states or Canadian provinces). Failing the identification of any such studies, the searches were further expanded to local studies (e.g. at the level of a city or organisational setting). The search engine Google Scholar was also used to identify such additional studies.

• The above approach was supplemented by a case study of one sub-national jurisdiction in the USA: California. This selection was based on the fact that California was the first major jurisdiction in the world to restrict smoking in the hospitality sector. This state is also a leader in smoke-free mass media campaigns and in outdoor SHS restrictions. As the third US state to adopt a smoke-free car law, it also has the second highest prevalence of smoke-free home rules in the USA (after Utah) (Centers for Disease Control and Prevention, 2007a), and has longitudinal data on public attitudes towards smoking restrictions that cover a long time period.

• For developing countries, searches included all published studies even if they were focused on a single state, city, or organisation. This was done due to the shortage of country level studies in such countries. This country grouping included all non-Organisation for Economic Cooperation and Development (OECD) countries, including Mexico, Poland, and Turkey.

The 1990 cut-off point for the start of the search period was somewhat arbitrary, but coincided with the

beginning of fairly comprehensive smoke-free laws at the country level (e.g. the 1990 smoke-free Environments Act in New Zealand). Substantive shifts in public attitudes towards SHS have been documented before this time in selected countries, probably in response to various key actions (see Chapter 3 for details). From 1969 on, for example, there was concern by flight attendants in the USA regarding SHS (Holm & Davis, 2004). The health-related evidence base concerning SHS continued to evolve from the first time it was discussed in a report of the US Surgeon General, though this was not a major focus of the report (U.S. Department of Health, Education, and Welfare, 1972).

Attitudes towards, and compliance with, smoking restrictions in workplaces

This subsection examines attitudes towards indoor workplace smoking restrictions, excluding hospitality venues and other special settings, which are detailed elsewhere in this Chapter. Smoking restrictions for indoor workplaces have become relatively common in developed countries (e.g. for the USA; Centers for Disease Control and Prevention, 2006a) and even some developing countries (e.g. in India and Indonesia in workplaces serving children, Mongolia, South Africa, and Uruguay (GTSS Collaborative Group, 2006); see Chapter 3 for details). Studies of attitudes are detailed in Table 5.1 and compliance data in Tables 5.2 and 5.3.

Table 5.1 Studies on public attitudes towards workplace smoking restrictions

Reference/Location	Study design and date	Results	Comments
Multi-country and country level studies			
Health Canada, 2006 Canada	Canadian Tobacco Use Monitoring Survey (CTUMS), (2006)	Majority support (86%) for some form of restriction on smoking in the workplace.	40% of respondents felt that smoking should not be allowed in any area of the workplace (indoor or outdoor); 46% felt that smoking should be allowed only in designated outdoor smoking areas.
U.S. Department of Health and Human Services, 2006 USA	Current Population Survey (CPS), (1991-93; 1998-99; 2001-02).	By 1992-93 majority public support (58.1%) for smoke-free indoor work-places in all geographic regions, age groups, both genders, education groups, income groups, and ethnic groups. Support has increased since this time.	Support rose from 58.1% in 1992-93 to 74.5% in 2001-02. In 1992-93 the only respondents who did not indicate majority favour (>50%) were smokers (30.6%) and blue collar workers (46.5%). By 2001-02 all groups had a majority in favour (>50%).
Fong *et al.*, 2006 Ireland, UK	Prospective cohorts (2003-04; 2004-05)	Among smokers: Overall, 67% of Irish smokers reported support for a total ban on smoking in work-places; for the UK, the support was just over 40% *.	The level of support among Irish smokers increased from 43%, prior to a smoke-free law (a statistically significant higher increase than for the UK). Overall, 83% of Irish smokers reported that the new smoke-free law (covering pubs and other places) was a "good" or "very good" thing (after its introduction).
Renaud, 2007 France	Opinion polls (2006, 2007)	Workplaces including restaurants & bars: Majority support (76% in 2006) for a law banning smoking in public areas and work-places; increased to 83% two months after the ban was enacted in 2007.	These polls related to a January 2007 law for public areas and workplaces. Relating to restaurants and cafés - law operational January 2008. The quality of these opinion polls was not documented in this report. No Medline-indexed national attitudinal studies for France were identified. However, other articles on France refer to "public opinion" supporting such a ban (Dubois, 2005).
European Commission, 2007 European countries**	Representative sampling, face-to-face interviews (2006)	High level of support (88%) for smoke-free workplaces.	Range of support for "totally in favour" - 46% for Austria to 93% for Sweden. The lowest for "totally in favour" plus "somewhat in favour" was 80% for Austria. Slight increase (+2 percentage points) compared to the 2005 survey. Increase was most marked among those "totally in favour" (+4 percentage points).
Edwards *et al.*, 2008 (with additional detail in Edwards *et al.*, 2007) New Zealand	Health Sponsorship Council (HSC) annual surveys (2003-2006)	Majority support for the right to work in a smoke-free environment (94.9% in 2006 - 92.3% in smokers).	Support increased from 90.7% in 2003 for all respondents; 82.6% for smokers (both significant). Support for non-office workers to work in a smoke-free environment was also high in 2006 at 94.7% and 89.8% (all respondents and smokers respectively). See Table 5.4 for data relating to bars and restaurants. Other national data for NZ also indicate negative attitudes towards SHS exposure (Ministry of Health, 2007).

Table 5.1 Studies on public attitudes towards workplace smoking restrictions

Reference/Location	Study design and date	Results	Comments
Studies in developing countries (Including sub-national and city studies)			
Bello *et al.*, 2004 Chile	Adults employed in the Chilean Ministry of Health (2001)	A majority (89%) agreed with smoking restrictions in work places.	Based only on the English translation of Medline abstract. This study may not be representative of the general population.
Barnoya *et al.*, 2007 Guatemala	Survey of workers in a convenience sample of settings in Guatemala City (2006)	A majority of groups of workers were in favour of smoke-free workplaces (but not in two of the five groups).	Majority support for smoke-free work-places among hospital workers (75%), school/university workers (67%), and government building workers (50%). Minority support among airport (39%) and bar/restaurant workers (30%).
Przewozniak *et al.*, 2008 Poland	Nationwide representative sample of adults (2007)	Majority level support for a complete ban in worksites (69%).	This level was a bit lower than for public places in general at 76% support (Smoking was restricted in worksites in 1995).

*These percentages are imprecise because they are based on graphically presented results and not on exact tabulated data (which were not in the published article)

** Austria, Belgium, Cyprus, Czech Republic, Denmark, Estonia, Finland, France, Germany, Greece, Hungary, Ireland, Italy, Latvia, Lithuania, Luxembourg, Malta, Netherlands, Poland, Portugal, Slovakia, Slovenia, Spain, Sweden, United Kingdom. Other jurisdictions: Bulgaria, Croatia, Romania

Discussion of the results

The findings from country level studies are suggestive of the following patterns:

• There are majority levels of public support for smoke-free workplaces in the developed countries for which data are available (including, since at least 1992-93, the USA). There is also majority public support in those developing countries that have attitudinal data, including those less developed European countries in the 29 country study detailed in Table 5.1.

• Smokers appear to be less supportive of restrictions than nonsmokers (particularly of complete restrictions), but in some studies a majority of them support workplace restrictions.

• There is a general pattern of increasing support by smokers and nonsmokers in the past two decades for such workplace restrictions. Support also increases after new laws designed to tighten restrictions on SHS exposure are enacted. This effect may relate to the law, or, in some cases, to mass media campaigns that precede, coincide with, and/or follow such new legislation.

• There is an overall pattern of higher support for smoke-free indoor workplace laws in general than for specific smoke-free workplaces in hospitality settings (e.g. for bars and restaurants, as detailed further in the next subsection).

The findings at the national level (Table 5.2) obscure some of substantive changes at the sub-national level. For example, California implemented a policy mandating smoke-free indoor workplaces in 1995 (with the law extending to all bars and clubs in 1998). Following the implementation of the smoke-free workplace policy, data from the California Tobacco Surveys (CTS) showed that the percentage of indoor workers reporting that their workplace was smoke-free increased markedly, from 46.3% in 1992 to 90.5% in 1996 (Gilpin *et al.*, 2002). The 1999 CTS data indicated a further increase in smoke-free workplaces (93.4%) after other venues became smoke-free.

Table 5.2 Country level and multi-country studies on compliance with indoor workplace smoking restrictions

Reference/Location	Study design and date	Results	Comments
Nebot et al., 2005 7 European countries	Measurements of airborne nicotine (multiple settings) (2001-2002)	In university settings: Some limited evidence for compliance, but nicotine was still found in most of the sites studied.	Nicotine levels were lower in the sites with smoking restrictions; also lower than other public places (e.g. transportation settings). Sweden had relatively low levels compared to Austria, France, Greece, Italy, Portugal, and Spain.
Health Canada, 2006 Canada	Canadian Tobacco Use Monitoring Survey (CTUMS) (2006)	Some possible evidence for incomplete compliance with restrictions.	23% reported SHS exposure at the workplace in the last month. Yet, 94% of those who worked at a job or business in the last 12 months reported that some kind of workplace smoking restriction was in place.
Pickett et al., 2006 USA	National Health and Nutrition Examination Survey (1999-2002)	Good scientific evidence from a biomarker (cotinine) study that smoke-free law coverage reduces exposure to SHS (indicating high compliance with such laws).	Blood cotinine levels were measured. Among nonsmoking adults living in counties with extensive smoke-free law coverage, 12.5% were exposed to SHS, compared with 35.1% with limited coverage, and 45.9% with no law. "These results support the scientific evidence suggesting that smoke-free laws are an effective strategy for reducing SHS exposure."
Fong et al., 2006 Ireland, UK	Prospective cohorts (2003-04; 2004-05)	Among smokers: Irish smokers reported that smoking had become uncommon in workplace settings after a smoke-free law.	The proportion of Irish smokers who observed smoking in these settings declined from 62% (pre-law) to 14% post-law. In the UK, levels were 37% and 34%, respectively, in this time period. See Chapter 6 for further details.
European Commission, 2007 29 European countries (25 in the EU)	Representative sampling, face-to-face interviews (2006)	Majority not exposed to SHS at work in all but one EU member state - suggestive of some compliance with laws that exist.	In all EU member states but one, the majority of respondents declared that they are never, or almost never, exposed to SHS at work in indoor workplaces or offices. The most likely to declare this were the Irish (96%); least likely were the Greeks (15%). Those claiming to be exposed to SHS for more than five hours a day ranged from 34% in Greece to 0% in Ireland. Despite the comprehensive restrictions in Italy, Malta, and Sweden, 30%, 19% and 6% respectively claimed to be exposed to SHS (for at least <1 hour per day).
Lund & Lindbak, 2007 Norway	Regular national surveys (most recently 2006)	Very low workplace exposure suggestive of good compliance.	In 1996, 9% of occupationally active adults reported workplace SHS exposure; this dropped to 2% in 2006. The new smoke-free hospitality law in 2004 may have been a factor in increased workplace restrictions, and provision of smoking cessation services at work.
Ministry of Health, 2007 New Zealand	National face-to-face survey (2006)	High compliance based on reported exposure to smoking (89.4% report no one smoking indoors at work).	There was no gradient by ethnicity (Maori versus non-Maori), deprivation level, or major occupational groupings. Also reported were attitudinal data indicating most respondents would be bothered by someone smoking near to them indoors (70.8%).

Table 5.2 Country level and multi-country studies on compliance with indoor workplace smoking restrictions

Reference/Location	Study design and date	Results	Comments
Edwards *et al.*, 2008 New Zealand	Health Sponsorship Council (HSC) annual surveys (2003-2006)	High compliance (only 8% of employed adults reported SHS exposure at work in the past week in 2006).	This figure fell from around 20% in 2003 (a new smoke-free law that tightened restrictions was introduced in 2004). There were greater reductions among Maori workers.

Table 5.3 Studies in developing countries on compliance with indoor workplace smoking restrictions (including country level, sub-national and city level studies)

Reference/location	Study design and date	Results	Comments
Yang *et al.*, 1999 China	Representative sample covering 30 Provinces (1996)	Workplaces: A quarter of respondents reported SHS exposure in their workplaces (25%) suggesting that restrictions in such areas are not fully complied with.	This was lower than for exposure at home (71%) and public places (32%).
McGhee *et al.*, 2002 Hong Kong, China	Telephone survey (circa 2001)	Some evidence for lack of workplace smoking restrictions (or compliance for any that exist).	Nonsmoking workers - 47.5% exposed to SHS in the workplace (compared with 26% exposed at home). Range (by occupational category): Men - 43.9% among financing/business workers to 80.1% for construction workers. Women - 24.0% for community/social services workers to 62.0% for transport/communication workers. Extent of restrictions was not documented.
Navas-Acien *et al.*, 2004 7 Latin American countries	Measurement of airborne nicotine in multiple settings in the capital cities (2002, 2003)	Government buildings: Some limited evidence for some compliance with smoking restrictions.	Smoking was usually restricted in these buildings. Median level of nicotine was lower than for hospitality settings in these countries, and was comparable to levels from studies of open US offices where smoking was restricted. The countries in this study were Argentina, Brazil, Chile, Costa Rica, Paraguay, Peru, and Uruguay.
Barnoya *et al.*, 2007 Guatemala, Honduras, Mexico, Panama	Measurement of airborne nicotine in multiple settings in the capital cities (2006)	Government buildings: Some evidence for compliance with smoking restrictions.	Nicotine levels were much lower than hospitality venues, but higher than schools and hospitals (the latter two comparisons were not statistically significant). Mexican component of this study noted nicotine levels in these offices "reflect the lack of compliance with mandatory nonsmoking official regulations in Mexico" (Barrientos-Gutierrez *et al.*, 2007b).
Stillman *et al.*, 2007 China	Nicotine sampling in urban and rural settings (2005)	Government buildings: No clear evidence for compliance with restrictions.	Airborne nicotine was detected in 97.7% of the locations. Median level was higher than hospitals and schools, but lower than transportation settings, restaurants, and entertainment settings.
Przewozniak *et al.*, 2008 Poland	Nationwide surveys based on random representative sample of adults (1995 and 2007)	Substantial decline in reported SHS exposure of adults at worksite after smoking restrictions in place.	Since 1995, when smoking in workplaces was restricted, the percentage of adult nonsmokers exposed to SHS in worksites declined in women from 37% to 14% and in men from 47% to 24%.

Compliance

The available country level data indicate fairly high compliance with smoke-free workplace laws in the countries with such data. The data presented in Chapter 6 also show that introducing smoke-free laws results in lower exposure to SHS, which suggests compliance with the law. There are, however, examples where such smoke-free laws have not been complied with. In 1991, for example, a law in France was considered to be unsuccessful: "Failure to properly implement Evin's law of 1991 explains why nonsmokers in France are still not protected" (Dubois, 2005). This lack of success resulted in a new law being introduced, which covered workplaces from 2007, and bars/restaurants from 2008.

The evidence in developing countries is also generally indicative of some compliance in workplaces; though results are more mixed than for developed countries. This is also the case in those less developed European countries in the 29 country study detailed in Table 5.3.

At the sub-national level compliance may be reported as problematic. For example, in California in 1999, there was an increase in the percentage (to 15.6%) of nonsmoking indoor workers reporting someone had smoked in their work area in the past two weeks (Gilpin *et al.*, 2002). This increase could have been due to poorer compliance with the law in venues that were covered by an expansion of it in the preceding year (i.e. to cover bars and clubs).

More recent reports for California still indicate incomplete compliance, with reports of smoke-free workplaces at 95.5% in 2002 and 94.8% in 2005, and with corresponding rates of reporting by respondents of exposure to someone smoking in their work area as 12.0% and 13.9%, respectively (Gilpin *et al.*, 2003; Al-Delaimy *et al.*, 2008). However, another factor may be that nonsmokers have become further aware of SHS over time, which may cause them to report this more than they would have previously.

Compliance with smoke-free laws may also be poorer in particular occupational settings. In California, daily exposure to SHS was about twice as common in factories, stores/warehouses, and restaurants/bars (10-13%), than in offices, hospitals, or classrooms (2-7%) (Gilpin *et al.*, 2003). This pattern may also reflect differing smoking prevalences among workers in these types of workplaces. For example, data from the 2005 CTS indicate that the people smoking were other employees (87%), customers or non-employees (63%), or supervisors (31%) (Al-Delaimy *et al.*, 2008).

Relevance for evidence-based tobacco control

Smoking restrictions in workplaces are likely to see a relatively high level of public support compared to most other settings. In general, workplaces have been one of the top priorities for smoke-free laws for any level of government that has relevant power to regulate them. However, policymakers and health workers should consider obtaining representative attitudinal data in their jurisdiction prior to implementing new laws. This will inform the need for the use of mass media campaigns that deal with the SHS hazard and highlight the rights of workers to be protected from a serious threat to their health. Attitudinal data may also justify the need for the resourcing of enforcement activities.

Taking a comprehensive approach to smoking restrictions in all workplaces (including in the hospitality sector) has advantages in terms of policy coherence and alerting the public of the seriousness of SHS as a workplace hazard. Another subsection of this Chapter gives further consideration to such workplaces as health care facilities, schools, and transportation settings.

Summary

There are generally majority levels of public support for smoke-free indoor workplaces in these developed countries for which country level data are available. Compliance with such smoking restrictions is usually fairly substantial and likely to be delivering significant public health benefits at a population level. However, in developing countries compliance generally appears to be poor in some settings.

Attitudes towards, and compliance with, smoking restrictions in hospitality settings (i.e. restaurants, bars, and pubs)

This subsection covers public attitudes towards, and compliance with, smoking restrictions in hospitality settings such as restaurants, bars and pubs, which have seen marked increases in smoking restrictions in the last few years (see Chapter 3).

Attitudinal studies are detailed in Table 5.4 and studies on compliance in Tables 5.5 and 5.6.

Discussion of the results – attitudes

The findings from the country level studies in Table 5.4 are suggestive of the following patterns:

• There are majority levels of public support for smoke-free restaurants in the developed countries studied. There is also generally majority support by smokers for at least partial smoking restrictions in restaurants, but not usually for fully smoke-free restaurants (though in some places, such as Australia, there was majority support (71%) among smokers; see Table 5.4).

• The support for totally smoke-free bars is generally lower than for smoke-free restaurants, and some countries do not have majority public support. However, in some settings (i.e. localities where extensive restrictions are already in place) smokers themselves may indicate majority support for these restrictions (e.g. in Australia, Canada, and the USA).

• A pattern of increasing support by smokers and nonsmokers in the past two decades for smoke-free hospitality settings is apparent. Other reviews have also identified these trends, for example, in Australia (Siahpush & Scollo, 2001; Walsh & Tzelepis, 2003).

• Though the attitudinal data from developing countries are more limited, there is still majority support for totally smoke-free policies in most of the studies identified (e.g. 68.9% for restaurants in Hong Kong). Also,

there was a pattern of majority public support in those less developed European countries in the 29 country study detailed in Table 5.4 (all countries had majority support for smoke-free restaurants and most had majority support for bars).

Detailed elsewhere in the literature are other reported patterns of note. These include evidence that levels of support for smoke-free hospitality settings increase before smoke-free laws are passed (Schofield & Edwards, 1995; Walsh *et al.*, 2000), perhaps as a result of the publicity surrounding the advocacy for such laws, and also after these laws come into force (Wakefield *et al.*, 1996; Tang *et al.*, 2003; Edwards *et al.*, 2008).

Discussion of the results – compliance

There are country level and multi-country studies that have collected observational data (from researchers and smokers), fine particulate data, and airborne nicotine data (Table 5.5). Collectively these results show fairly high levels of compliance with smoking restrictions in all the hospitality settings with smoking restrictions. They also show that in the comparison countries, without such restrictions, the indoor air pollution from SHS is at hazardous levels. The data presented in Chapter 6 also show that introducing smoke-free laws into hospitality settings results in lower exposure to SHS, which suggests compliance with the law.

Of particular note is the apparent high compliance with smoke-free pubs in Ireland given the strong

traditional pub culture in this society. Similarly, Norway achieved very high compliance despite the cold and wet climate making outdoor smoking much more difficult. However, one multi-country study in Europe reported that nonsmoking areas within restaurants had similar air nicotine levels to smoking areas in cities in France, Italy, and Austria (Nebot *et al.*, 2005).

In comparison, the studies in developing countries indicate poorer compliance and even an apparent absence of any compliance in some settings (Table 5.6). Despite this, in some settings no smoking was observed in the smoking-restricted parts of restaurants, and there was sometimes evidence of modest benefits in terms of air quality from partial smoking restrictions (e.g. the studies in Hong Kong, Beijing, and seven Latin American countries).

It is important to note that by focusing on country level studies this Chapter has not examined a wealth of literature at the sub-national level. For example, one review of the Australian literature identified 31 sub-national attitudinal studies on hospitality settings and smoking restrictions, in addition to the three national ones mentioned in Table 5.4 (Walsh & Tzelepis, 2003). Similarly, in the area of compliance and attitudes towards smoke-free laws in hospitality settings, there is a substantial body of literature at the state level in the USA (e.g. California), with studies covering direct observation in bars and interviews with staff (Weber *et al.*, 2003; Tang *et al.*, 2004; Moore *et al.*, 2006), and population telephone surveys that identified and interviewed bar patrons (Tang *et al.*, 2003; Friis & Safer, 2005).

Table 5.4 Studies on public attitudes towards smoking restrictions in hospitality venues (restaurants, bars, pubs, etc.)

Reference/location	Study design and date	Results	Comments
Country level and multi-country studies			
Walsh & Tzelepis, 2003 Australia	Three national studies (1993, 1998, 2001)	All licensed premises: Majority support in most recent national survey (60.8%). This was the case for all but one of the eight states/territories in 2001.	1993 - 41% support for smoking bans in pubs/clubs (versus 35% opposed). 1998 - 49.9% support for smoking bans in pubs/clubs. 2001 - majority support at 60.8% (range by state: 48.5% to 63.4%). This analysis (which studied 34 community surveys) reported that from 2000 all state level surveys with the ban option alone had majority support for bars (52-68%) and gambling areas (64-76%). A survey in Victoria in 2002 also reported 88% support for having a smoke-free room.
Lund, 2006; Lund & Lund, 2006; Lund & Lindbak, 2007 Norway	National annual surveys (2003 -2006)	Hospitality venues: Majority support (76%) which increased after a new smoke-free law became operational in 2004.	In 2005, support was 84% among nonsmokers and 45% among daily smokers (up from 25% in 2003). After the ban, a minority of daily smokers reported a reduction in satisfaction when visiting smoke-free pubs and restaurants (38% and 32%, respectively). Among nonsmokers, higher satisfaction was reported at 81% and 82%, respectively. Majority support amongst young people aged 16-20 years (73%) and employees (60% - up from 48% before the law).
- Just restaurants			
U.S. Department of Health and Human Services, 2006 USA	Current Population Survey (CPS) (1991-93; 1998-99; 2001-02)	By 2001-02 there was widespread public support (>50%) for smoke-free restaurants in all geographic regions, age groups, both genders, education groups, income groups, main occupational groups, and ethnic groups.	Support rose from 45.1% in 1992-93 to 57.6% in 2001-02. In 2001-02 the only respondents who did not indicate majority favour (>50%) were those living in the Midwest (49.9%) and smokers (26.6%). In the 1992-93 survey only some population groups favoured smoke-free restaurants overall (those in the West, nonsmokers, those with higher education, and those who were Hispanic or non-Hispanic Asian).
Borland et al., 2006b Australia, Canada, UK, USA	Prospective cohorts (2002)	Among smokers: A large majority of smokers accepted at least some restrictions in restaurants (all >94%). But only in Australia (out of four countries) did most support total bans in indoor areas (71.4%).	Support for total bans: Australia (71.4%), the UK (24.2%), Canada (29.7%), and the USA (26.7%). Associates of support for bans (on logistic regression) were: reported presence of a total ban, documented extensive restrictions, thinking about the harms of passive smoking more frequently, and the belief that SHS can cause lung cancer in nonsmokers. Female smokers, and those with heavier cigarette consumption, were less supportive of bans.
Fong et al., 2006 Ireland, UK	Prospective cohorts (2003-04; 2004-05)	Among smokers (restaurants/fast food outlets): Most Irish smokers (77%) supported a total ban on smoking, in restaurants; the UK smokers support was lower (just over 40%*).	The level of support for Irish smokers increased from 45% prior to a smoke-free law (a statistically significant higher increase than for the UK). The support for a total ban in fast food outlets was around 90% among Irish smokers and over 75% for UK smokers.*

Table 5.4 Studies on public attitudes towards smoking restrictions in hospitality venues (restaurants, bars, pubs, etc.)

Reference/location	Study design and date	Results	Comments
- Just restaurants			
European Commission, 2007 29 European countries	Representative sampling, face-to-face interviews (2006)	Majority support (77%) for banning smoking in restaurants. A majority of smokers (59%) also support this.	77% supported restrictions; 55% completely in favour. Majority support in all countries: Malta (95%), Ireland (95%), Sweden (93%), and Italy (90%). Proportion completely supportive of restrictions was highest in Ireland (88%) and lowest in Austria (31%). Least support was in Czech Republic (59%), though support had increased from the 2005 survey by +10 points. Most in favour of smoke-free restaurants were nonsmokers (87%) compared to smokers (59%). Those who work in restaurants were also generally in favour (64%). Of note was that the respondents with the least level of education were more "totally in favour" of restrictions than those with higher educational levels.
Health Canada, 2006 Canada	Canadian Tobacco Use Monitoring Survey (CTUMS) (2006)	Majority support for no smoking in any section of a restaurant (69%).	An increase from 2001 (also a CTUMS survey), where only 42% believed that smoking should not be allowed in any section of a restaurant. Even in 2001 most (57%) of current smokers wanted some kind of restriction (25% wanted no smoking at all and 32% wanted smoking only in an enclosed area).
Edwards et al., 2008 New Zealand		Majority support for smoking bans in restaurants (80% in 2006). Majority support for the right of restaurant workers to work in a smoke-free environment (95.6% in 2006; 93.4% in smokers).	Support for a ban increased from 61% in 2001 to 80% by 2006 (UMR data). HSC data reported it at 90% in 2006 (up from 73% in 2004). Among smokers it was 78% (up from 48% in 2004). The level of support increased for the rights of restaurant workers from 84.4% in 2003 for all respondents and from 67.8% for smokers (both significant). Support increased after a law banning smoking in bars in 2004.
- Just bars / pubs			
U.S. Department of Health and Human Services, 2006 USA	Current Population Survey (CPS) (1991-93; 1998-99; 2001-02)	By 2001-02 there was still limited public support (<50%) for smoke-free bars in all geographic regions, age groups, smokers and nonsmokers, both genders, education groups, income groups, main occupational groups, and ethnic groups.	Support rose from 24.2% in 1992-93 to 34.0% in 2001-02. In 2001-02 the only respondents who indicated favour in the 40%+ category were: those living in the West, where smoke-free bars were more common (43.3%); those aged 65+ (44.8%); nonsmokers (40.2%); Hispanics (46.1%); and non-Hispanic Asians (45.2%).
U.S. Department of Health and Human Services, 2006 USA	Current Population Survey (CPS) (1991-93; 1998-99; 2001-02)	Parts of bars: In all surveys there was only minority support for smoking being allowed in "some areas of bars."	Attitude over time: 44.2% in 1992-93 to 40.6% in 2001-02.
Borland et al., 2006b Australia, Canada, UK, USA	Prospective cohorts (2002)	Among smokers: Majority support for total bans where extensive bans were in place (all >51%), but only minority support where there were no or limited bans in place (range: 20.9% to 54.2%).	Where there were extensive bans the support was: Australia (71.6%), UK (not applicable), Canada (51.1%), and USA (63.0%). Logistic regression analysis showed that the same variables related to support for bans in restaurants also applied to bars (see above in this Table). In addition, "both reported and documented restrictions in restaurants were also significantly related to support for bans in bars."

Table 5.4 Studies on public attitudes towards smoking restrictions in hospitality venues (restaurants, bars, pubs, etc.)

Reference/location	Study design and date	Results	Comments
- Just bars / pubs			
Fong *et al.*, 2006 Ireland and UK	Prospective cohorts (2003-04; 2004-05)	Among smokers: A minority (46%) of Irish smokers supported a total ban on smoking in bars/pubs; for the UK smokers support was lower (at just over 10%*).	Level of support for Irish smokers (which reached 46%) was substantially up from 13% prior to a smoke-free law (a statistically significant higher increase than for the UK). A more direct question about support for the total ban in pubs produced a higher result (64% of Irish smokers versus 25% of UK smokers).
European Commission, 2007 29 European countries	Representative sampling, face-to-face interviews (2006)	Majority support (62%) for banning smoking in bars/pubs (only a minority of smokers (38%) supported this).	As in a 2005 survey, the attitudes are divided across the European countries. Level of support exceeds 80% in Ireland (92%), Italy (89%), Sweden (88%) and Malta (81%). Only a minority are supportive in Austria (45%), the Czech Republic (42%), Denmark (46%), and in the Netherlands (46%). The majority of nonsmokers (77% totally) support a smoking ban when compared to a minority of smokers (38%).
Health Canada, 2006 Canada	Canadian Tobacco Use Monitoring Survey (CTUMS) (2006)	Around half (49%) felt that smoking should not be permitted in a bar or tavern.	This represented an increase from 26% in 2001 (also the CTUMS survey).
Edwards *et al.*, 2008 New Zealand	Health Sponsorship Council (HSC) annual surveys (2003-2006) & UMR Research Ltd surveys	Majority support for smoking bans in bars (74% in 2006). Majority support for the right of bar and pub workers to work in a smoke-free environment (91.5% in 2006; 82.7% in smokers).	Support for a ban increased from 38% in 2001 to 74% by 2006 (UMR data). HSC data reported it at 82% in 2006 (up from 61% in 2004). Among smokers it was 58% (up from 25% in 2004). The level of support increased for the rights of bar workers went from 79.1% in 2003 for all respondents and from 56.9% for smokers (HSC data). Support in all these areas increased after a law banning smoking in bars (in 2004).
Studies in developing countries - including sub-national and city studies			
Lam *et al.*, 2002 Hong Kong, China	A population-based, random digit dialing telephone survey of adults (1999, 2000)	Restaurants: Majority support (68.9%) for a totally smoke-free policy in restaurants.	Multivariate analyses concluded nonsmokers (among other groups) were more likely to support a totally smoke-free policy in restaurants. This comprehensive survey - the first in Asia - shows strong community support for smoke-free dining.
Barnoya *et al.*, 2007 Guatemala	Survey of workers in Guatemala City (2006)	Bar/restaurants (workers): Only a minority of bar and restaurant workers (30%) supported smoke-free workplaces	Results were lower than for the four other groups of workers studied. Study involved a convenience sample in the capital city - may not be representative.
Non-English language data sources reviewed in Sebrie *et al.*, 2008 Argentina and Brazil	Probabilistic telephone surveys in Argentina and convenience sampling in Brazil (both 2006)	Various hospitality settings: Majority support in all the various settings.	Argentina - 76.5% support for smoke-free restaurants and bars Brazil - 83% support for smoke-free restaurants, 79% for luncheonettes, 67% for bingo venues, 63% for bars, and 62% for night clubs.
Przewozniak *et al.*, 2008 Poland	Nationwide representative sample of adults (2007)	Various hospitality settings: Majority level support for bans in four types of venues (range: 54% to 66%).	Support for bans: restaurants (66%), coffee bars (60%), pubs (55%) and disco and dancing clubs (54%). There were bigger differences between smokers and nonsmokers and between different social strata for support of a ban in the hospitality sector than for bans in other public places and worksites in Poland.

*These percentages are imprecise because they are based on graphically presented results and not on exact tabulated data (which were not in the published article)

Table 5.5 Country level and multi-country studies on compliance with smoking restrictions in hospitality venues

Reference/location	Study design and date	Results	Comments
Connolly et al., 2006 13 countries / jurisdictions	Air quality study in Irish pubs, convenience samples (2004-2006)	Irish pubs: Air pollution was much lower in the pubs in smoke-free cities. In other smoking-permitted settings there was always evidence of serious pollution from SHS.	$PM_{2.5}$ levels in Irish pubs in smoke-free cities were 93% lower than in pubs in smoking-permitted cities. This study mainly covered pubs in Ireland, the USA, and Canada, but also in Armenia, Australia, Belgium, China, England, France, Germany, Greece, Lebanon, Northern Ireland, Poland, and Romania. See Chapter 6 for further details.
Lund, 2006; Lund & Lund, 2006 Norway	National annual surveys (2003-2006)	Hospitality venues: Improved self-reported air quality by customers after a new smoke-free law in 2004, suggestive of compliance. Customer and hospitality staff reports also indicate high compliance.	Reports by nonsmokers of "very good air quality" increased after the law (from 9% to 58% for pubs and 36% to 70% for restaurants). Hospitality industry employees also reported improved air quality with a decline in problems due to SHS from 44% to 6% at five months post-law. Customers with high patronage rarely observed serious enforcement problems (3% for pubs and 2% for restaurants in the first 18 months). No indication of a change in patronage levels, so no evidence for smoking being displaced into home settings. A 1998 survey in one city also indicated compliance with an earlier law in hospitality settings (Emaus et al., 2001).
European Commission, 2007 29 European countries	Representative sampling, face-to-face interviews (2006)	Restaurants and bars: High exposure probably reflects the low prevalence of smoking restrictions and the low use of voluntary restrictions in these settings in 2006.	The largest segment of European citizens who say they are exposed to SHS on a daily basis (70%), work in restaurants, pubs, and bars.
Hyland et al., 2008a 32 country study (18 developing countries, including former Soviet Union countries)*	International cross-sectional air quality study (2005-2006)	Various settings: Air pollution from SHS was substantially lower in all settings where smoking was not permitted compared to where it was (for 30 relevant countries). Levels were much lower in the two countries with national smoke-free laws.	Fine particulate ($PM_{2.5}$) levels were 9.9 times greater in establishments where smoking was permitted than in places where it was not (most settings were either bars or restaurants). New Zealand and Ireland had the lowest levels of indoor air pollution (consistent with their national smoke-free policies). Average levels were far greater than what the US Environmental Protection Agency (EPA) and the WHO have concluded is harmful to human health. See Chapter 6 for further details.
Travers et al., 2007 USA	Air quality study in 20 states and Puerto Rico (2003-2006)	Various settings: Observed compliance was high; air quality data supported this.	Observed compliance with new smoke-free laws: 96%. Venues that had gone smoke-free had a 91% reduction in $PM_{2.5}$ levels (before/after study); they included bars, restaurants, pool halls, bingo halls, bowling centres, dance clubs, and casinos. (This large study (790 venues in many jurisdictions), was not designed to be fully nationally representative). See Chapter 6 for further details.
Lopez et al., 2008 10 European cities of eight countries	Air nicotine sampling in 167 hospitality venues	Hospitality venues: Evidence for compliance with smoking restrictions in public places.	Lower air nicotine concentrations in countries with strong smoke-free policy (i.e. Ireland) and venues where smoking is not allowed or restricted.

Table 5.5 Country level and multi-country studies on compliance with smoking restrictions in hospitality venues

Reference/location	Study design and date	Results	Comments
Country level studies - smokers only			
Borland *et al.*, 2006b Australia, Canada, UK, USA	Prospective cohorts (2002)	Restaurants: Most smokers complied with total bans in restaurants (when last visited).	The incidence of smoking in restaurants by respondents (on the last visit and where there was a total ban on smoking): 2.5% (Australia); 20.4% (UK); 5.5% (Canada), and 4.2% (USA). Logistic regression analysis revealed that reported compliance was higher where there were also documented bans and among those supportive of total bans. It varied significantly by country (higher in the UK).
Fong *et al.*, 2006 Ireland and UK	Prospective cohorts (2003-04; 2004-05)	Restaurants: Irish smokers reported that smoking had become rare in these venues after a smoke-free law.	The proportion of Irish smokers who observed smoking in these venues declined from 85% (pre-law) to 3% post-law. In the UK, levels were 78% and 62%, respectively, in this time period. See Chapter 6 for further details.
Borland *et al.*, 2006b Australia, Canada, UK, USA	Prospective cohorts (2002)	Bars: Majority compliance by smokers in two out of the four countries (for total bans in bars and when last visited).	The incidence of smoking in bars by respondents (on the last visit and where there was a total ban on smoking) was: 52.1% (Australia); 85.1% (UK); 31.2% (Canada), and 27.1% (USA). In the USA, reported compliance was higher (82.5%) where there were also documented bans (mainly California).
Fong *et al.*, 2006 Ireland and UK	Prospective cohorts (2003-04; 2004-05)	Bars/pubs: Irish smokers reported that smoking had become rare in these venues after a smoke-free law.	The proportion of Irish smokers who observed smoking in these venues declined from 98% (pre-law) to 5% (post-law). In the UK, the level remained at 97%+ in this time period. Also, at post-law, 98% of Irish smokers said that there was less smoke in pubs than one year before (pre-ban), and 94% reported that pubs were enforcing the law "totally" ("somewhat" was 5%; "not at all" was 2%). See Chapter 6 for further details.
Country level studies - nonsmokers and smokers			
Ministry of Health, 2007 New Zealand	National face-to-face survey (2006)	Pub, club, or restaurants: High compliance with majority of respondents reporting no exposure to smoking indoors (only 7.4% report such exposure).	Where smoking was identified it was most common in: pubs (pubs=39.2%; restaurants=39.0%; clubs=14.4%; night clubs=14.1%; other public venue=6.8%).
Edwards *et al.*, 2008 New Zealand	Review of multiple and geographically distributed studies (2003-2006)	Bars and restaurants: High compliance suggested by the collective findings of five relevant studies.	Three observational studies detailed (one including restaurant data) and reports from participants in a bar managers cohort study. All indicated high compliance, as did cotinine and air quality studies (with some restaurant data). When considered collectively, these studies were not necessarily nationally representative.

Table 5.5 Country level and multi-country studies on compliance with smoking restrictions in hospitality venues

Reference/location	Study design and date	Results	Comments
Multi-country air quality studies			
Nebot et al., 2005 Seven European countries	Measurements of airborne nicotine (multiple settings) (2001-2002)	Restaurants: Some limited evidence for compliance; nicotine still found in most of the sites studied.	Nicotine levels lower in sites with smoking restrictions. Nonsmoking areas within restaurants had similar levels to smoking areas in Vienna, Paris, and Florence. The countries were Austria, France, Greece, Italy, Portugal, Spain, and Sweden.
Nebot et al., 2005 Seven European countries	Measurements of airborne nicotine (multiple settings) (2001-2002)	Discos or bars: No evidence for lower levels of SHS (no sites had restrictions).	These settings had the highest levels in the study of multiple public places. The countries were Austria, France, Greece, Italy, Portugal, Spain, and Sweden.

* Jurisdictions in this study included: Argentina, Armenia, Belgium, Brazil, Canada, China, Faroe Islands, France, Germany, Ghana, Greece, Ireland, Laos, Lebanon, Malaysia, Mexico, New Caledonia, New Zealand, Pakistan, Poland, Portugal, Romania, Singapore, Spain, Syria, Thailand, Tunisia, United Kingdom, USA, Uruguay, Venezuela, Viet Nam

Table 5.6 Studies in developing countries on compliance with smoking restrictions in hospitality venues (including country level, sub-national and city level studies)

Reference/location	Study design and date	Results	Comments
Navas-Acien et al., 2004 Seven Latin American countries	Measurement of airborne nicotine in multiple settings in the capital cities (2002, 2003)	Restaurants: General evidence for some level of compliance based on lower nicotine levels in the non-smoking areas in restaurants.	The median level of nicotine in nonsmoking areas was around half that in smoking areas of restaurants (but some levels were even higher than in adjacent smoking areas). The countries in this study were Argentina, Brazil, Chile, Costa Rica, Paraguay, Peru, and Uruguay.
Navas-Acien et al., 2004 Seven Latin American countries	Measurement of airborne nicotine in multiple settings in the capital cities (2002, 2003)	Bars: No clear evidence for any compliance at this time.	Median level of nicotine was generally higher in bars than restaurants, but this was at a time when there were minimal restrictions in these countries for smoking in bars (since then there have been new laws that relate to bars in Uruguay and Buenos Aires, Argentina) (Barnoya et al., 2007). The countries in this study were Argentina, Brazil, Chile, Costa Rica, Paraguay, Peru, and Uruguay. More recent survey reports are suggestive that nearly 90% of respondents in Uruguay considered that enforcement with the recent comprehensive smoke-free law was "high or very high" (reviewed in Sebrie et al., 2008).
Lung et al., 2004 Taiwan, China	Observational and air quality study of coffee shops (2001)	Coffee shops: Some evidence for compliance (i.e. no smoking observed in the nonsmoking sections).	High levels of $PM_{2.5}$ detected in the nonsmoking areas of these shops. Divisions between smoking and nonsmoking sections were not effective in preventing SHS exposure. See Chapter 6 for further details.
Fidan et al., 2005 Turkey	Surveys of workers and hair nicotine sampling in the City of Izmir (2000-2001)	Coffee houses: No evidence that any smoking restrictions are operational in this setting (high hair nicotine levels found in workers).	Levels of hair nicotine in nonsmoking coffee house workers were 5.2 times higher than nonsmoking hospital worker controls, but the sample sizes in this study were small.

Table 5.6 Studies in developing countries on compliance with smoking restrictions in hospitality venues (including country level, sub-national and city level studies

Reference/location	Study design and date	Results	Comments
Hedley et al., 2006 Hong Kong, China	Cotinine measurements among workers (2000-2001)	Restaurants and bars: Some evidence for compliance with full smoking restrictions.	Among nonsmoking catering workers working in smoke-free areas there were higher levels of urinary cotinine than a control group (of university workers). This was explained by SHS exposure during break times. Levels of cotinine were much higher among workers in those workplaces with unrestricted smoking.
Barnoya et al., 2007 Guatemala, Honduras, Mexico, Panama	Measurement of airborne nicotine in multiple settings in the capital cities (2006)	Restaurants/bars: No evidence for compliance with smoking restrictions.	Nicotine levels in each of these settings were high (relative to hospitals, schools, government buildings, and airports). In Guatemala, there was no clear evidence that the law covering restaurants was substantially reducing levels in bars (where there is no smoke-free law).
Stillman et al., 2007 China	Nicotine sampling in urban and rural settings (2005)	Restaurants: No clear evidence of restrictions or compliance with restrictions.	Airborne nicotine was detected in 100.0% of the locations. The median level was higher than four other types of settings, but was three times lower than for "entertainment settings".
Stillman et al., 2007 China	Nicotine sampling in urban and rural settings (2005)	Entertainment settings: No evidence for voluntary restrictions or compliance with any such restrictions (including internet cafés, karaoke bars, and mahjong parlours).	Airborne nicotine detected in 100.0% of the locations. Median level was >3 times higher than for restaurants. China did not have smoke-free regulations for these settings at this time.
Based on English language abstract of Chinese language article: Kang et al., 2007 China	Telephone survey and PM$_{2.5}$ measurements in restaurants and bars in Beijing (no year given).	Restaurants and bars: Some evidence for compliance with smoking restrictions.	Surveyed 305 restaurants and bars: 27.9% had either complete or partial smoking restrictions. Average indoor PM$_{2.5}$ levels were less than half the levels in the restaurants and bars without smoking ban regulations. Levels in western fast-food restaurants were much lower than the levels in bars.
Lazcano-Ponce et al., 2007 Mexico	Cotinine study among disco attendees (Central Region) (circa 2005)	Discos: Evidence of a lack of smoking restrictions or compliance for any that exist.	Large increases in urinary cotinine levels among nonsmokers (pre- versus post-exposure to the discos). Evidence that the average urinary cotinine value was higher in subjects who reported SHS exposure at home. This study did not indicate that any official restrictions were operational.

It appears that the general patterns at the sub-national level in Australia and the USA are fairly reflective of the national level results described above.

Relevance for evidence-based tobacco control

Policymakers and health workers need to be aware that smoking restrictions in hospitality settings may often have lower levels of public support relative to other workplaces. This suggests the desirability for obtaining representative attitudinal data in the relevant jurisdiction prior to implementing new laws. Such information can inform the need for relevant mass media campaigns and even for resourcing of enforcement activities (especially in the first few months of the operation of a new law). There are examples of successful mass media and educational campaigns, such as in California (California Department of Health Services, 2006), which have helped shift public attitudes before a new law was introduced. Norwegian data also indicate successful mass media campaigns around a new smoke-free law covering hospitality venue workplaces (Lund & Rise, 2004). Although mass media campaigns associated with new smoke-free laws have not been systematically reviewed, there is good evidence that tobacco control mass media campaigns are effective in changing attitudes and behaviour (Hopkins *et al.*, 2001; Friend & Levy, 2002; Farrelly *et al.*, 2003).

For some countries there is evidence that majority support for smoke-free restaurants and bars

may quickly develop; as a result, new legislation could be part of a comprehensive workplace law. In settings where these laws are already in place, there may be a need for ongoing monitoring or periodic research studies to evaluate compliance, or at least the extent of self-policing of the law. If compliance is low, then an option is for this to be addressed by mass media campaigns (to educate the public), improved policing of the law (by authorities or by self-policing), and increasing fines paid by venue owners (or customers) for violations. In many jurisdictions these measures can also be promoted by public health authorities through the use of media opportunities to obtain unpaid publicity (i.e. earned media).

Summary

In general, there are majority levels of public support for smoking restrictions for indoor hospitality settings in developed countries for which country level data are available. Compliance with such smoking restrictions in these settings is usually fairly substantial. In developing countries, there are fewer studies, but they generally indicate majority support. In contrast, the studies in these countries indicate poorer compliance and even apparent complete non-compliance in some settings.

Attitudes towards, and compliance with, smoking restrictions in other public places (health care facilities, schools, public transport, shopping malls, and indoor sports arenas)

This subsection covers public attitudes towards, and compliance

with, smoking restrictions in a diverse range of other indoor settings. These settings are generally workplaces, but workers may often be out-numbered by other members of the public. Some of these settings, such as schools and child day-care centres, may also have restrictions on smoking in outdoor areas as well.

Studies of these public places with country level samples are detailed in Table 5.7. Subsequent tables discuss studies on compliance with smoking restrictions in various settings (Tables 5.8 and 5.9).

The main findings from the country level studies indicate that in countries with attitudinal data there is:

- Majority public support in developed countries for smoking restrictions in hospitals, indoor sporting arenas/events, and shopping malls (with a majority of the public giving support for at least the past 15 years for some settings).
- Majority support by smokers in developed countries for some of these restrictions (e.g. for shopping malls, trains/train stations, and indoor sporting events).
- Where trend data are available, the pattern is for increasing support for such restrictions over time.

The patterns around compliance indicate fairly variable levels with smoking restrictions for schools and hospitals. However, studies of smokers indicate that smoking is rarely observed in shopping malls and public buses (where restrictions apply).

Table 5.7 Studies on public attitudes towards smoking restrictions in a range of other public settings (those not previously covered in this chapter and focusing on just multi-country and country level studies except for developing countries)

Reference/location	Study design and date	Results	Comments
Schools			
Reeder & Glasgow, 2000 New Zealand	Survey of primary and intermediate school representatives (1997)	Most school representatives (62%) thought school staff would support completely smoke-free schools.	Majority support apparent in other NZ data (see below). Survey was limited by reliance on only one school representative in each school.
Darling & Reeder, 2003 New Zealand	Survey of secondary school representatives (2002)	Most school representatives (74.1%) thought school staff would support completely smoke-free schools.	Survey was limited by reliance on only one representative per school. Views are consistent with the low smoking rates amongst teachers (Census data indicated only 8.8% of secondary school teachers were current smokers). Introduction of fully smoke-free schools in 2004 appears to have been successful (but no studies have been published).
Wold et al., 2004a Eight European countries/ jurisdictions	Survey of policies and key informant interviews (1998/1999)	This study reported a lack of systems for monitoring, reporting, and evaluating smoke-free legislation relating to schools; hence a lack of attitudinal data.	Jurisdictions with smoke-free legislation: Austria, French-speaking Belgium, Finland, and Norway. Those without were: Denmark, North Rhine Westphalia region of Germany, Scotland, and Wales.
Przewozniak et al., 2008 Poland	Nationwide survey based on random representative sample of adults (2007)	Majority of adults (89%) support complete ban of smoking in schools and other educational premises.	The ban on smoking in schools and other educational premises began in 1995.
Hospitals			
Joseph et al., 1995 USA	Survey of hospitals (1993)	There was evidence that patient and employee complaints about new smoking restrictions were uncommon.	Managers of smoke-free hospitals reported that patient complaints had either never occurred (33%) or occurred <1 time per month (47%). No employee disciplinary measures (74%); 1-4 (21%) since policy implemented.
National Cancer Institute, 2000; U.S. Department of Health and Human Services, 2006 USA	Current Population Survey (CPS) (1991-93; 1998-99; 2001-02).	By 1992-93 widespread public support (74.8%) for smoke-free hospitals.	The overall support rose from 74.8% in 1992-93 to >83% in 2001-02.
Przewozniak et al., 2008 Poland	Nationwide survey based on random representative sample of adults (2007)	Majority support (88%) for a complete ban of smoking in hospitals and other health care settings.	1995 - Smoking banned in health care facilities. There was no significant difference in support between smokers and nonsmokers and between different social strata.
Other settings			
McMillen et al., 2003 USA	National telephone survey (Social Climate Survey of Tobacco Control (CSTC)) (2000, 2001)	Indoor sporting events: High levels of support (80.4% in 2001).	Support increased significantly between surveys (from 77.5% in 2000). Support in 2001 among smokers: 69.5%; nonsmokers: 83.5%.
McMillen et al., 2003 USA	Social Climate Survey of Tobacco Control (CSTC) (2000, 2001)	Shopping malls: High level of support (75.3% in 2001).	Support increased significantly between surveys (from 71.4% in 2000). Support in 2001 among smokers: 60.0%; nonsmokers: 75.5%.

Table 5.7 Studies on public attitudes towards smoking restrictions in a range of other public settings (those not previously covered in this chapter and focusing on just multi-country and country level studies except for developing countries)

Reference/location	Study design and date	Results	Comments
Other settings			
U.S. Department of Health and Human Services, 2006 USA	Current Population Survey (CPS) (1991-93; 1998-99; 2001-02).	Indoor sports arenas: By 1992-93 there was majority public support (67.0%) and up to 77.2% in 2001-02.	By 1992-93 there was majority support in all geographic regions, age groups, both genders, education groups, income groups, main occupational groups, and ethnic groups. Support rose from 67.0% in 1992-93 to 77.2% in 2001-02. In 1992-93 the only respondents who did not indicate majority favour (>50%) were smokers (48.7%).
U.S. Department of Health and Human Services, 2006 USA	Current Population Survey (CPS) (1991-93; 1998-99; 2001-02).	Shopping malls: By 1992-93 majority public support (54.6%) for smoke-free malls.	Majority support in all geographic regions, both genders, education groups, income groups, main occupational groups, and ethnic groups. Support rose from 54.6% in 1992-93 to 76.4% in 2001-02. In 1992-93 the only respondents who did not indicate majority favour (>50%) were: 18-24 year olds (49.9%) and smokers (31.8%).
Fong *et al.*, 2006 Ireland and UK	Prospective cohorts (2003-04; 2004-05)	Shopping malls - smokers: Most Irish and UK smokers supported a total smoking ban in these settings (around 80% and 70% respectively*).	Level of support among Irish smokers increased after the smoke-free law at a higher rate than for UK smokers, but not statistically significantly different.
Fong *et al.*, 2006 Ireland and UK	Prospective cohorts (2003/4 & 2004/5)	Trains/train stations - smokers: Most Irish and UK smokers supported a total smoking ban in trains (at around 80%*). For train stations it was around 60% and 30% respectively.*	Level of support among Irish smokers increased for both trains and train stations after the smoke-free law; a statistically significant higher increase than for the UK for both settings.
Non-English language data sources reviewed in Sebrie *et al.*, 2008 Argentina and Mexico	Probabilistic telephone surveys in Argentina (2006) and Mexico (2006-2007)	Majority support for smoke-free health care and educational facilities.	Support in Argentina - 96.7%. In Mexico, support for hospitals was mixed in with other public settings for which there was 75% support.
Przewozniak *et al.*, 2008 Poland	Nationwide survey based on random representative sample of adults (2007)	Indoor cultural and art events: Majority support (84%).	1999 - Smoking banned in cultural institutions. Only slight differences in levels of support between smokers and nonsmokers and between different social strata.
California case study - other settings			
Gilpin *et al.*, 2003; Al-Delaimy *et al.*, 2008 California, USA	Regular surveys (1996 to 2005)	Schools: Vast majority (91.6%) of students support a complete ban on smoking on school grounds (69.8% for current smokers).	Support 90.5% in 2002; up from 55.8% in 1996. In 2005, 69.8% of current student smokers supported a ban.
Gilpin *et al.*, 2004; Al-Delaimy *et al.*, 2008 California, USA	Population surveys (2002)	Majority public support for smoking not being allowed (range of settings).	Common areas of hotels and motels (88.8%); common areas of apartments/-condominiums (87.1%); on-campus university housing (79.2%); hotel rooms (65.7%); Indian gambling casinos (60.1%).

*These percentages are imprecise because they are based on graphically presented results and not on exact tabulated data (which were not in the published article)

In developing countries there is a general lack of attitudinal data on these settings. Some compliance data are available and provide a more mixed picture of compliance with the smoking restrictions that exist.

With regard to "other" settings of note, this review identified few country level studies on restrictions relating to special traditional or cultural settings (e.g. just for Poland as detailed in Table 5.7). But there were no country level studies of major smoke-free religious settings (such as Mecca in Saudi Arabia) and of "smoke-free villages" adopted in some Pacific Island countries. In New Zealand, where the indigenous Maori people have increasingly adopted smoke-free marae (communal meeting places), these have been at a local tribal level and have not involved legal policies.

Discussion – public transport

There appears to be little attitudinal and compliance data relating to public transport (at least at a country level). This may partly reflect the acceptance of current practice with nearly all airlines in the world providing smoke-free aircraft. Airlines have likely become smoke-free for a mixture of reasons: to reduce the risk of fires, minimise nuisance effects to passengers, and due to health concerns by aircrew and passengers (including associated risks of legal action). Similarly, public attitudes towards smoking in trains and buses may also be influenced by this wide range of health and non-health issues, particularly where the transportation is crowded or underground (e.g. urban subway trains). These safety

issues have been important in the past, as detailed in Chapter 3. The situation may well be different in many parts of the developing world given data on the lack of compliance in transportation settings in China (Table 5.9).

Discussion – health care settings

Of all public settings, support for smoke-free hospitals may be one of the highest. National survey data for the USA reported that hospitals were the venue with the most support for being smoke-free in all three national surveys (i.e. ahead of indoor work areas, indoor sports venues, indoor shopping malls, restaurants, and bars) (U.S. Department of Health and Human Services, 2006). Despite this, compliance with smoking restrictions in health care facilities appears to be variable from the data presented in Tables 5.8 and 5.9. Yet there is other evidence suggesting improvements in air quality from smoking restrictions in such settings (see Chapter 6).

Policies for smoke-free hospitals, that include long-term residential care and acute psychiatric facilities, have been successfully introduced (Lawn & Pols, 2005; Kunyk et al., 2007). But there are complex issues to address, which may potentially improve attitudinal support and compliance for the policies by health workers.

Discussion – schools

Smoke-free schools can be justified as a workplace health protection issue; both shielding the health of students and staff from SHS exposure. Some also argue that

schools and school grounds should be completely smoke-free, to not only provide smoke-free role models for students, but also to ensure consistency with the messages in school-based health education programmes (Pickett et al., 1999; Reeder & Glasgow, 2000; Darling & Reeder, 2003; Darling et al., 2006).

The data in Tables 5.8 and 5.9 indicate mixed compliance with smoke-free school legislation. Some studies indicate problems with compliance, for instance schools in New York State (Stephens & English, 2002), and in five US states (Wakefield & Chaloupka, 2000). Also of note is a study from Scotland that showed evidence of compliance where complete restrictions on teacher smoking existed, and students perceived smoking among teachers less often in the staff rooms (Griesbach et al., 2002). However, in these schools with complete restrictions, the students observed teachers smoking more often outside on the school premises.

Teacher/staff attitudes may be a factor in the adoption of smoke-free school policies, with several studies suggesting that staff smokers may not favour smoke-free schools (e.g. three studies described in Wold et al., 2004a). Logistic regression analysis of survey data from Ontario, Canada also indicated that teachers/staff who believed the restriction on smoking on school property was not effective, opposed it and desired a repeal of the restrictions (Pickett et al., 1999).

Compliance in smoke-free schools might be improved by appropriate enforcement. An indirect indicator of this comes from a study that found that although the existence of school policies that restricted smoking was not related to smoking uptake among students, when there was evidence that these policies were enforced, they were effective in reducing smoking uptake, regardless of smoking stage (Wakefield *et al.*, 2000a).

Another issue reported in the literature is that poorly designed smoke-free school legislation may hinder its acceptability and effectiveness. For example, there was evidence to suggest that in Finland, the legislation prohibiting smoking "has been interpreted to mean that smoking is permitted if certain conditions are fulfilled, even though the intention was quite clearly the creation of smoke-free schools" (Wold *et al.*, 2004a). Also, in New Zealand, the sub-optimal design of an earlier 1990 law (that just treated schools no differently from other workplaces) meant that the law did not lead to completely smoke-free environments for students (Reeder & Glasgow, 2000; Darling & Reeder, 2003). This was ultimately addressed when a new law required schools to become completely smoke-free on all school property and at all times.

Relevance for evidence-based tobacco control

There are a number of special issues that policymakers and health workers can consider when proposing smoking restrictions in settings covered here. These include:

• The crowded nature of some transportation settings (which may exacerbate risks to health and also nuisance effects).
• The special fire risks from smoking in some modes of

transportation (e.g. on aircraft, trains, subway trains, and ships), which may provide strong additional safety reasons for smoking restrictions (see Chapter 3 for safety arguments for smoking restrictions).
• The special status of health care facilities and arguments around these providing a pro-health example in the community. Some patients may also be especially vulnerable to the harm of SHS exposure. However, it may be necessary to consider special issues regarding acute psychiatric inpatient facilities and long-term residential care facilities when designing and implementing such policies.
• The special status of schools in the community, and therefore the need for coherence between teacher role modelling behaviour and smoke-free health education messages. The case is strengthened when considering that children are more vulnerable to SHS exposure than other populations (see Chapter 2). These arguments also apply to child day-care centres.

Further jurisdiction-specific data on all these issues can be obtained from conducting attitudinal studies and considering relevant research published in other settings (e.g. particularly neighbouring states, provinces, or countries).

Summary

For countries that have country level data, the available evidence indicates majority public support in developed

countries for smoking restrictions in a number of settings (e.g. hospitals, indoor sporting arenas/events, and shopping malls). A majority of smokers also support restrictions in most of these settings. The patterns around compliance indicate fairly variable levels of compliance with smoking restrictions for schools and hospitals. However, studies of smokers indicate that smoking is rarely observed in shopping malls and public buses (where restrictions apply and such studies have been conducted). In developing countries there are fewer attitudinal studies on these settings and available compliance data provides a general picture of mixed compliance with the smoking restrictions that exist. The range of settings covered here are diverse, and so policymakers and health workers should ideally consider many of the setting-specific issues involved in determining public attitudes and compliance with smoking restrictions.

Table 5.8 Studies in developed countries on compliance with smoking restrictions in a range of other public settings (those not previously covered in this chapter and focusing on just multi-country and country level studies)

Reference/location	Study design and date	Results	Comments
Schools - compliance			
Reeder & Glasgow, 2000 New Zealand	Survey of primary and intermediate school representatives (1997)	Variable compliance in primary and intermediate schools with the national legislation at the time.	Most schools (97%) reported having a current, written school smoking policy. Only 49% had policy on display, which was required. While not required by law at this time, 82% of respondents reported school buildings were totally smoke-free; 54% said schools were smoke-free in buildings and grounds.
Based on an English language abstract by Hernandez-Mezquita *et al.*, 2000 Spain	Large survey of school principals	Evidence of reduced teacher smoking in the presence of pupils (suggestive of some compliance). Suboptimal use of signage reported.	80.9% of principals claim "the fulfilment of the legislation is demanded in their centres." Only 64.9% reported having posters in theirs schools that warn about the smoking ban. Level of teacher smoking in the presence of pupils in schools where anti-tobacco legislation was demanded was lower compared to other schools (5.9% versus 12.9%).
Wakefield *et al.*, 2000a USA	Survey of high school students (14-17 years) (1996)	Generally poor compliance based on student perception of how many students obeyed the rule.	Based on student perceptions, enforcement was graded "weak" or "no enforcement" for 71.7% of respondents. 91.8% of respondents stated that a smoking ban existed at their school.
Darling & Reeder, 2003 New Zealand	Survey of secondary school representatives (multistage cluster sampling survey of schools) (2002)	Variable compliance in secondary schools with the national legislation at the time.	Most schools (87.7%) reported having a current, written school smoking policy. Only 25.9% had policy on display, which was required. 56.9% of school policies included guidelines regarding nonsmoking signage.
Wold *et al.*, 2004a Eight European countries / jurisdictions	Survey of policies and key informant interviews (1998/1999)	This study reported a lack of systems for monitoring, reporting and evaluating smoke-free legislation relating to schools.	See the preceding table for a list of the jurisdictions covered.
Wold *et al.*, 2004b Seven European countries / jurisdictions	Student and teacher surveys (1997-1998)	Evidence of reduced exposure to indoor smoke from teachers suggestive of some level of compliance.	Both national and school level laws restricting smoking by teachers were associated with a reduced probability of students reporting that they are exposed to teachers who smoke indoors. Conversely, there was a greater probability of students being exposed to teachers smoking outdoors. There was a clear relationship between a restrictive national policy and higher proportions of smoke-free schools.
Nebot *et al.*, 2005 Seven European countries	Measurements of airborne nicotine (multiple settings) (2001-2002)	Some evidence for compliance, though nicotine still detected in most sites.	Nicotine levels were lower in sites with smoking restrictions. Schools had lowest concentrations compared to all other public places sampled. Sweden had relatively low levels compared to the other countries (Austria, France, Greece, Italy, Portugal, and Spain).

Table 5.8 Studies in developed countries on compliance with smoking restrictions in a range of other public settings (those not previously covered in this chapter and focusing on just multi-country and country level studies)

Reference/location	Study design and date	Results	Comments
Schools - compliance			
Eaton *et al.*, 2006 USA	Annual Youth Risk Surveillance System (including national, state, and local surveys) (2004-06)	Only 6.8% of students had smoked cigarettes on school property on one of the 30 days preceding the survey (nationwide).	The prevalence of having smoked cigarettes on school property ranged from 1.7% to 10.7% across state surveys (median: 6.8%) and from 2.5% to 6.4% across local surveys (median: 4.5%).
European Commission, 2007 29 European countries	Representative sampling, face-to-face interviews (2006)	Educational facilities: Majority not exposed to SHS in educational facilities (87%) suggesting some compliance.	This level of no exposure (87%) was better than in government facilities (78%) and health care facilities (81%). Another 5% reported exposure of <1 hour per day.
Health care facilities and hospitals - compliance			
Joseph *et al.*, 1995 USA	Survey of hospitals (1993)	Survey data provided general evidence that hospitals had implemented and enforced smoking restrictions.	Most (65%) hospitals were compliant. Only <1% had no restrictions on smoking anywhere in the hospital. It was reported that the "the standard is well accepted by most patients and employees."
Longo *et al.*, 1996 USA	Natural experiment (hospitals and corresponding community samples) (1993-1994)	The higher quit ratios for smoke-free hospital employees provide some indirect evidence of the restrictions having an impact; hence compliance.	Employees of smoke-free hospitals had significantly higher post-ban quit ratios. This finding has been supported in subsequent work (Longo *et al.*, 2001).
Based on an English language abstract by Nardini *et al.*, 2003 Italy	Survey of hospital managers (1998)	Suboptimal compliance reported.	Insufficient or no compliance reported in 25.4%; majority (50.7%) reported no support services (e.g. smoking cessation clinic). National survey indicated 33.3% of hospital staff are active smokers and "up to 80% of them admit to smoking in the workplace." Poor response rate limits the value of this study.
Nebot *et al.*, 2005 Seven European countries	Measurements of airborne nicotine (multiple settings) (2001-2002)	Some evidence for compliance, though nicotine was still found in most of the sites studied.	Nicotine levels were lower than other public places (e.g. universities). Sweden had relatively low levels compared to the other countries (Austria, France, Greece, Italy, Portugal, and Spain). Austria had high levels due to measurements in "smoking rooms."
Other settings - compliance			
Nebot *et al.*, 2005 Seven European countries	Measurements of airborne nicotine (multiple settings) (2001-2002)	Train stations and airports: Some evidence for compliance in both these settings.	Nicotine levels were lower in sites with smoking restrictions. Despite most of these sites having smoking restrictions, appreciable concentrations of nicotine were still found. The countries were: Austria, France, Greece, Italy, Portugal, Spain, and Sweden.
Fong *et al.*, 2006 Ireland and UK	Prospective cohorts (2003-04; 2004-05)	Shopping malls - smokers only: Irish smokers reported that smoking had become rare in these settings after a smoke-free law.	Proportion of Irish smokers who observed smoking in these settings declined from 40% (pre-law) to 3% post-law. In the UK the levels were 29% and 22%, respectively, in this time period. See Chapter 6 for further details.

Table 5.8 Studies in developed countries on compliance with smoking restrictions in a range of other public settings (those not previously covered in this chapter and focusing on just multi-country and country level studies)

Reference/location	Study design and date	Results	Comments
Other settings - compliance			
Fong *et al.*, 2006 Ireland and UK	Prospective cohorts (2003-04; 2004-05)	Public buses - smokers only: Irish and UK smokers reported that smoking continued to be uncommon in these settings (both <10%).	The proportion of Irish and UK smokers who observed smoking in public buses (last ride) remained uncommon; changes between countries over time did not differ at a statistically significant level.
Hyland *et al.*, 2008a 32 country study*	International cross-sectional air quality study ($PM_{2.5}$) (2005-2006)	Various transportation settings: Air pollution from SHS was 8.3 times lower in those transportation settings with smoking restrictions.	Suggestive of compliance. Average levels of air pollution in settings with smoking were far greater than what the US EPA and WHO have concluded is harmful to human health.
California case study - other settings			
Gilpin *et al.*, 2003; Al-Delaimy *et al.*, 2008 California, USA	Regular surveys (1996-2005)	Schools: High level of compliance based on student reports of smoker compliance with school smoke-free policies.	2005 - 74.5% among nonsmokers; 67.6% among smokers (up from 40.7% for all students in 1996). 2002 - only 20.8% of students reported seeing smoking on school property in the past two weeks; declined in 2005 to 19.6%. 2005 - only 13.3% perceived that teachers smoked at school.

* Jurisdictions in this 32-country study included: Argentina, Armenia, Belgium, Brazil, Canada, China, Faroe Islands, France, Germany, Ghana, Greece, Ireland, Laos, Lebanon, Malaysia, Mexico, New Caledonia, New Zealand, Pakistan, Poland, Portugal, Romania, Singapore, Spain, Syria, Thailand, Tunisia, United Kingdom, USA, Uruguay, Venezuela, Viet Nam.

Table 5.9 Studies in developing countries on compliance with smoking restrictions in a range of other public settings (those not previously covered in this chapter and including country level, subnational and city level studies)

Reference/location	Study design and date	Results	Comments
Schools / educational facilities			
Navas-Acien *et al.*, 2004 Seven Latin American countries	Measurement of airborne nicotine in multiple settings in the capital cities (2002, 2003)	Evidence suggestive of some level of compliance based on lower nicotine levels in schools relative to other public settings.	Smoking was banned in schools in most of these countries. Nicotine was still detected in 78% of secondary school samples (some with substantial amounts). Median level of nicotine was lower than for hospitals and government buildings. The countries in this study were Argentina, Brazil, Chile, Costa Rica, Paraguay, Peru, and Uruguay.
Barnoya *et al.*, 2007 Guatemala, Honduras, Mexico, Panama	Measurement of airborne nicotine in multiple settings in the capital cities (2006)	Some evidence for compliance with smoking restrictions.	Nicotine levels below the limit of detection in three countries (and very low in the other one). Levels were much lower than hospitality venues and lower than government buildings and hospitals; the latter two comparisons were not statistically significant.
Stillman *et al.*, 2007 China	Nicotine sampling in urban and rural settings (2005)	Evidence for some compliance with restrictions.	Airborne nicotine was detected in 78.6% of the school locations (the lowest out of all types of settings). Median level was 2-7 times lower than those for hospitals, government buildings, and transportation settings. Some Beijing schools had levels that were similar to restaurants and bars.

Table 5.9 Studies in developing countries on compliance with smoking restrictions in a range of other public settings (those not previously covered in this chapter and including country level, subnational and city level studies)

Reference/location	Study design and date	Results	Comments
Schools / educational facilities			
Przewozniak *et al.*, 2007 Poland	Air quality ($PM_{2.5}$) study in 60 venues in four Polish towns (2005-2006)	Some evidence of compliance with smoke-free policies.	This study was part of the 32 country study detailed in Table 5.5, but it also collected data on schools. Much lower $PM_{2.5}$ levels were observed in schools where smoking is banned when compared with non-restricted hospitality venues.
Hospitals / health facilities			
Tsai *et al.*, 2000 Thailand	Indoor air quality sampling in venues in Bangkok (1996)	Some evidence for the lack of air pollution from smoking in nurse's dormitories associated with a hospital.	There were lower $PM_{2.5}$ and PM_{10} levels of particulates indoors than ambient outdoor levels. This contrasted with the levels in shops and homes found in this study; however, these settings had other sources of pollutants (e.g. from cooking).
Navas-Acien *et al.*, 2004 Seven Latin American countries	Measurement of airborne nicotine in multiple settings in the capital cities (2002, 2003)	Some limited evidence for some compliance with smoking restrictions.	Though smoking was banned in hospitals in these seven countries, nicotine was regularly detected. Median level of nicotine was lower than for hospitality settings and was comparable to levels from studies of open US offices where smoking was restricted. The countries in this study were Argentina, Brazil, Chile, Costa Rica, Paraguay, Peru, and Uruguay.
Fidan *et al.*, 2005 Turkey	Surveys of workers and hair nicotine sampling in the City of Izmir (2000-2001)	Some limited evidence for compliance based on relatively low hair nicotine levels in non-smoking workers.	Smoking is restricted in Turkey's hospitals to special smoking rooms. Nicotine hair levels among hospital nonsmoking staff were much lower (5.2 times) than in nonsmoking coffee house workers. Sample sizes in this study were small.
Barnoya *et al.*, 2007 Guatemala, Honduras, Mexico, Panama	Measurement of airborne nicotine in multiple settings in the capital cities (2006)	Some evidence for compliance with smoking restrictions.	Nicotine levels were below limit of detection in three countries (and very low in the other one). Levels were much lower than hospitality venues and lower than government buildings; the latter was not statistically significant.
Stillman *et al.*, 2007 China	Nicotine sampling in urban & rural settings (2005)	Limited evidence for some compliance with restrictions.	Airborne nicotine was detected in 91.4% of the locations. Median level was 2-3 times lower than those for government buildings and transportation settings. Some Beijing hospitals had levels that were similar to those in restaurants and bars.
Przewozniak *et al.*, 2007 Poland	Air quality ($PM_{2.5}$) study in 60 venues in four Polish towns (2005-2006)	Some evidence of compliance for smoke-free policies.	This study was part of the 32-country study detailed in Table 5.5, but it also collected data on hospitals. Much lower $PM_{2.5}$ levels were observed in hospitals where smoking is banned when compared with non-restricted hospitality venues. Another study reported a decline in the proportion of physicians who smoke at hospital worksites (Przewozniak & Zatonski, 2002).
Other settings			
Li *et al.*, 2001 Hong Kong, China	Indoor air quality sampling in shopping malls (1999)	Shopping malls: some evidence for non-compliance with the law (from observational and air quality data).	Despite the smoke-free laws, it was reported that "during the air sampling work, illegal smoking was always found inside these malls." Conclusion: "the increased PM_{10} levels could be attributed to illegal smoking inside these establishments." Another Hong Kong study also found high PM_{10} levels at some local shopping malls with tobacco smoking (Lee *et al.*, 1999).

Table 5.9 Studies in developing countries on compliance with smoking restrictions in a range of other public settings (those not previously covered in this chapter and including country level, subnational and city level studies)

Reference/location	Study design and date	Results	Comments
Other settings			
Navas-Acien *et al.*, 2004 Seven Latin American countries	Measurement of airborne nicotine in multiple settings in the capital cities (2002, 2003)	Airports: Limited evidence for some compliance with smoking restrictions.	Lower nicotine levels in airports in Argentina (domestic airport) and Costa Rica (that had smoke-free initiatives in place) were reported. Median level of nicotine lower than for hospitality settings, and was comparable to levels from studies of open US offices where smoking was restricted. The countries in this study were Argentina, Brazil, Chile, Costa Rica, Paraguay, Peru, and Uruguay.
Barnoya *et al.*, 2007 Guatemala, Honduras, Mexico, Panama	Measurement of airborne nicotine in multiple settings in the capital cities (2006)	Airports: Some evidence for compliance with smoking restrictions.	Nicotine levels were much lower than hospitality venues and lower than government buildings; the latter comparison was not statistically significant. The Mexican component of this study stated that the nicotine levels in the airport "reflect the lack of compliance with mandatory non-smoking official regulations in Mexico" (Barrientos-Gutierrez *et al.*, 2007b).
Stillman *et al.*, 2007 China	Nicotine sampling in urban & rural settings (2005)	Transportation settings: Evidence for general non-compliance with restrictions.	Airborne nicotine was detected in 91.7% of the locations. Median level was higher than three other types of settings, but lower than restaurants and entertainment settings, despite a smoking ban in public transportation vehicles and waiting rooms throughout the whole of China.

Attitudes towards, and compliance with, outdoor smoking restrictions (e.g. parks, sports grounds, and facility grounds)

Outdoor smoking restrictions around the world cover such settings as parks, beaches, bus stops, partly enclosed streets, grounds of health care facilities, sports stadiums and grounds, university campuses, and within specific distances from public building entryways (e.g. 20 feet of a main exit, entrance, or operable window of a public building in California). Outdoor areas within hospitality venues are also completely or partially smoke-free in some jurisdictions. Many residents also impose voluntary restrictions on smoking on their properties, but this is considered in Chapter 8 on smoke-free homes.

This review identified few country level studies in outdoor settings; therefore, the searches were expanded to include sub-national and local studies. This identified more studies, as the focus of such restrictions appears to generally be at a local level (i.e. by local city and district governments, or at the level of specific organisations which own sports venues). Data from the limited number of published studies identified are detailed in Table 5.10.

These data indicate a wide range of levels of support for outdoor smoking restrictions. For example, for smoke-free parks, the range was from 25% for smoke-free parks in the USA in 2001 up to 83% among park users in a New Zealand city in 2007 (Table 5.10). There is some evidence for overall support for smoke-free sports grounds in the settings where these have been studied.

While the available data are limited, there is some indication that support for restrictions on smoking in outdoor settings is less than for restrictions in indoor settings (McMillen *et al.*, 2003; Kunyk *et al.*, 2007).

All of the studies relating to compliance were suggestive of at least some level of compliance with outdoor smoking restrictions. In some settings this compliance reached high levels (e.g. sporting events in Western Australia) (Giles-Corti *et al.*, 2001).

Discussion of the results

Consideration of public attitudes concerning restrictions on outdoor smoking is particularly complex given the diversity of reasons as to why such restrictions may exist. For example, the Minnesota study (Klein *et al.*, 2007) found that reasons cited by the public for supporting smoke-free park policies included: to reduce litter (71%), to reduce youth opportunities to smoke (65%), to avoid SHS (64%), and to establish positive role models for youth (63%).

The New Zealand study also found that the main reasons people gave for supporting the policy were: positive role modelling, reducing SHS, and that 'parks are for children' (Arcus *et al.*, 2007). In contrast, the chief explanations people gave for opposing the policy were: smoking outdoors is acceptable, smokers should have the right to autonomy, and the policy will not work or cannot be enforced. Furthermore, the respondents who agreed with the policy thought the Council had implemented it because 'parks are for children,' and it reduces negative role modelling and litter. The respondents who disagreed with the policy most frequently stated that the Council implemented it for political reasons.

Other reasons cited in the literature for outdoor smoking restrictions include decreasing fire risk and protecting people from nuisances (Bloch & Shopland, 2000). But some of the public may think these reasons do not ethically justify legal controls, as some tobacco control experts have themselves suggested (Chapman, 2000, 2007).

The context of the outdoor restrictions is also likely to be important in determining attitudes and compliance. For example, in the Minnesota study where only 32% of smokers supported the policy, 59% of smokers supported smoking restrictions at youth activities, and 51% supported restrictions in areas used by children. Only 19% of smokers supported a total outdoor smoke-free requirement at all times. Furthermore, it is likely that perceptions of crowding may influence attitudes (e.g. smoking in a crowded outdoor stadium versus smoking in a park with few other people present).

Another contextual factor is the degree of signage that informs the public of the smoking restrictions. For example, the New Zealand study reported that only 62% knew that the parks were covered with a smoke-free policy, and that there was the capacity for improving the type and location of the signage. The fact that the New Zealand "policy" was not an actual bylaw that was enforced and had penalties, may also contribute to reduced compliance by the public.

In general, there appears to be a shortage of evaluation studies on smoke-free outdoor settings, despite an apparent growth of such restrictions in recent years. In particular there are little data on the following smoke-free outdoor settings: the entrances to public buildings, beaches, semi-enclosed streets, bus stops, and outside of apartment blocks.

Relevance for evidence-based tobacco control

Policymakers and health workers may find that there are already

settings in their country with majority public acceptance of outdoor smoking restrictions (e.g. in sports stadiums, child-orientated parks, and the grounds of hospitals (especially in developed countries)). Nevertheless, given the lack of data in this area, there is a strong case for obtaining representative attitudinal data in jurisdictions prior to implementing new laws (or at least data for specific groups, such as park users or hospital patients). This could then guide the need for educational campaigns, appropriate signage, and the resourcing of enforcement activities.

It is plausible that widespread restrictions on smoking outdoors may create smoker resistance to restrictions in indoor and more confined outdoor areas (i.e. if smokers consider the restrictions to lack adequate justification in a setting where societal norms are not particularly anti-smoking). There is no evidence for this type of reaction to date (at least from the studies reviewed here). Additional research on the role modelling effect of adults, on children who see them smoking in public places, is also needed to help guide the appropriate control of smoking in outdoor settings not dominated by other factors (e.g. SHS levels, nuisance effects, litter, or fire hazard).

Summary

The evidence concerning public attitudes towards outdoor smoking restrictions is limited and needs to be interpreted with care given the diversity of settings (e.g. from crowded outdoor stadiums to large

Table 5.10 Country level, sub-national and city studies on attitudes towards, and compliance with, legal smoking restrictions in a range of outdoor settings

Reference/location	Study design and date	Results	Comments
National and sub-national studies			
McMillen *et al.*, 2003 USA	Random digit dialing telephone surveys of adults (2000, 2001)	Parks: Low public support (25% overall) for smoking bans in outdoor parks.	Support in 2001 was 10% in smokers; 30% in nonsmokers. Figures for the 2000 survey were not significantly different. These levels of support were much lower than for indoor settings, which all had majority support.
Gilpin *et al.*, 2004; Al-Delaimy *et al.*, 2008 California, USA	Population surveys (2002, 2005)	Various settings: Majority support for smoking restrictions in four out of six settings.	2002 and [2005] results: Child play yards (90.5%); immediately outside building entrances (62.7% [67.1%]); outdoor restaurant dinning patios (62.5% [70.0%]); outdoor bar/club patron patios (39.7%); outdoor public places (52.2% [52.4%]); outdoor work areas (42.7%). Among young adults aged 18-29 years in 2005, 30.9% supported smoke-free outdoor areas at restaurants and bars (25.5% among current smokers).
California Department of Health Services, 2006 California, USA	Population surveys (2006)	Beaches: Majority support (58.6%).	At this time 25 California beaches had smoke-free laws.
Health Canada, 2006 Canada	Canadian Tobacco Use Monitoring Survey (CTUMS) (2006)	Various settings: Outdoor exposure to SHS frequently reported which may partly relate to incomplete compliance.	Respondents reported SHS exposure in the last month at an entrance to a building (51%) and on an outdoor patio of a restaurant or bar (31%). Restrictions apply to some of these settings in some parts of Canada.
Klein *et al.*, 2007 Minnesota, USA	Mail survey of a random selection of adults (plus survey of park directors)	Parks: Among the general public, 70% favoured tobacco-free park policies. Only 32% of smokers supported the policy compared with 77% of nonsmokers.	Recreation directors, in cities without a policy, expressed a high level of concern over enforcement issues (91%). However, few problems with enforcement were reported (26%) in communities with a tobacco-free park policy. Park and recreation directors supported such policies (75%).
Studies in cities and of specific organisations			
Nagle *et al.*, 1996 Newcastle, Australia	Before and after observational study (with control hospital) (1991)	Hospital grounds: Some evidence for compliance with a new smoke-free zone around a hospital.	Statistically significant decline in observed outdoor smoking in the intervention setting (from 32% to 28%). This was slightly more than the decline in the control hospital (from 48% to 46%). See Chapter 6 for further details.
Corti *et al.*, 1997 Western Australia, Australia	Survey of organisations funded by a health promoting organisation (1993-1994)	Sports, racing, and arts venues: Majority official adoption of voluntary smoke-free area policies (average of 85%) by organisations supported by a health promotion agency.	Adoption among arts organisations (90%), sports organisations (84%), racing organisations (61%) (n=296 organisations). The extent of compliance was not detailed, but all venues had the potential for reducing outdoor exposures (especially racing venues, but also arts venues, such as music concerts).
Pikora *et al.*, 1999 Perth, Australia	Surveys and observational studies (and butt count study) (1997)	Sports grounds: There was a majority level of awareness (81%+) and agreement (79%+) with the smoke-free policies among attendees at the cricket grounds.	Policies involved smoke-free grounds with designated smoking areas (of 20% or less of the total area). Acceptance of the policies was lower among smokers (40.0% and 47.4% for the two venues). Results of the observational study and the butt count indicated that there was high compliance.

Table 5.10 Country level, sub-national and city studies on attitudes towards, and compliance with, legal smoking restrictions in a range of outdoor settings

Reference/location	Study design and date	Results	Comments
Studies in cities and of specific organisations			
Giles-Corti *et al.*, 2001 Western Australia, Australia	Various surveys and observational studies (1994-1998)	Sports grounds: Majority support by football spectators for an existing outdoor smoke-free policy. Compliance was very high.	Majority awareness of policy (81.4%); majority support (78.6%). Support less among smokers (40.0%). Observed smoking was very rare (supported with a butt count study).
Thompson *et al.*, 2006 Idaho, Oregon, Washington, USA	Survey of students in 30 colleges and universities (circa 1995)	College grounds: Majority support for some type of outdoor restriction (86.7%), but only 33.0% favoured a completely smoke-free outdoor policy.	Nonsmokers favoured some outdoor restrictions compared to smokers (91.9% versus 61.8%) and complete restrictions (38.5% versus 6.9%). (These percentages calculated from the published numbers).
Arcus *et al.*, 2007 Upper Hutt, New Zealand	Face-to-face survey of park users (plus observation study and butt study) (2007)	Parks: 83% of park users were for a "smoke-free parks policy." Most smokers (73%) also agreed with this. Some non-compliance was reported (17% of smokers who knew about the policy still smoked in the parks).	The attitudinal survey was limited to users of two parks only and may have been subject to social desirability bias (the interviewees were identified as medical students). Of smokers who did not know about the policy, 32% reported smoking in the parks. Collection of cigarette remnants over one week showed that "there is still frequent smoking in all of these parks." Observational data also indicated smoking among adults (8/488 observed) but not children (0/1013).
Kunyk *et al.*, 2007 Edmonton, Canada	Description of policy implementation (2005)	Health facility grounds: Suggested compliance with outdoor smoking ban in a large regional health authority (89 facilities).	Outdoor smoking restriction was one of many changes including closing some smoking rooms in facilities. Despite minor violations, during the early stages of its implementation and challenges in enforcing it at several sites, Capital Health has found no compelling reason to reverse the policy and now considers it to have been safely and effectively implemented in all of its facilities.
Wilson *et al.*, 2007 Hong Kong, China	Observational study (2007)	Parks and beaches: High compliance with the law on smoke-free parks and beaches (no smoking observed).	Limited validity - study involved only one observer and a small sample. An absence of cigarette butts was also noted and smoke-free signage was very prominent.

parks). There is, however, evidence of majority public support in some developed country jurisdictions for restricting outdoor smoking in select settings (e.g. on sports grounds and some parks where children or youth activities are present). The evidence relating to compliance with such restrictions is also limited, but the available data indicate that some level of compliance occurs and that this is not perceived as a major practical problem for area administrators (e.g. park managers).

Given the growth of outdoor smoking restrictions in many developed countries in recent years, this would appear to be a priority area for further attitudinal research and studies that evaluate compliance.

Attitudes towards, and compliance with, smoking restrictions in public places in general

Attitudes towards smoking restrictions that encompass the broad domain of "public places," and which are not just workplaces, are examined here. The largest such studies have been from the Global Youth Tobacco Surveys (GYTS) (GTSS Collaborative

Group, 2006; Centers for Disease Control and Prevention, 2008). These surveys of 13-15 year olds who attend school, use a standard methodology and have had good response rates (a median response rate of 88.6%) (GTSS Collaborative Group, 2006). Overall the results indicate that there is widespread and strong support by students for restrictions on smoking in public areas all over the world. The first major compilation of these surveys for 221 jurisdictions in 123 countries (data from 1999 to 2005) put this level of support at 76.1%. The findings were in the context of students being heavily exposed to SHS (43.9% exposed at home and 55.8% exposed in public places) (GTSS Collaborative Group, 2006).

More recent results from the GYTS are summarised in Table 5.11 and demonstrate even higher levels of support at 78.3% (Centers for Disease Control and Prevention, 2008). The results demonstrate that there is a wide range of attitudinal support by jurisdiction. In three of the WHO regions, there was majority support for bans on smoking in public places within all jurisdictions surveyed. Overall, in only 8.6% of 151 jurisdictions, in which surveys were conducted, was there not majority support for such bans (with this proportion being highest in the Africa region). Indeed, majority support levels of over 80% were apparent in four out of the six WHO regions. In general, the GYTS attitudinal results

give the impression of lower levels of support in rural jurisdictions relative to more urban jurisdictions, but no formal analysis by rurality appears to have been done.

A number of countries have undertaken a second GYTS (see Table 5.12). In seven out of 10 of these countries there was an increase in attitudinal support between the two survey periods. In the Philippines, student support for bans on smoking in public places increased substantially during the 2000 to 2003 period (from 39.2% to 88.7%) (Centers for Disease Control and Prevention, 2005b).

Table 5.11 Attitudinal results from the Global Youth Tobacco Survey for 151 jurisdictions worldwide* from 2000-2007 (abstracted and calculated from Centers for Disease Control and Prevention, 2008)

WHO Region	Percent supporting ban on smoking in public places	95%CI	Range for jurisdictions within each region	Percentage of jurisdictions with <50% support (n)
African	58.9	53.0-64.6	Swaziland (26.0%) to Addis Ababa, Ethiopia (95.7%)	24.1% (7/29)
Americas	82.0	79.0-84.6	Belize (52.2%) to Suriname (91.0%)	0.0% (0/39)
Eastern Mediterranean	83.6	81.0-85.9	United Arab Emirates (71.2%) to Islamabad, Pakistan (94.5%)	0.0% (0/23)
Europe	83.1	81.2-84.7	Bulgaria (62.5%) to Albania (93.7%)	0.0% (0/29)
South East Asia	77.5	74.2-80.4	East Timor (39.9%) to Dhaka, Bangladesh (94.4%)	20.0% (2/10)
Western Pacific	83.6	81.6-85.5	Micronesia (32.5%) to Hanoi, Viet Nam (91.7%)	19.0% (4/21)
Total	78.3	75.3-81.1	Swaziland (26.0%) to Addis Ababa, Ethiopia (95.7%)	8.6% (13/151)

* GYTS data from 140 WHO member states, six territories (American Samoa, British Virgin Islands, Guam, Montserrat, Puerto Rico, and U.S. Virgin Islands), two geographic regions (Gaza Strip and West Bank), one United Nations administrative province (Kosovo), one special administrative region (Macau), and one Commonwealth (Northern Mariana Islands); nine study sites (three in the Pan-American Region and six in the Western Pacific).

Table 5.12 Changes in attitudes towards bans on smoking in public places with a comparison of results from the first and second round of the Global Youth Tobacco Survey (GYTS) for selected countries* (abstracted and calculated from Warren *et al.*, 2000 and Centers for Disease Control and Prevention, 2008)

Country by WHO regions	Study years and percent of students favouring a ban on smoking in public places				% Annual change
	Year	% (95% CI)	Year	% (95% CI)	
Africa					
South Africa	1999	53.4 (44.3-62.5)	2002	59.4 (55.3-63.5)	+2.0
Zimbabwe, Harare	1999	43.2 (32.1-54.3)	2003	43.7 (36.4-51.4)	+0.1
Americas					
Barbados	1999	79.4 (77.2-81.4)	2002	77.2 (71.6-82.0)	-0.7
Costa Rica	1999	73.5 (71.6-75.4)	2002	81.6 (78.8-84.1)	+2.7
Eastern Mediterranean					
Jordan	1999	78.3 (76.2-80.4)	2007	82.6 (80.7-84.4)	+0.5
Europe					
Poland (urban)	1999	76.5 (74.5-78.5)	2003	75.0 (72.7-77.1)	-0.4
Russian Federation, Moscow	1999	71.0 (68.9-73.1)	2004	82.6 (80.9-84.1)	+2.3
Ukraine, Kiev	1999	66.9 (64.2-69.6)	2005	83.2 (81.5-84.7)	+2.7
South East Asia					
Sri Lanka	1999	91.4 (89.0-93.8)	2003	93.0 (90.0-94.7)	+0.4
Western Pacific					
Fiji	1999	54.0 (45.8-62.2)	2005	39.1(35.4-43.0)	-2.5

*Countries which conducted the Global Youth Tobacco Survey (GYTS) in 1999 and then took part in the second round of the study; data from China were not included in the comparative analysis as surveys were conducted in different sites.

This change occurred at the time of a large reduction in exposure to SHS in public places (from 74.6% in 2000 to 59.0% in 2003). An editorial comment on these changes suggested that, "During the same period, major changes in tobacco-control policies in the Philippines might have contributed to these changes" (Centers for Disease Control and Prevention, 2005b).

In some cases the GYTS data has been analysed in more detail. For example, in Kurdistan, Iraq, the results for supporting a ban on smoking in public places were significantly higher for never smokers than current smokers (81.2% versus 59.8%) (Centers for Disease Control and Prevention, 2006b). Ideally countries will eventually have GYTS equivalent data for adults (from the Global Adult Tobacco Surveys (GATS)), but such surveys are still fairly rare in developing countries.

Population studies on adult public attitudes towards smoking restrictions in public places at the national level (all countries) and other levels (for developing countries) are detailed in Table 5.13. All these surveys indicate majority support for such restrictions, even amongst the smokers. This was also the case for the Chinese population (at 74% for the national survey). In a survey of 29 European countries, the lowest levels of support were in Romania (79%) and Austria (80%).

Table 5.13 Additional studies on public attitudes towards smoking restrictions in public places (where multiple public places are considered or were not otherwise specified)

Reference/location	Study design and date	Results	Comments
Multi-country and country level studies			
Yang *et al.*, 1999 China	Representative sample covering 30 Provinces (1996)	Most respondents supported bans against smoking in public places (74%).	This finding was consistent with majority support for most of the other tobacco control measures asked about (i.e. 64% for advertising bans and 83% for bans against sales to minors).
Environics Research Group, 2001 India, Argentina, Russia, Japan and Nigeria	Nationally representtative samples, face-to-face interviews (2000-01)	Majority support in five countries (89% overall) including majority support by smokers.	The 89% total was comprised of strong support (72%) or somewhat supportive (17%). Only 8% were opposed. The overall levels of support were 98% for Indian respondents overall (smokers [s]=98%), 94% for Argentina (s=89%), 90% for Russia (s=80%), 85% for Japan (s=73%) and 79% for Nigeria (s=64%). There was higher support by women and slightly higher support among those with higher education. The exception to the nationally representative sampling was urban sampling in Argentina and India.
Based on an English language abstract by Gallus *et al.*, 2006 Italy	National face-to-face survey (2004)	Majority support for restrictions on smoking in public places.	> 85% of Italian adult population favoured restrictions of smoking in public places (such as cafés and restaurants), and to banning smoking in workplaces.
Hammond *et al.*, 2006 Australia, Canada, UK, USA	Prospective cohorts (2002, 2003)	Smokers only: Majority agreement that: "There are fewer and fewer places I feel comfortable smoking" (81% overall for four countries).	Agreement with this statement by smokers was: 77% (UK), 78% (USA), 84% (Canada), and 84% (Australia).
European Commission, 2007 29 European countries	Representative sampling, face-to-face interviews (2006)	Majority support (70%) for smoke-free indoor public places (including subways, airports, shops, etc.).	Support highest in Finland (96%) and Sweden (95%) and lowest in Romania (79%) and Austria (80%). Resistance to laws strongest in Lithuania, where 9% totally opposed such restrictions. Citizens in countries where comprehensive smoke-free policies have already been introduced, such as Ireland, Sweden, and Italy, were most in favour of them. When compared to the 2005 survey, there was a slight increase in the proportion of people favouring a smoking ban in any indoor public space (+4 percentage points).
Young *et al.*, 2007 Australia, Canada, UK, USA	Prospective cohorts (2004)	Smokers only: Overall favourable support for either partial or full smoke-free restrictions in each of the four countries.	Level of support was based on total, partial, or no restrictions on indoor workplaces, bars/pubs, restaurants. Australian smokers were most supportive of restrictions at 2.49/3; smokers in Canada (2.30), the UK (2.20), and the USA (2.16). This was consistent with agreement by these smokers that tobacco products should be more tightly regulated (range: 61.7% in the USA to 68.9% in Australia).

Table 5.13 Additional studies on public attitudes towards smoking restrictions in public places (where multiple public places are considered or were not otherwise specified)

Reference/location	Study design and date	Results	Comments
Multi-country and country level studies			
Non-English language data sources reviewed in Sebrie *et al.*, 2008 Argentina, Brazil, Mexico, Uruguay	Probabilistic telephone and home surveys (except for Brazil which used convenience sampling) (2006-2007)	Majority support in these four countries of 80% and higher.	Argentina (2006) - 93.4% support for smoke-free government offices, private offices, banks, and shopping malls. Brazil (2006) - 85% support for covered public places in general. Mexico (2006-07) - 81% of smokers preferred smoke-free environments in all types of facilities (with >75% supporting smoke-free hospitals, public transportation, museums, cinemas and theatres). Uruguay (2006) - 80% support for the "100% smoke-free country" policy covering all types of facilities. In Argentina, another study reported highest support in the two smoke-free provinces, which suggested that once these laws are passed support for them grows. All other surveys reported in this review article indicated majority public support for smoke-free public places.
Studies at the sub-national and local level (developing countries)			
Yang *et al.*, 2007 China	Face-to-face survey of adults in two cities (provincial capitals) (year of survey not described)	Majority support (81.8%) for banning smoking in public places. Majority support from smokers (61.0% for heavy smokers).	81.8% supported banning smoking in public places (versus 85.7% favouring banning tobacco advertising). Significant predictors to support bans in public places: female, younger than aged 50+ years, being a professional (in occupation), and a nonsmoker. Most smokers supported bans (67.8% of light smokers and 61.0% of heavy smokers).
Bird *et al.*, 2007 Mexico	Students (11-13 years old) from randomly selected schools, Ciudad Juarez (2000)	Majority of the students favoured banning smoking in public places (85.1%).	Support was lowest in students from public low-socioeconomic status (SES) schools (79.2%) versus private high-SES schools (93.1%); this gradient was statistically significant.

Compliance with restrictions

The GYTS is also the largest international study that provides information of the general level of smoking exposure in public places outside the home (GTSS Collaborative Group, 2006; Centers for Disease Control and Prevention, 2008). "Public places" are described in a broad sense by the GYTS: restaurants, buses, streetcars, trains, schools, playgrounds, gyms, sports arenas, and discos. The overall result was that a majority (55.8%) of students reported SHS exposure in the last seven days (see Chapter 7).

It is difficult to interpret the GYTS figures in terms of specific settings as such details were not collected in the surveys. Therefore these results could possibly reflect SHS exposure in settings with smoking restrictions (indicating poor compliance or various exemptions to the laws), but also exposure in numerous public settings not covered by restrictions. Although many countries now have at least some restrictions on where smoking can occur (as detailed in GTSS Collaborative Group, 2006) few of these are particularly comprehensive (e.g. few cover outdoor settings, such as streets, and a minority cover outdoor hospitality settings, such as cafés and restaurants).

Other studies relating to compliance are shown in Table 5.14. These suggest that compliance is generally poor in public places in the countries that have been studied, and in some cases it appears to be nearly non-existent. Nevertheless, the multi-country European study of nicotine in air did provide evidence for lower levels of nicotine in some smoking-restricted settings.

Discussion of the results

The general nature of the term "public places" may limit the extent to which some of the findings can be interpreted. The more setting-specific results elsewhere in this Chapter are therefore of more value in guiding decisions by policymakers and health care workers. Nevertheless, the majority support for smoking restrictions in public places (including majority support from smokers) among adults is notable. The only surveys reviewed for this setting that did not indicate a majority of attitudinal support for smoking restrictions in public places were some of the student GYTS surveys. However, only 8.6% of all the GYTS surveys (out of surveys conducted in 151 jurisdictions) had minority support (<50%). Student attitudes may potentially differ from those of adults on the basis of poorer or different knowledge of the hazards of SHS, or on perceptions of vulnerability to harm and reaction to laws passed by authorities.

The public's desire for smoking restrictions contrasts with the high level of exposure to SHS in public places around the world (with the GYTS results showing this clearly). Other studies indicate negligible or otherwise fairly poor compliance with smoking restrictions. Also of note are some of the general comments that come from the GTSS Collaborative Group (GTSS Collaborative Group, 2006) with regard to smoking restrictions that are not enforced:

• In Egypt: "the ban is not being enforced" (for legislation adopted in 2002). A factor here may be that the implementation "depends largely on the administration in each facility and public place."
• In Mongolia: "the ban and restrictions are widely ignored and unenforced."
• In Samoa: "Smoking is banned in all government buildings and hospitals, but enforcement is weak."

Sub-optimal compliance with the law may also be partly explained by some jurisdictions having no sanctions for violations of the law. An example given here was Austria's smoke-free law (GTSS Collaborative Group, 2006).

Summary

To date, the largest study on attitudes towards smoking restrictions in public places is the GYTS, which has examined student attitudes in 221 national and sub-national jurisdictions (with 151 jurisdictions in the most recent updated review). Overall the results indicated that there was widespread and strong support by these students for restrictions on smoking in public areas all over the world (at 76.1%; 78.3% in the more recent review). All the other studies detailed in this subsection reported majority support for smoking restrictions in public places, including by smokers.

The GYTS study gives little clear information on compliance with existing smoking restrictions in public places, but it does show that SHS exposure is common with a majority (55.8%) of students reporting this in the last seven days. Other studies indicate negligible or otherwise fairly poor compliance with smoking restrictions in public places. Elsewhere in this chapter, attitudinal and compliance data are examined that is more setting-specific and therefore easier to interpret.

Attitudes towards, and compliance with, voluntary and legal restrictions on smoking in cars

This subsection considers both legal restrictions regarding smoking in cars, as well as the use of voluntary "restrictions" or "rules" that relate to decisions by individuals or families. When voluntary, such restrictions are likely to reflect beliefs that SHS poses a health hazard, or at least, significant nuisance effects. Similarly, the adoption of voluntary practices potentially provides some indication of the extent and strength of public attitudes towards SHS and its control. This is especially the case when smokers report having a smoke-free car. There has recently been an increase in the number of jurisdictions adopting smoke-free car laws (when children are present), because of the very high levels of SHS that can occur in the car environment (see Chapter 6); this is an area that could benefit from ongoing development.

Table 5.14 Studies on compliance with smoking restrictions in public places in developing and developed countries

Reference/location	Study design and date	Results	Comments
Multi-country and country level studies			
Yang et al., 1999 China	Representative sample covering 30 Provinces (1996)	32% of respondents reported SHS exposure in public places suggesting restrictions are minimal or not complied with.	This was lower than for exposure at home (71%) but higher than for workplaces (25%).
Navas-Acien et al., 2004 Seven Latin American countries	Measurement of airborne nicotine in multiple settings in the capital cities (2002, 2003)	General evidence for poor compliance in many public settings (out of those with some type of smoking restriction).	All countries had some national smoking regulations in public places (except for Argentina at the national level). The countries in this study were Argentina, Brazil, Chile, Costa Rica, Paraguay, Peru, and Uruguay. Specific results for select settings are detailed elsewhere in this Chapter (for hospitals, schools, government buildings, airports, restaurants and bars).
Nebot et al., 2005 Seven European countries	Measurements of airborne nicotine (multiple settings) (2001-2002)	Some evidence for compliance overall; nicotine still found in most of the public places studied.	Nicotine levels were lower in sites with smoking restrictions. The countries were Austria, France, Greece, Italy, Portugal, Spain, and Sweden. (See other sections in this Chapter for data from this study relating to hospitals, transportation settings, restaurants, schools, workplaces and hospitality settings).
Stillman et al., 2007 China	Nicotine sampling in urban and rural settings (2005)	Evidence for limited levels of compliance with restrictions in multiple settings.	Airborne nicotine was detected in 91% of the locations sampled (including hospitals, secondary schools, city government buildings, train stations, restaurants, and entertainment establishments). This was despite smoking restrictions in 34% of all the settings studied. Overall, sites which had written smoke-free regulations had statistically significantly lower nicotine concentrations.
European Commission, 2007 29 European countries	Representative sampling, face-to-face interviews (2006)	Majority view (54%) that compliance with the law occurs.	90% of European citizens believe that smoke-free laws exist in their country. 54% believe that the laws are respected; 36% believe that smokers do not respect these laws. The range for stating these beliefs: 21% in Slovakia, up to 91% in Ireland (and generally higher in Scandinavian countries as a group). The figure for laws existing that are respected was 4% higher overall compared to a 2002 survey in 15 EU countries. Also, the proportion saying existing laws were not respected was 6% lower.
Sub-national and city studies (developing countries only)			
Martinez-Donate et al., 2005 Mexico	Household survey in Tijuana (2003-2004)	Evidence for limited compliance with restrictions overall.	Most adults (53.9%) reported chronic exposure to SHS, despite 44.4% stating that there was a nonsmoking policy in their workplace, and 65.8% had smoke-free households.
Bird et al., 2007 Mexico	Students (11-13 years old) from randomly selected schools, Ciudad Juarez (2000)	No evidence of compliance with the existing smoking restrictions.	53.2% were exposed to smoking outside their homes in the past seven days (higher than exposure in the home at 41.3%). Exposure was highest in students from public low-socioeconomic status (SES) schools (72.2%) versus private high-SES schools (48.6%). With regard to smoking restrictions in public places, "the law is rarely, if ever, enforced."

The evidence from studies detailed in Table 5.15 indicates that there is majority adoption of voluntary smoke-free car policies in all the jurisdictions studied (including the smokers in most studies). One study even reported fairly high levels of smoke-free cars among smokers (70% for UK smokers) (Fong *et al.*, 2006).

The data from 29 European countries in Table 5.15 does not specifically identify adoption of smoke-free cars. Instead it indicates that a majority of respondents who are smokers in these countries claim to not smoke in the presence of nonsmokers (especially children). In particular, only 24% of smokers claimed to smoke in a car in the company of nonsmokers, which contrasted with the 49% who smoke in a car when alone. This is suggestive of either some compliance with a type of smoke-free car rule or episodic restraint in smoking behaviour.

In jurisdictions that have passed laws restricting smoking in cars there is evidence for majority support for this, for example, in the state of South Australia and for California (albeit, before the law was passed for the latter). No other studies were identified in the other states or provinces that had adopted such laws by the end of 2007 (i.e. Arkansas, Louisiana, Nova Scotia, Puerto Rico, and Tasmania). Given the recent increase in the number of such laws, this would appear to be a priority area for further research. Children are most likely to be exposed to the highest levels of SHS from others smoking in cars, and they have no easy way of avoiding it.

Relevance for evidence-based tobacco control

Policymakers and health workers, concerned about SHS exposure in cars, can probably expect to see attitudinal shifts towards smoke-free car adoption if educational levels in their country improve and they enhance tobacco control activities in general. Potential laws calling for smoke-free cars may benefit if legal restrictions are introduced on smoking in a range of other settings, such as workplaces and hospitality settings. Smoke-free schools may also alert parents to the need to protect their children from SHS in cars (and in homes). However, to appropriately inform the need for smoke-free car campaigns it is desirable that jurisdiction-specific attitudinal data and prevalence data are collected.

There remains insufficient data on the acceptability and compliance with legal interventions requiring smoke-free cars (e.g. when children are present). Nevertheless, such research is likely to be forthcoming, as a number of jurisdictions have recently adopted such laws (and states such as California have a strong record for evaluating all tobacco control interventions). There is also some suggestion of a diffusion effect here with smoke-free car laws in cities in Maine (USA) and Nova Scotia preceding state and province level laws for these two jurisdictions. Also of note is that research in the injury prevention area could also inform country-specific policymaking on smoke-free car legislation (e.g. acceptability/compliance with seat belt laws, child safety seat laws, and laws restricting mobile phone use in cars).

Summary

The available data indicates majority public adoption of smoke-free cars (or at least reduced smoking in cars when others are present), and, in some settings, there is also majority smoker adoption of smoke-free cars. A high level of support for a law restricting smoking in cars has been reported in one setting, but further data are likely to be forthcoming as these laws are increasingly being enacted.

Discussion of chapter findings

Main findings and their level of evidence

The main findings are summarised below and are considered in terms of the level of evidence supporting them. Firstly, the evidence from developed countries is considered:

• Public attitudes towards smoking restrictions: In developed countries, there is considerable evidence to indicate that there are, in most cases, majority levels of public support for smoke-free workplaces, smoke-free hospitality settings (restaurants and bars/pubs), and various other settings (i.e. schools, health care facilities, indoor sporting arenas/events, and shopping malls).

• Smoker attitudes: While smokers are usually less supportive of restrictions than nonsmokers, there is evidence that the majority of smokers do support some

Table 5.15 Studies on the prevalence of smoke-free cars along with attitudes and compliance (country level studies plus other types of studies in jurisdictions with smoke-free car laws and in developing countries)

Reference/location	Study design and date	Results	Comments
Gillespie *et al.*, 2005 New Zealand	Telephone survey of adults (2004)	Among smokers: Minority prevalence of the adoption of, or compliance with, full smoke-free cars among smokers (29.2%) based on reported smoking behaviour. Mixed attitudinal data on acceptability of smoking in cars.	40.2% thought smoking should not be allowed in private cars; 46.0% of nonsmokers, 23.2% of smokers. 75.8% disagreed that it is "okay" to smoke around nonsmokers inside cars when there are windows open.
Fong *et al.*, 2006 Ireland, UK	Prospective cohorts (2003-04; 2004-05)	Among smokers: Majority prevalence for full smoke-free cars (range: 55% to 70%).	Adults surveyed before/after a law banning smoking in public places in Ireland; prevalence changed from 58% to 55% (not significant). For the UK, it changed from 62% to 70% (a significant increase). See Chapter 6 for further details.
European Commission, 2007 29 European countries	Representative sampling, face-to-face interviews (2006)	Compliance among smokers: Majority claim to not smoke in the presence of nonsmokers (especially children). This is suggestive of either compliance with a smoke-free car rule or episodic restraint in smoking behaviour.	24% of smokers smoke in a car in the company of nonsmokers. Range: 42% (Austria) to 87% (Sweden). 9% smoke in this situation when they are with children. Range: 1% (Estonia and Sweden) to 17% (Denmark), and 19% (Croatia). These figures contrast with the 49% who smoke in a car when alone. The proportion of smokers smoking in a car in the company of nonsmokers decreased by 4 percentage points relative to 2005 (decrease in Ireland - 16 points). Proportion who smoke in cars in the company of children also decreased by 5 percentage points (decrease in Spain - 17 points).
Health Canada, 2006 Canada	Canadian Tobacco Use Monitoring Survey (CTUMS) (2006)	Compliance (voluntary): Frequent exposure to SHS suggestive of incomplete adoption of, or compliance with, voluntary smoke-free cars.	A quarter (25%) of respondents reported SHS exposure inside a car or other vehicle in the last month.
Ministry of Health, 2007 New Zealand	National face-to-face survey (2006)	Majority prevalence of smoke-free cars based on reported behaviour (15% of population smoke around others inside cars).	Maori (indigenous New Zealanders) reported others smoking in the car (30.1%) compared to non-Maori (12.6%). A gradient by deprivation level was also reported, as it was in a separate observational study (Martin *et al.*, 2006).
Healton *et al.*, 2007 USA	National survey (American Legacy Foundation) (2003)	Exposure/compliance (voluntary): Significant exposure of young people to SHS in cars was suggestive of incomplete use of voluntary measures or voluntary rule compliance.	7% of young people aged 12-17 were exposed to SHS daily in a car.
Przewozniak *et al.*, 2008 Poland	Nationwide survey based on random representative sample of adults (2007)	Majority support for a complete ban of smoking in cars (64%).	No restrictions on smoking in cars existed in 2007. There were significant differences between smokers (50%) and nonsmokers (70%) in support of a ban.

Table 5.15 Studies on the prevalence of smoke-free cars along with attitudes and compliance (country level studies plus other types of studies in jurisdictions with smoke-free car laws and in developing countries)

Reference/location	Study design and date	Results	Comments
Studies in settings that have legal bans on smoking in cars (with children)			
Roberts *et al.*, 1996 South Australia, Australia	Representative survey of adults in the state (circa 1995).	Prior to the new law: A majority of adults (73%) had smoke-free cars a decade before the new law.	Among those who smoked and had children, 27.5% had a ban; an additional 6.9% said they did not smoke in the car.
Norman *et al.*, 1999 California, USA	Telephone survey of adults using random digit dialing (1996-97)	Prior to the new law: A majority (65.5%) of adults had car smoking bans (a decade before the new law).	16% of adults said smoking was sometimes allowed in cars. For smokers the prevalence of car smoking bans was 28.6%. A lower prevalence of car smoking bans was associated with being a smoker or African American, not having children in the home, having more friends who smoke, and lower household income.
Miller, 2002 South Australia, Australia	Pre- and post-campaign telephone surveys of parents (2000 & 2001)	Prior to the new law: A majority of parents (of those with cars and with children living with them) reported that they had smoke-free cars (88.4% in 2001).	Between surveys: a non-significant increase in smoke-free car prevalence (87.1% to 88.4%). Among smokers the change was from 58.0% to 63.8% (p=0.05). Other survey data indicating 81% of cars were smoke-free in 2001.
Tobacco Control Research and Evaluation, 2008 South Australia, Australia	Telephone survey of adults (random sample of the state) (2007)	Around the time of the new law: High public support on restricting smoking in cars (92%; 87% among smokers).	Law passed - 28 March 2007. Survey conducted - March/April 2007 (before it was implemented on 31 May 2007). Law relates to smoking in cars where children under the age of 16 years are present.
Al-Delaimy *et al.*, 2008 California, USA	Population survey (2005)	Prior to the new law: A majority (92.3%) were in favour of smoking bans.	The figure for smokers was 85.1%. Results were before the new law became operational in January 2008.

"Partial" refers to smoking being allowed in some parts of the home. "Full" refers to smoking not being allowed in any part of the home (or at any time in a car).
* That is excluding county and city level bans in other countries (e.g. Canada).

smoking restrictions (including hospitality settings) in a number of countries.

• Trends in attitudes: There is evidence of a pattern of increasing support by the general public and by smokers for smoking restrictions over time and after smoke-free laws are in place. No evidence was found for a reduction in public support after enacting a smoke-free law in any setting. When such laws are accompanied by public education campaigns, there appears to be increased support for the smoke-free policy.

• Attitudes towards smoke-free cars: There is evidence for a majority voluntary adoption of smoke-free cars in developed countries, and increased willingness to legislate smoke-free cars in the presence of children.

• Attitudes towards smoke-free outdoor areas: Although there are only a few studies addressing this issue, there is evidence for majority support for many settings (e.g. smoke-free parks, sports facilities, transition areas such as entryways, and beaches).

• Compliance with smoking restrictions: There is evidence that moderate to high levels of compliance generally occur with smoke-free laws. Nevertheless, when laws are enacted prior to mobilisation or activation of popular support, poor compliance can occur (e.g. some laws in the 1990s). International experience suggests that compliance is higher in countries that conduct public education campaigns accompanying the law.

In developing countries there are some differences in the main findings:

• Public attitudes towards smoking restrictions: Most developing and developed countries have attitudinal data from the Global Youth Tobacco Surveys (GYTS) that indicate majority student support for smoking restrictions in public places. There are a number of studies of adult attitudes in developing countries, with most showing majority support for smoking restrictions in public places and workplaces. The Global Adult Tobacco Survey (GATS) should improve the evidence base in the future.

• Trends in attitudes: The GYTS surveys suggest a general pattern of increasing support by students over time. There is emerging evidence that new smoke-free policies increase support in some developing countries.

• Compliance with smoke-free policies: For most of the smoke-free policies in developing countries, there is evidence that meaningful compliance occurs in some settings. In settings with poor compliance, it may be that lack of awareness of the existence of the law is a factor.

Recommendations for advancing evidence-based tobacco control

Issues have been raised for informing evidence-based tobacco control. Specific recommendations for consideration by policymakers and health professionals include the following:

1. Assessing attitudinal data among the general public, smokers, and any relevant population groups (e.g. hospitality workers) prior to new smoke-free policies being introduced can be helpful in policy development. If there is a shortage of recent representative data, then consideration should be given to undertaking attitudinal surveys within the relevant jurisdiction (e.g. the GATS). For example, such data can inform public education campaigns, use of media advocacy, and the extent of signage and enforcement activities.

2. Once smoke-free laws are passed, further monitoring of attitudes and compliance is helpful in guiding implementation, enforcement, and future policy development.

3. Public health professionals should be prepared to respond to inaccurate or misleading information regarding the effect of smoke-free policies (see Chapter 4).

Possible priorities
for further research

This review has identified many areas in which further research could be undertaken. Major ones include:

• Research to address the shortage of attitudinal and compliance studies in developing countries, including the ones with the largest populations (China and India). For India, in particular, relatively few studies were identified. Such studies are particularly desirable before new smoking restrictions are considered so that policymakers can determine the optimal scope of the new laws and the need for mass media campaigns and resourcing for signage and enforcement.

• Research to more fully analyse the existing attitudinal and SHS exposure data in the GYTS studies (e.g. ecological analyses across all the countries). Also how student attitudes compare to adult attitudes in countries with data for both. This may be increasingly possible once data are available from Global Adult Tobacco Surveys.

• Research into why public support for smoking in hospitality venues is lower than for other workplaces and how this gap can be reduced (e.g. by educating the public on workers' rights for clean air).

• Research into compliance in the many countries that have introduced new smoke-free laws covering hospitality settings in 2006-2008.

• Research into attitudes and compliance in settings that have introduced smoke-free car laws (where children are present in the car).

• Research into attitudes and compliance in smoke-free outdoor areas, which have been another area of rapid development in recent years (particularly smoke-free parks and beaches).

Countries could finance such research by introducing dedicated tobacco taxes (an approach that is already used by some developed and developing countries to fund various aspects of tobacco control). Other funding possibilities are via international research collaborations, as already seen with the successful GYTS surveys around the world.

Role of beliefs and knowledge in determining attitudes

Some of the studies in this review have touched on explanations for public support for smoke-free laws. These include public education and mass media campaigns on the hazard of SHS and on workers' rights. There is also some suggestion of spill-over effects from one area of tobacco control to another (e.g. smoke-free laws for workplaces may facilitate the adoption of smoke-free homes). More comprehensive and better re-sourced tobacco control activities in general may also facilitate support for expanding smoke-free laws. Indeed, once the public perceives the successful implementation of one new smoke-free law (e.g. in work-places) they may increase support for extensions of smoke-free laws into new domains (e.g. hospitality settings).

Below the issue of beliefs in the health effects of SHS exposure is discussed. In countries for which data are available, a majority of the public now believe that SHS exposure is a health hazard for nonsmokers (Table 5.16). Also, in settings where the trend in beliefs about SHS harm have been studied, there is evidence of an increase over time in such beliefs

(U.S. Department of Health and Human Services, 2006). An additional example is California, where since 1992 the California Tobacco Surveys (CTS) have included two questions to assess the population's beliefs with respect to the dangers of SHS: "Smoke from someone else's cigarette causes lung cancer in a nonsmoker" and "Inhaling smoke from someone else's cigarette harms the health of babies and children." Agreement with the first statement increased from 62.4% in 1992 to 72.2% in 2005, and agreement with the second statement increased from 85.3% to 90.3% over this period (Al-Delaimy et al., 2008).

Limitations of this review

As detailed in the Introduction, the literature search particularly focused on country level and multi-country studies for developed countries (albeit all types of studies in developing countries). Some unique settings were not substantively examined, given that public attitudes are less critical in these areas (e.g. prisons and long-term residential care settings). However, there is some consideration of the impact of smoke-free prison laws and smoke-free residential care homes in Chapter 6.

The review did not undertake a rigorous methodological critique of all the cited studies. There are limitations with questionnaire-based studies and some methods used for measuring compliance. In general, readers should put most weight on the results from the prospective cohort studies for attitudes and on large repeated cross-sectional surveys using the same methods and questions. For

compliance studies, the most robust are those that use experimental designs or objective measures (i.e. airborne particulates, airborne nicotine, biomarkers such as serum cotinine, or number of cigarette butts counted). Multi-country or country level studies are also likely to have higher methodological quality, due to study size and the need to meet quality control requirements of the funder, than small city level studies.

A general issue is that many of the reported studies rely on self-reports, which may be subject to various limitations. One of these is social desirability bias which could lead respondents to over-report smoke-free workplace or car status as social norms make smoking in these settings less socially acceptable. Smokers themselves may fear social sanction for violating legal restrictions and hence deny non-compliance. Other problems with self-reports are the ability of respondents to remember exposure to SHS in various settings (e.g. over the past week or month) or their observations of smoking in restricted settings.

There is also the more specific issue concerning the unknown generalisability of the GYTS to the attitudes held by the general adult population. Indeed, students may plausibly have stronger pro-smoke-free attitudes if they themselves have been exposed to effective school-based educational programmes, have been targeted by youth-orientated mass media campaigns (such as the "Truth" campaign in the USA), or have lower smoking rates than the adult population. This deficit in our understanding may be better addressed once Global

Table 5.16 Selected study results on beliefs about SHS and health in adults and adolescents (country level studies)

Reference / location	Study design and date	Results	Comments
Warren et al., 2000 17 sites of 12 countries* representing all WHO regions	First round of the Global Youth Tobacco Surveys (GYTS) (1999)*	Majority belief by students that SHS from others is harmful to them (in 14 out of the 17 surveys).	Three survey areas where level of belief was <50%: Kiev (Ukraine), and Harare and Manicaland (both in Zimbabwe). The full range of results was from 31% in Manicaland to 81.4% in Tianjin, China.
Borland et al., 2006b Australia, Canada, UK, USA	Prospective cohorts (2002)	Smokers only: Majority of smokers believe that SHS causes lung cancer in nonsmokers (all four countries >72%).	There was statistically significant variation across countries (lowest in the USA at 72.1% and highest in the UK at 82.6%).
U.S. Department of Health and Human Services, 2006 USA	National Health Interview Survey (NHIS) (1992, 2000)	80%+ believe that SHS is harmful to health.	Variation in beliefs by educational level (those with more years of education were more likely to believe that SHS was harmful).
U.S. Department of Health and Human Services, 2006 USA	Various national surveys	Majority of public consider SHS harmful.	54% considered SHS to be "very harmful" and 32% "somewhat harmful." There is some evidence that such beliefs are more common among women, younger adults, and among Hispanic/Latino and African Americans (for the latter see Yañez, 2002).
European Commission, 2007 29 European countries	Representative sampling, face-to-face interviews (2006)	Majority belief that SHS can cause health problems in all of these European countries.	Only 3% of European citizens believe that SHS exposure has no dangers at all. This figure was highest for Poland (14%) and Lithuania (8%). In Sweden, 23% reported that SHS exposure can lead to some health problems; 65% believe it can lead to cancer. Only 24% of Romanians and 17% of the Cypriot Turks believed that SHS exposure can lead to cancer. In all but two countries there were increasing proportions of people who think that cancer may result from SHS exposure (relative to the 2005 survey).
Baska et al., 2007 Czech Republic, Hungary, Poland, Slovakia	Global Youth Tobacco Surveys (GYTS) (2002-2003)	Majority belief by students that SHS from others is harmful to them.	Nonsmokers: range was 65.1% to 78.0% (for boys and girls by country). Smokers: 49.5% to 55.7%.

* The 12 countries: Barbados, China, Costa Rica, Fiji, Jordan, Poland, the Russian Federation (Moscow), South Africa, Sri Lanka, Ukraine (Kiev), Venezuela, and Zimbabwe.

Adult Tobacco Survey (GATS) data become available.

Research on smoke-free homes provides some indication of the reliability of self-reports and of the impact of variation in survey methods. For example, one study in California in 1996 found a reported smoke-free home prevalence of 76% (Norman et al., 1999), while another in this year reported a prevalence of 63% (the California Tobacco Survey). The difference was because the latter survey only considered a home to be smoke-free if all household adults interviewed said that it was (Gilpin et al., 2002). Similarly, a study of the Current Population Survey (CPS) in the USA found that an estimated 12% of sample households provided inconsistent reports about home smoking restrictions. In particular, multimember households with smokers were substantially less likely to consistently report strict home rules; there were discrepancies by smoking behaviour, socioeconomic status, and race/ethnicity (Mumford et al., 2004). Nevertheless, there is work that is suggestive that self-reports by parents on smoke-free home rules are reasonably accurate (based on correlations with child cotinine levels) (Spencer et al., 2005). Another study has reported that simple surveys inquiring about home smoking restrictions were probably adequate compared to more detailed questionnaires (Wong et al., 2002). More recently one study concluded that "parental reports of household smoking alone fail to capture all youth secondhand smoke exposures, but they correlate well with cotinine levels when expressed as the number of household smokers or the number of cigarettes smoked in the household" (Wilkinson et al., 2006).

Question wording is also important and attitudes around the "rights" of workers can be particularly favoured over other attitudinal questions relating to smoking restrictions (Thomson & Wilson, 2004).

Some of the compliance studies have various limitations with regard to the measurements taken. These include problems with other sources of pollutants (e.g. fine particulates are influenced by air pollution from vehicles and from cooking) and even for the source of smoking-specific pollutants (e.g. hair nicotine levels reflect total exposure).

Chapter 6
Reductions in exposure to secondhand smoke and effects on health due to restrictions on smoking

Introduction

Earlier chapters have reviewed the evidence that secondhand smoke (SHS) is harmful to health, and have described the range and extent of smoking restrictions that have been applied around the world. Chapter 6 attempts to answer these questions: do smoking restrictions reduce the exposure of nonsmokers to SHS, and if so by how much? And, do these reductions in exposure to SHS lead to evident improvements in health? We look first at smoking restrictions in the workplace, since this has been a major focus of tobacco control activities around the world in the last 20 years. Initially restrictions were voluntary and partial, covering some workplaces (such as white collar offices) more thoroughly than others, but in the last decade many countries have introduced legal restrictions on where smoking is permitted (as described in Chapter 3). This Chapter also includes an account of the much smaller body of scientific work conducted on smoking restrictions in cars and public settings other than workplaces.

Methods

A variety of searches were undertaken to identify studies reporting on the effects of smoking restrictions. The Web of Science was searched from 1990 to 2007 using the terms "Smoke Free" SAME ban*, "Smoke Free" SAME polic*, "Smoke Free" SAME law*, and "Smoke Free" SAME legislation. Other databases, including Google Scholar, PubMed, and the National Library of Medicine, were searched in a similar fashion using expressions such as "legislation" and "tobacco smoke pollution." Relevant material was also sought from the European Network for Smoking Prevention's GLOBALink.

Effects of restrictions on smoking in the workplace

The first comprehensive assesments of the damage caused to health by SHS appeared in the mid-1980s (National Research Council, 1986; U.S. Department of Health and Human Services, 1986; National Health and Medical Research Council, 1987). In many countries smoking was already restricted in buildings such as theatres and cinemas (due mostly to concerns about fire risks), and the Civil Aeronautics Board required nonsmoking sections on US commercial flights beginning in 1973. However, reports by authoritative agencies, such as the US Department of Health and Human Services, added considerable impetus to the spread of bans on smoking in public places and worksites (Rigotti, 1989; Fielding, 1991). These restrictions were, at first, adopted on an industry-by-industry basis (U.S. Department of Health and Human Services, 2006). For example, the Australian Federal Government banned smoking in all offices in 1986, several years ahead of the first smoke-free laws in that country. The New Zealand Smoke-free Environments Act of 1990 was one of the first pieces of national legislation that aimed to protect the health of nonsmoking employees by banning smoking in the workplace (although this particular law had many loop-holes) (Laugesen & Swinburn,

2000). Since that time, laws have been passed in many jurisdictions and the pace at which new restrictions are being introduced has increased recently (see Chapter 3 for a more detailed account of the history of smoking restrictions). In some jurisdictions, laws have been passed that prohibit smoking in almost all occupational settings. For example, in early 2004, Ireland was the first country to pass comprehensive smoke-free legislation, and many more jurisdictions have introduced partial bans.

Partial bans have contributed to a substantial reduction in population exposures to SHS in many countries. In California throughout the early 1990s, the spread of community level ordinances was associated with a diminishing proportion of the population exposed to cigarette smoke at work (e.g. 29% of nonsmokers were exposed in indoor workplaces in 1990, compared with 22.4% in 1993) (Pierce et al., 1994). In New Zealand in 1991, 39% of indoor workers were exposed to SHS during tea and lunch breaks. Five years later that proportion fell to 24% as a result of the increasing number and extent of voluntary smoking restrictions in workplaces not covered by the Smoke-free Environments Act (Woodward & Laugesen, 2001). Since 1980, most of the reduction in population exposure to smoking at work in Australia has occurred prior to the introduction of legislation. Court cases and legal rulings on the issue of liability highlighted the risk of litigation for employers if they continued to permit smoking at work, and thus voluntary adoption of smoke-free policies

was rapid in most workplaces, but with important exceptions. In many countries, it was the continuing high levels of exposure to SHS in blue collar workplaces, and in bars, restaurants, and gaming venues that led to pressure for comprehensive, statutory restrictions.

It is clear from Table 6.1 that countries now vary widely in the nature and extent of prohibitions on smoking. It is important to note that the so-called "total bans," in countries like Ireland and New Zealand, in fact do not apply to absolutely all workplaces. In New Zealand, for example, prisons, hotel and motel rooms, and long-term nursing establishments have partial exemption. Smoking is still permitted in outdoor dining and drinking areas, which means employees remain at risk of exposure to SHS (albeit much less than indoors). In some countries there are nationwide restrictions; elsewhere the responsibility for smoke-free legislation rests at the level of provincial or city authorities. There may be considerable variation in tobacco policies within countries (e.g. in Canada, such laws are the business of provincial governments and there is not a common view between the provinces on smoking bans). In some countries, like the USA, laws and regulations have been passed by multiple levels of government.

Studies also vary considerably in design and the methods used to measure exposure to SHS. These include direct observation of smoking and the smokiness of venues, questionnaires eliciting perceptions of exposure to SHS, air sampling, and biomarkers (mostly cotinine in

saliva and urine, and nicotine in hair). The most common study type has been the cross-sectional survey with population samples drawn before and after the implementation of legislation. There have also been panel studies, in which the same participants are questioned at numerous points in time, and multiple cross-sectional representative samples of the population (e.g. the California Tobacco Surveys). A minority of studies have included geographic controls - study populations drawn from jurisdictions not affected by legislation and followed over the same period of time (Fong et al., 2006; IARC, 2008).

Despite the heterogeneity of smoking restrictions and study designs, the results listed in Table 6.1 show some common patterns. In every country included in the table, the introduction of comprehensive legislation banning smoking in workplaces has been associated with a substantial reduction in exposure to SHS. Similar results have been obtained in studies of comprehensive smoking restrictions applied at levels of states and municipalities. For instance, an 80-90% reduction in polycyclic aromatic hydrocarbons (PAHs) in six Boston bars following implementation of smoke-free ordinances was observed (Repace et al., 2006b). A study of 14 bars and restaurants from western New York State found a 90% reduction in $PM_{2.5}$ levels from a mean of 412 µg/m^3 to 27 µg/m^3 post-legislation (Travers et al., 2004).

Evidence from Europe

Reference/location	Study participants	Study design	Restriction on smoking	Measure of exposure to SHS	Levels of exposure reported	Comments
Heloma et al., 2001 Finland	Pre-Act: 967 employees Winter 1994-1995 Post-Act: 1035 employees Winter 1995-1996	Repeated cross-sectional studies	March 1995 - Reformed Tobacco Control Act: Smoking prohibited on all public premises of workplaces	Vapour-phase nicotine	1994-1995: $PM_{2.5}$ in Industrial places 1.2 $\mu g/m^3$ Service sector 1.5 $\mu g/m^3$ Offices 0.4 $\mu g/m^3$ 1995-1996: $PM_{2.5}$ in Industrial places 0.05 $\mu g/m^3$ Service sector 0.2 $\mu g/m^3$ Offices 0.1 $\mu g/m^3$	
				Self-reported SHS exposure	1994-1995: SHS 18.6% 1995-1996: SHS 9.1 (p<0.001)	Proportion of employees reporting daily exposure to SHS for 1-4 hours
				Self-reported daily smoking prevalence	1994-1995: prevalence 30% 1995-1996: prevalence 25% (p=0.021)	Prevalence of daily smoking among employees
Heloma & Jaakkola, 2003 Finland	1994-95: 880 1995-96: 940 1998: 659 (post-law) Studied in eight workplaces in the Helsinki metropolitan area	Repeated cross-sectional studies	March 1995 - Reformed Tobacco Control Act: Smoking prohibited on all public premises of workplaces	Indoor air nicotine concentrations	Median indoor airborne nicotine concentrations: 1994-95: 0.9 $\mu g/m^3$ 1995-96 and 1998: 0.1 $\mu g/m^3$	Indoor air nicotine: 41 sites in 1994-95, 40 sites in 1995-96, 18 sites in 1998
				Self-reported exposure to SHS	1994: 51% 1995: 17% 1998: 12%	Employees exposure to SHS for at least one hour daily. Respondents' daily smoking prevalence
				Self-reported smoking behaviour	From 30% to 25%: remained at 25% in the last survey three years later (1998)	

Johnsson et al., 2006
 	
Finland
	20 restaurants and bars with a serving area larger than 100 m² from three Finnish cities	1999 - Indoor air quality assessed (six months Pre-act)
		
		2000 - six months Post-act
		
		2002 - when 50% of clientele area should be smoke-free
			1 March 2000 - Finnish Tobacco Act amended to include restrictions on smoking in all Finnish restaurants and bars with certain exceptions	Indoor air nicotine concentration, 3-EP, and TVOC by thermo-desorption-gas chromatography-mass spectrometry	Geometric mean (GM) nicotine concentration
					All Pre-ban: 7.1 $\mu g/m^3$
					        Post-ban: 7.3 $\mu g/m^3$
					
					Dinning Pre-ban: 0.7 $\mu g/m^3$
					        Post-ban: 0.6 $\mu g/m^3$
					
					Bars/Taverns Pre-ban: 10.6 $\mu g/m^3$
					        Post-ban: 12.7 $\mu g/m^3$
					
					Disco Pre-ban: 15.2 $\mu g/m^3$
					        Post-ban: 8.1 $\mu g/m^3$
						In this study, partial smoking restrictions did not reduce SHS concentrations in workplaces

Table 6.1 Studies that report the effect of legislation restricting smoking in the workplace on exposure to SHS

Reference/location	Study participants	Study design	Restriction on smoking	Measure of exposure to SHS	Levels of exposure reported	Comments
Evidence from Europe						
Johnsson et al., 2006 Finland		2004 - when entire Act was in force			3-ethenylpyridine (3-EP) concentration Pre-ban: 1.2 µg/m³ Post-ban: 1.7 µg/m³ Total Volatile Organic Compounds (TVOC) Pre-ban: 250 µg/m³ Post-ban: 210 µg/m³	
			Ventilation rate		All establishments in the survey had mixed ventilation (i.e. dilution ventilation and none had displacement ventilation)	
Allwright et al., 2005 Ireland	329 bar staff from three areas of the Republic and one area in Northern Ireland (UK) Pre-ban: Sep 2003-March 2004 Post-ban: Sep 2004-March 2005	Comparisons	2002 Public Health (Tobacco) Act (Commencement) Order 2004: Smoking is forbidden in enclosed places of work in Ireland, including office blocks, various buildings, public houses/bars, restaurants, and company vehicles (cars and vans)	Salivary cotinine concentration	*In the Republic:* 80% reduction Pre-ban: 29 nmol/l (95% CI=18.2-43.2 nmol/l) Post-ban: 5.1 nmol/l l (95% CI=2.8-13.1 nmol/l) *In Northern Ireland:* 20% reduction Pre-ban: 25.3 nmol/l (95% CI=10.4-59.2 nmol/l) Post-ban: 20.4nmol/l l (95% CI=13.2-33.8 nmol/l)	
				Respiratory and sensory irritation symptoms	*In the Republic* - *Respiratory symptoms* Pre-ban (baseline): 65% (one or more respiratory symptoms) Post-ban: 25%-49% (p=0.001) - *Sensory symptoms* Pre-ban: 67% Post-ban: 45% (p<0.001) *In Northern Ireland* - *Respiratory symptoms* Pre-ban (baseline): 45% (one or more respiratory symptoms) Post-ban: 45% - *Sensory symptoms* Pre-ban: 75% Post-ban: 55% (p=0.13)	

Evidence from Europe

Reference/location	Study participants	Study design	Restriction on smoking	Measure of exposure to SHS	Levels of exposure reported	Comments
Allwright et al., 2005 Ireland				Self-reported exposure to SHS	*Work-related exposure* *In the Republic* Pre-ban: 40 hours Post-ban: 0 hours (p<0.001) *In Northern Ireland* Pre-ban: 42 hours Post-ban: 40 hour (p=0.02) *Outside work* *In the Republic* Pre-ban: 4 hours Post-ban: 0 hours (p<0.001) *In Northern Ireland* Pre-ban: 0 hours Post-ban: 2.5 hour (p=0.41)	
Mulcahy et al., 2005 Ireland	Cohort study, 35 workers in 15 city hotels, a random sample from 20 city centre bars (range 400-5000 square feet)	Repeated measures of exposures before and after legislation. Saliva samples obtained 2-3 weeks before and 4-6 weeks after smoking ban. Airborne nicotine was measured for 7-10 hours on the Friday preceding the ban and six weeks later	29 March 2004 - Act effective. Smoking banned in all bars, restaurants, cafes, and hotels (excluding bedrooms, outdoor areas, and properly designed smoking shelters)	Salivary cotinine concentration Air nicotine concentration Duration of self-reported exposures to SHS	69% reduction Pre-ban: 1.6 ng/ml Post-ban: 0.5 ng/ml (SD: 1.29; p < 0.005) Overall: 74% reduction (range 16-99%) 83% reduction Pre-ban: 35.5 mg/m³ Post-ban: 5.95 mg/m³ (p < 0.001) Pre-ban: 30 hours Post-ban: 0 hours (p < 0.001)	
Fong et al., 2006 Ireland and UK	1679 adult smokers aged >18 years from Ireland (n=1071) and UK (n=608); 1185 completed the survey Pre-ban: Dec 2003-Jan 2004 Post-ban: Dec 2004-Jan 2005	Prospective cohort study	29 March 2004 - Republic of Ireland implemented comprehensive smoke-free legislation in all workplaces, including restaurants and pubs, with no allowance for designated smoking rooms and few exemptions	Respondents' reports of smoking in key public venues	Bars/pubs, *Ireland* Pre-ban: 98%; Post-ban: 5% (p < 0.0001) Bars/pubs, *UK* Pre-ban: 98%; Post-ban: 97% (p=0.462) Restaurants, *Ireland* Pre-ban: 85%; Post-ban: 3% (p < 0.0001)	

Table 6.1 Studies that report the effect of legislation restricting smoking in the workplace on exposure to SHS

Reference/location	Study participants	Study design	Restriction on smoking	Measure of exposure to SHS	Levels of exposure reported	Comments
Evidence from Europe						
Fong et al., 2006 Ireland and UK					Bars/pubs, *UK* Pre-ban: 78%; Post-ban: 62% (p<0.001) Shopping malls, *Ireland* Pre-ban: 40%; Post-ban: 3% (p < 0.0001) Bars/pubs, *UK* Pre-ban: 29%; Post-ban: 22% (p=0.012) Workplaces, *Ireland* Pre-ban: 62%; Post-ban: 14% (p < 0.0001) Bars/pubs, *UK* Pre-ban: 37%; Post-ban: 34% (p=0.462) (adjusted OR=8.89; 95% CI=8.14-9.33, p < 0.0001)	
Valente et al., 2007 Italy	40 establishments in the city of Rome (14 bars, six fast food restaurants, eight restaurants, six video game parlours, six pubs)	Repeated measures of indoor air quality were taken in Nov/Dec (before the law was in effect), and again in March/April 2005 and Nov/Dec 2005 (after the law was in effect)	10 January 2005 - A smoking ban in all indoor public places was enforced in Italy	Exposure to environmental tobacco smoke was measured by determining $PM_{2.5}$ and the number of ultrafine particles (UFP) Urinary cotinine concentration	$PM_{2.5}$ Pre-ban (Jan 2005): 119.3 mg/m³ (95% CI=75.7-162.8) Post-ban (Mar/Apr 2005): 38.2 mg/m³ (95% CI=27.5-48.8) (Nov/Dec 2005): 43.3 mg/m³ (95% CI=33.2-53.3) UFP Pre-ban (Jan 2005): 76 956 pt/cm³ (95% CI=59 723-65 354) Post-ban (Mar/Apr 2005): 38 079 pt/cm³ (95% CI=25 499-50 658) (Nov/Dec 2005): 51 692 pt/cm³ (95% CI= 38 030-65 354) Urinary cotinine Pre-ban (Jan 2005): 17.8 ng/ml (95% CI=14-21.6)	

Reference/location	Study participants	Study design	Restriction on smoking	Measure of exposure to SHS	Levels of exposure reported	Comments
Evidence from Europe						
Valente *et al.*, 2007 Italy				Subjective exposure to passive smoke in the workplace and at home	Post-ban (Mar/Apr 2005): 5.5 ng/ml (95% CI=3.8-7.26) (Nov/Dec 2005): 3.7 ng/ml (95% CI=1.8-5.6) There was a reduction in subjective exposure to SHS at the workplace in the post-law periods (p<0.0005) (data not shown)	
Ellingsen *et al.*, 2006 Norway	93 employees from 13 bars and restaurants in Oslo during the last month before the smoking ban (1 June 2004), and three months after implementation (Sep 2004-Feb 2005)	Prospective study with exposure measures one month before and three months after legislation	1988 - Norway enacted comprehensive legislation on smoking in public places; restaurants and bars exempt Revision of Environmental Tobacco Smoke Act was proposed. Total smoking ban in bars, nightclubs, and restaurants enacted 1 June 2004	Level of airborne contaminants (airborne nicotine, airborne dust) Urinary cotinine concentration	Total dust Pre-ban: 262 $\mu g/m^3$ (range 52-662) Post-ban: 77 $\mu g/m^3$ (range Nd-261) (p<0.001) Nicotine Pre-ban: 28.3 $\mu g/m^3$ (range 0.4-88.0) Post-ban: 0.6 $\mu g/m^3$ (range Nd-3.7) (p<0.001) Non-snuffing nonsmokers Pre-ban: 9.5 $\mu g/mg$ creatinine (95% CI=6.5-13.7) Post-ban: 1.4 $\mu g/mg$ (95% CI=0.8-2.5) (p < 0.001) Non-snuffing smokers Pre-ban: 1444 $\mu g/mg$ (95% CI=957-2180) Post-ban: 688 $\mu g/mg$ (95% CI=324-1458) (p < 0.05)	Nd: not detected
Akhtar *et al.*, 2007 Scotland	2559 primary school children surveyed before the smoke-free legislation (January 2006) 2424 surveyed after implementation (January 2007)	Repeated cross-sectional survey	2005 - Smoking, Health and Social Care (Scotland) Act: Smoking is not permitted in most fully and substantially enclosed public places in Scotland (implemented 26 March 2006)	Salivary cotinine concentrations Reports of parental smoking Self-reported exposure to tobacco smoke in public and private places before and after legislation	39% reduction 2006: 0.36 ng/ml (95% CI=0.32-0.40) 2007: 0.22 ng/ml (95% CI=0.19-0.25) 51% reduction in households with no parental smoking 2006: 0.14 ng/ml (95% CI=0.13-0.16) 2007: 0.07 ng/ml (95% CI=0.06-0.08) Cafes/restaurants 2006: 3.2%; 2007: 0.9%; p<0.001 Buses and trains 2006: 1.5%; 2007: 0.6%; p=0.015	Adjusted for age and family affluence Lack of a comparison group to control for secular changes in exposure to SHS No evidence of displacement of adult smoking from public places into home

Table 6.1 Studies that report the effect of legislation restricting smoking in the workplace on exposure to SHS

Evidence from Europe

Reference/location	Study participants	Study design	Restriction on smoking	Measure of exposure to SHS	Levels of exposure reported	Comments
Haw & Gruer, 2007 Scotland	Adults 18-74 years contacted at home Pre-ban: n=1815 1 Sept - 20 Nov 2005 9 Jan - 25 March 2006 Post-ban: n=1834 1 Sept - 10 Dec 2006 8 Jan - 2 Apr 2007	Repeated cross-sectional survey	2005 - Smoking, Health and Social Care (Scotland) Act: Smoking is not permitted in most fully and substantially enclosed public places in Scotland (implemented 26 March 2006)	Salivary cotinine concentration Self-reported exposure to SHS in public and private places Self-reported smoking restriction in homes and in cars	39% reduction (95% CI= 29%-47%) 2005-2006: 0.43 ng/ml (95% CI=0.39-0.47) 2006-2007: 0.26 ng/ml (95% CI=0.23-0.29) Pub: OR=0.03; 95% CI=0.02-0.05 Work: OR=0.32; 95% CI=0.23-0.45 Public Transport: OR=0.29; 95% CI=0.15-0.57 Other enclosed public place: OR=0.25; 95% CI=0.17-0.38 (not in homes or in cars) Reference: Self-reported exposure to SHS before legislation Complete/partial ban in homes: OR=1.49; 95% CI=1.26-1.76	Lack of a comparison group to identify secular trends unrelated to legislation No evidence of displacement of adult smoking from public places into home ORs adjusted for sex, education, and deprivation category Exposure to SHS significantly reduced only in enclosed public places (not private) covered by the law
Semple *et al.*, 2007a,b Scotland	41 randomly selected pubs in two cities Pre-ban : 26 March 2006 Post-ban: eight weeks later	Repeated measures of indoor air quality before and after legislation	2005 - Smoking, Health and Social Care (Scotland) Act: Smoking is not permitted in most fully and substantially enclosed public places in Scotland (implemented 26 March 2006)	PM$_{2.5}$ was measured for 30 minutes in each bar in 1 or 2 visits in eight weeks prior to and 8 weeks after legislation	Pre-ban: PM$_{2.5}$ 246 $\mu g/m^3$ (range 8-902 $\mu g/m^3$) Post-ban: PM$_{2.5}$ 20 $\mu g/m^3$ (range 6-104 $\mu g/m^3$)	
Galan *et al.*, 2007 Spain	1750 participants from the non-institutionalised population aged 18-64 years prior to the law (Oct-Nov 2005), and 1252 participants immediately after the law was enacted (Jan-July 2006)	Cross-sectional population-based study	January 2006 - A national tobacco control law introduced in Spain. Includes a total ban of smoking in workplaces and a partial limitation of smoking in bars and restaurants	Self-reported questionnaire to gather levels of passive exposure to SHS at home, work, in bars, and restaurants	At home: OR=0.84 (95% CI=0.11-0.19) (p < 0.001) 2005 Pre-ban: 34.3% (95% CI=32.1-36.6) 2006 Post-ban: 30.5% (95% CI=27.9-33.2)	

Reference/location	Study participants	Study design	Restriction on smoking	Measure of exposure to SHS	Levels of exposure reported	Comments
Evidence from Europe						
Galan et al., 2007 Spain					At work: OR=0.14 (95% CI=0.71-1.00)(p=0.044) 2005 Pre-ban: 40.5% (95% CI=37.5-43.6) 2006 Post-ban: 9.0% (95% CI=7.0-11.3) Bars and restaurants: OR=0.54 (95% CI=0.37-0.80) (p<0.001) 2005 Pre-ban: 0.30% (95% CI=0.20-0.44) 2006 Post-ban: 0.16% (95% CI=0.10-0.24) Results were similar for smoking and nonsmoking populations	
Fernandez et al., 2008 Spain	Air quality measured in 44 hospitals before and after a national ban on smoking in the workplace	Before and after environmental measures	January 2006 - Spanish Smoking Control Law. Exemptions apply for some hospitality venues	Vapour phase nicotine in multiple locations Sep-Dec 2005 and Sep-Dec 2006	56.5% reduction 2005: 0.23 $\mu g/m^3$ (IQR 0.13-0.63) 2006: 0.10 $\mu g/m^3$ (IQR 0.02-0.19)	IQR: Inter-quartile range
Evidence from Australia and New Zealand						
Cameron et al., 2003 Australia	A stratified random sample of 1078 members of the Victorian Branch of the Australian Liquor, Hospitality, and Miscellaneous Workers Union interviewed by telephone in September 2001	Cross-sectional survey	Four main categories of smoking restrictions were constructed based on the participants' responses: total ban, ban at usual work station, no ban at usual workstation, and no restrictions	Self-reported exposure to SHS (hours per day)	Total bans: No exposure: 100% > 0-≤7.5 hours of exposure: 0% > 7.5 hours of exposure: 0% Banned at workstation: No exposure: 76% > 0-≤7.5 hours of exposure: 20% > 7.5 hours of exposure: 4% No ban at workstation: No exposure: 4% > 0-≤7.5 hours of exposure: 51% > 7.5 hours of exposure: 45% No restriction: No exposure: 4% > 0-≤7.5 hours of exposure: 49% > 7.5 hours of exposure: 47%	

Table 6.1 Studies that report the effect of legislation restricting smoking in the workplace on exposure to SHS

Evidence from Australia and New Zealand

Reference/location	Study participants	Study design	Restriction on smoking	Measure of exposure to SHS	Levels of exposure reported	Comments
Al-Delaimy et al., 2001a New Zealand	117 workers from 62 workplaces (restaurants or bars) from two cities (Wellington and Auckland) were surveyed from Dec-March 1997/98 and 1998/99, respectively	Cross-sectional survey	1990 - New Zealand introduced smoke-free environment legislation which prohibited smoking in most workplaces. Restaurants could elect to prohibit smoking, but were required to designate only 50% of seating as smoke-free; bars were exempt	Geometric means of hair nicotine level in nonsmoking workers (tested by high performance liquid chromatography)	Smoke-free policy (nonsmoking workers) 100% smoke-free restaurants: 0.62 ng/mg (95% CI=0.5-0.7) In bars with no restriction: 6.69 ng/mg (95% CI=4.1-10.5) In places with partial restriction: 2.72 ng/mg (95% CI=1.9-4) In places with no restriction: 6.69 ng/mg (95% CI=4.1-10.5) Smoke-free policy (smoking workers): 7.92 ng/mg (95% CI=5-12)	
Bates et al., 2002 New Zealand	Three categories of non-smoking subjects (n=92): 1) employees in bars and restaurants that permitted smoking by customers; 2) employees in hospitality premises that did not permit customers to smoke; 3) employees in smoke-free government ministries and departments	Repeated cross-sectional survey. All interviews took place between June-Oct 2000	1990 - New Zealand introduced smoke-free environment legislation which prohibited smoking in most workplaces. Restaurants could elect to prohibit smoking, but were required to designate only 50% of seating as smoke-free; bars were exempt	Salivary cotinine concentration was measured pre- and post-shift or work day	Government employees: Pre-shift: 0.12 ng/g; Post-shift: 0.08 ng/g Hospitality workers (smoke-free workplaces) Pre-shift: 0.37 ng/g; Post-shift: 0.28 ng/g Hospitality workers (smoking only in designated area) Pre-shift: 1.12 ng/g; Post-shift: 1.68 ng/g Hospitality workers (no smoking restrictions) Pre-shift: 1.60 ng/g; Post-shift: 3.38 ng/g	The permissiveness of the smoking policy of a workplace was directly associated with the likelihood of an increase in salivary cotinine concentration at work.

Reference/location	Study participants	Study design	Restriction on smoking	Measure of exposure to SHS	Levels of exposure reported	Comments
Evidence from Australia and New Zealand						
Fernando *et al.*, 2007 New Zealand	Nonsmokers living or working in a nonsmoking environment aged 24-45 years, randomly selected bars in three cities. Pre-ban: July-Sept 2004-Winter and again in Oct/Nov-Spring Post-ban: Same times in 2005	Panel study with exposure measures before and after legislation	10 Dec 2004 - Smoking not permitted in any indoor place of work including bars, restaurants, and hotels	Count of the number of cigarettes lit in three 10 min intervals Salivary cotinine levels were measured before and after a three hour visit Subjective assessment of ventilation was measured by a questionnaire	Pre-ban 2004 (Winter): 889 (Spring): 928 Post-ban 2005 (Winter): 0 (Spring): 1 Pre-ban 2004 (Winter): 0.76 ng/ml (SE 0.05 ng/ml) (Spring): 0.54 ng/ml (SE 0.41 ng/ml) Post-ban 2005 (Winter): 0.10 ng/ml (SE 0.01 ng/ml) (Spring): 0.07 ng/ml (SE 0.01 ng/ml) Increases in cotinine strongly correlated with the volunteers' subjective observation of ventilation, air quality, and counts of lit cigarettes.	Study controlled for secular trends in exposure to SHS at home and in outdoor public places SE: standard error of mean
Evidence from USA						
Eisner *et al.*, 1998 California, USA	53 daytime bartenders from 25 bars and taverns in San Francisco Baseline: 1 Dec - 31 Dec 1997 Follow-up: 1 Feb - 28 Feb 1998	Panel study with exposure measures before and after legislation	1 Jan 1998 - California State Assembly Bill 13 amended the California Labour Code to prohibit smoking in bars and taverns	Respiratory and sensory irritation symptoms Self-reported SHS exposure	1997 Pre-ban: 39 bartenders (74%) with respiratory symptoms, 77 % with at least one sensory irritation 1998 Follow-up: 17 bartenders (32%) still symptomatic, 19% with sensory irritation 1997 Pre-ban: All 53 bartenders reported SHS exposure (A median exposure of 28 hours per week) 1998 Follow-up: Median SHS exposure per week: 2 hours (P<0.001) Despite the prohibition of smoking, 29 subjects (55%) continued to report some SHS exposure (≥1 hour/wk) while working as bartenders.	

Table 6.1 Studies that report the effect of legislation restricting smoking in the workplace on exposure to SHS

Reference/location	Study participants	Study design	Restriction on smoking	Measure of exposure to SHS	Levels of exposure reported	Comments
Evidence from USA						
Pion & Givel, 2004 Missouri, USA	Airports: Lambert, St Louis and Seattle-Tacoma (Sea-Tac) International	Measures of indoor SHS with varying levels of restrictions on smoking. Testing in nonsmoking areas adjacent to a designated smoking room conducted at Lambert Airport in 1997-98 and again in 2002. Tests also performed in 1998 inside nominally smoke-free Sea-Tac.	Lambert Airport: smoking is allowed in shops, restaurants, cocktail lounges, gate areas, and airline clubs; restricted smoking in the terminal and concourses	Ambient nicotine vapour level	Lambert Airport 1997-1998: 0.46 $\mu g/m^3$ 2002: 0.72 $\mu g/m^3$ Inside nonsmoking Sea-Tac Airport 1998: 0.15 $\mu g/m^3$	Smoking rooms in airport are a source of SHS exposure for nonsmokers in adjacent nonsmoking areas
Repace, 2004 Delaware, USA	A casino, six bars, and a pool hall in Wilmington metropolitan area Pre-ban: 15 Nov 2002 Post-ban: 24 Jan 2003	Cross-sectional air quality survey before/ after enactment of statewide Clean Indoor Air law	27 Nov 2002 - Delaware Clean Indoor Air Act was amended to ban smoking in restaurants, bars, and casinos (hospitality venues that were excluded in the original Act)	Real-time measurements were made of RSP-$PM_{2.5}$ and PPAH	2002 Pre-ban: Outdoor of hotel room, RSP=9.5 $\mu g/m^3$ Indoor of hospitality, RSP=231 $\mu g/m^3$ (SD: 208 $\mu g/m^3$) 2003 Post-ban: RSP (range = 2.5%-25%, mean 9.4%) 2002 Pre-ban: PPAH= 134 ng/m^3 2003 Post-ban: (range = 0.5%-11%, mean 4.7%)	RSP: respirable size particles PPAH: particulate polycyclic hydrocarbons
Farrelly *et al.*, 2005 New York, USA	104 nonsmoking workers aged ≥18 years, recruited from restaurants, bars, and bowling facilities.	Panel study	26 March 2003 - New York State legislature passed the statewide Clean Air Act prohibiting smoking in	Saliva cotinine concentration	2003 Pre-ban: 3.6 ng/ml (95% CI=2.6-4.7 ng/ml) 2004 Post-ban: 0.8 ng/ml (95% CI=0.4-1.2 ng/ml)	Half of baseline sample lost to follow-up, due to changes in employment and moving out of state.

Evidence from USA

Reference/location	Study participants	Study design	Restriction on smoking	Measure of exposure to SHS	Levels of exposure reported	Comments
Farrelly et al., 2005 New York, USA	Pre-ban: In the period of recruitment (before legislation) Post-ban: 12 months later		all places of employment, including restaurants, bars, and bingo and bowling facilities. 24 July 2003 – law went into effect	Self-reported exposure to SHS in the workplace and other settings in the previous four days	2003 Pre-ban: Mean hours of exposure to SHS in hospitality jobs: 12.1 hours (95% CI=8–16.3 hours) 2004 Post-ban: Mean hours of exposure to SHS in hospitality jobs: 0.2 hours (95% CI=0.1–0.5 hours)	However, comparing baseline statistics for those who participated across all waves to those who dropped out of the study shows no substantial difference, suggesting no bias was introduced due to attrition
Hahn et al., 2006 Kentucky, USA	105 bar and restaurant workers aged ≥18 years from 44 restaurants, and six bars in Lexington Pre-ban: 27 April 2004 Post-ban: three and six months later	Panel study	July 2003 – Lexington-Fayette Urban County Council passed Kentucky's first smoke-free law. It prohibited smoking in most public places, including, but not limited to, restaurants, bars, bowling alleys, bingo halls, convenience stores, Laundromats, and other businesses open to the public. 27 April 2004 – law went into effect	Hair nicotine samples were obtained from subjects as an objective measure of SHS exposure Self-reported exposure to SHS	2004 Pre-ban: 1.79 ng/mg (SD: 2.62) 2004 Post-ban: 1.30 ng/mg (SD: 2.42) Comparing nonsmokers and smokers on change in hair nicotine, the average decline was significant among nonsmokers (t=2.3, p=0.03), but smokers did not exhibit a significant change over time (t=0.3, p=0.8) 2004 Pre-ban: (in past 7 days): 31 hours/wk 2004 Post-ban: (in past 7 days): 1–2 hours/wk	High attrition rate (43% at six months follow-up) Intention to treat analysis was used to account for the potential effects of attrition
Pickett et al., 2006 USA	5866 nonsmoking adults (≥ 20 years) sampled from the National Health and Nutrition Examination Survey (NHANES)	Repeated cross-sectional studies	Survey locations were categorised into: Extensive coverage if at least one smoke-free law (work, restaurant, bar) existed at the county or state level and covered the entire county; limited coverage if there was not	Serum cotinine level	The median cotinine level was below the limit of detection (<0.05 ng/ml) for all three groups Adults at locations with extensive coverage of smoking restrictions showed no detection of cotinine up through the 75th centile. The 90th [0.07 ng/ ml (95% CI=0.03–0.12)] and 95th centile [0.16 ng/ ml (95% CI=0.11–1.49)] values in the extensive coverage group were 80% lower than for the no coverage group	Smoke-free law classification scheme is not part of the sample design of NHANES, which limits the generalisability of the study findings

Table 6.1 Studies that report the effect of legislation restricting smoking in the workplace on exposure to SHS

Evidence from USA

Reference/location	Study participants	Study design	Restriction on smoking	Measure of exposure to SHS	Levels of exposure reported	Comments
Pickett et al., 2006 USA			a state or county smoke-free law, but there was at least one municipality within the county with a smoke-free law (work, restaurant, bar); no smoke-free law coverage at the state, county, or city level		After adjusting for confounders (race, age, education, restaurant visit), men and women residing in counties with extensive coverage had 0.10 (95% CI=0.06–0.16) and 0.19 (95% CI=0.1-0.34) times the odds of SHS exposure compared to those residing in counties without a smoke-free law	
Alpert et al., 2007 Massachusetts, USA	27 hospitality venues were selected from five Massachusetts towns that either did not have a smoking policy or had a very weak one Pre-ban: 23-29 June 2004 Post-ban: 27 Oct-1 Dec 2004	Repeated cross-sectional survey	5 July 2004 - Massachusetts Smoke-free Law went into effects smoking completely banned in all workplaces, including restaurants and bars	To assess indoor air quality: Change in RSP less than 2.5 microns in diameter ($PM_{2.5}$) from pre-law to post-law Observations were made to determine the number of people present and the number of burning cigarettes	93% reduction 2004 Pre-ban (Jun): $PM_{2.5}$ 206 $\mu g/m^3$ Post-ban (Oct-Dec): $PM_{2.5}$ 14 $\mu g/m^3$ 2004 Pre-ban (Jun): smoking density: 0.89 burning cigarettes per 100 m³ Post-ban (Oct-Dec): smoking density: 0.00 burning cigarettes per 100 m³	Small sample - less likely to be representative
Biener et al., 2007 Massachusetts (MA), USA	Smokers and recent quitters (aged 18–30 years) from Boston (n=83), and another 203 Massachusetts cities and towns (n=903) that did not adopt smoking bans prior to July 2004 Pre-ban: Jan 2001 and June 2002 Post-ban: 5 May 2003 and before 5 July 2004	Panel study with measure of exposure	May 2003 - City of Boston implemented a smoke-free workplace ordinance that extended the existing ban on smoking in restaurants to all workplaces in the city, including bars	Self-reported exposure to SHS measured by proportion of respondents who reported seeing smoking by other people when they went out to a bar or a nightclub Self-reported exposure to SHS at home	In Boston: 69.2% (95% CI=51.0-82.9) In other MA town: 25.1% (95% CI=18.9-32.6) (p=0.000) In Boston: 66.9% (95% CI=57.1-79.7) In other MA town: 62.5% (95% CI=58.5-66.4) There was no significant difference in exposure to SHS at home.	Small sample - less likely to be representative Older nonsmokers were not included in the research design

Reference/location	Study participants	Study design	Restriction on smoking	Measure of exposure to SHS	Levels of exposure reported	Comments
Evidence from USA						
Centers for Disease Control and Prevention, 2007b New York, USA	2008 nonsmokers age ≥18 years who participated in New York Adult Tobacco Survey (NYATS). Pre-ban: 26 June 2003 (<1 month before implementation of the statewide law) Post-ban: 30 June 2004 (1 week after implementation)	Repeated cross-sectional survey with measures of exposure before and after implementation of the 2003 New York state ban on smoking	24 July 2003 - New York City amended its anti-smoking law to include all restaurants, bars, and private clubs	Salivary cotinine concentration Self-reported exposure to SHS	47.4% reduction 2003: 0.078 ng/ml (95% CI=0.054-0.111) 2004: 0.041ng/ml (95% CI=0.036-0.047) Restaurant/bar respondents 2003: 19.8% (95% CI=15.6-24.1) 2004: 3.1% (95% CI= 2.0-4.2) Restaurant patrons 2003: 52.4% (95% CI=41.5-63.4) 2004: 13.4% (95% CI= 9.5-17.3)	Relatively low exposures to SHS in workplaces likely attributed to local smoke-free laws and voluntary workplace smoking restrictions in place before implementation of the state law
Lee et al., 2007 Kentucky, USA	Nine hospitality venues and one bingo hall in Georgetown that allowed smoking before the enforcement of the law. Pre-ban: 10 July 2005 Post-ban: 1-week, 2-weeks, and 3-months after the legislation	Measures of indoor air quality	July 2005 - Georgetown, Kentucky City Council passed a 100% smoke-free public and workplace law. It was implemented 1 October 2005	Average indoor $PM_{2.5}$ concentration was measured using a Sidepak monitor	*In hospitals* Pre-ban: 84 $\mu g/m^3$ Post-ban (1 week later): 18 $\mu g/m^3$ (21% of the mean) *In bingo mall* Pre-ban: 226 $\mu g/m^3$ Post-ban (2 weeks later): 748 $\mu g/m^3$ (3 months later): 43 $\mu g/m^3$	

Partial restrictions have been less effective than wide-reaching statutes. By way of illustration: in Spain, reductions in airborne nicotine were observed in hospitality venues that applied smoking bans, but not in venues that allowed smoking to continue (as permitted by the legislation implemented in 2006 (Luschenkova et al., 2008). Amongst Spanish hospitality workers, salivary cotinine levels fell overall, but the drop was more marked among workers in venues where smoking was totally prohibited (55.6% fall compared with 10.6% where smoking continued) (Fernandez et al., 2009). Comparable studies from countries with comprehensive bans report much larger reductions in salivary cotinine levels among hospitality workers (Allwright et al., 2005; Semple et al., 2007a).

Another example of partial bans is Georgia: in 2003 the country restricted smoking in health care facilities to designated smoking areas. In 2007, a study of airborne nicotine and $PM_{2.5}$ levels found evidence of smoking in many areas that were theoretically smoke-free; the highest levels of nicotine were observed in medical staff offices (Schick et al., 2008). In Finland, no improvement in air quality was found after legislation in March 2000 that introduced nonsmoking areas in some bars and restaurants (Johnsson et al., 2006).

What might explain the reduction in exposures to SHS following the implementation of comprehensive smoke-free legislation? This reduction is typically an 80-90% decrease from levels observed pre-legislation. The size of the changes and the consistency with which this result is reported effectively rules out chance. Biases in reporting and publishing may favour the dissemination of positive studies over those with equivocal or negative results, but it is not plausible that systematic error of this kind explains the full picture seen here. For instance, comprehensive national assessments have been reported from the 3 countries that were first to implement smoke-free legislation (Ireland, Norway and New Zealand) with remarkably similar findings, which very closely match observations from long running state level evaluations, such as in California.

In many countries there has been a gradual reduction in exposures to SHS over the course of the last decade, or in some instances, longer. This has resulted from a range of tobacco control measures, other than smoke-free legislation, which have contributed to a fall in the prevalence of smoking, a reduction in the average number of cigarettes smoked per day, and changing social norms on smoking in the home. The effects have been substantial; a 20% drop in mean saliva cotinine levels was seen in Northern Ireland in the 12 months prior to smoke-free legislation (Fong et al., 2006). Studies with geographic controls have shown the decline in SHS exposure was even more marked in the presence of legislation. A study in New Zealand used internal controls, measured the change in SHS biomarkers associated with visits to bars in the same study participants (before and after legislation), and reported effects very similar to those observed in times series studies (Fernando et al., 2007). Lastly, the rapidity, consistency, and magnitude of the reduction in SHS exposure associated with legislation all but rule out confounding as an explanation.

The effect of legislation tended to be less noticeable where there were local authority regulations and voluntary restrictions already, as in New York. Improvements in air quality were generally greater in pubs and bars than in other entertainment venues (such as bingo halls and video parlours), though findings varied between studies. For instance, air samples were taken from 31 public premises in Florence and Belluno, Italy and a 77% reduction in $PM_{2.5}$ (0.47 to 0.11 µg/m³) was found in offices, a 42.5% reduction (0.40 to 0.23 µg/m³) in industrial premises, a 95% reduction (35.59 to 1.74 µg/m³) in pubs, and a 94% reduction (127.16 to 7.99 µg/m³) in discos, two to three months post-legislation (Gasparrini et al., 2006). However, a study in 40 public places in Rome (Valente et al., 2007) found only a 28% reduction in bars (46.8 to 33.7 µg/m³), and a 16% reduction in fast food restaurants (29.8 to 25.1 µg/m³) at one year post-legislation. Larger reductions were found in other settings in Rome: a 67% reduction in restaurants (111.0 to 36.5 µg/m³), a 56% reduction in video game parlours (150.1 to 65.7 µg/m³), and an 84% reduction in pubs (368.1 to 57.7 µg/m³). In other countries similar relative changes have been observed (e.g. in Scotland, there was a reduction of 86% in $PM_{2.5}$ readings in bars following the smoking ban) (Semple et al., 2007b). Post-legislation levels of particles in the hospitality venues in Rome were considerably higher than those reported in either Northern Italy or in Ireland and Scotland, but this may reflect variations in background levels of particulate matter from sources other than SHS.

It is important to note the effect of smoking restrictions on inequalities in exposures to SHS in the workplace. Voluntary restrictions were most effective in white collar occupational groups and workplaces with a large number of employees (Pierce *et al.*, 1998a). Comprehensive smoking restrictions have reduced this bias, and therefore have tended to be socially progressive, benefiting particularly disadvantaged groups. In New Zealand a similar effect was noted following the 2004 legislation, when it was apparent that inequalities had been reduced between Maori (the indigenous people) and non-Maori. The post-legislation fall in SHS exposure at work was greater among Maori, since they were over-represented in elements of the work force that were poorly served by voluntary restrictions (Edwards *et al.*, 2008). In the general population, the effect on SHS exposures overall has tended to be greatest among nonsmokers from nonsmoking households (Adda & Cornaglia, 2005; Haw & Gruer, 2007). In the USA, serum cotinine levels of working age adults participating in the US National Health and Nutrition Examination Survey (NHANES) fell by approximately 80% from 1988 to 2002. This was during a period when an increasing proportion of the population was covered by indoor clean air legislation, and the largest reductions occurred in blue collar and service occupations, construction and manufacturing industrial workers, and

non-Hispanic black male workers - the groups that historically were most heavily exposed to SHS (Arheart *et al.*, 2008).

The balance of the research to date indicates that legislation restricting smoking in the workplace does *not* lead to increased exposures to SHS in other settings. Studies in New Zealand, Ireland, and Scotland examined contemporaneous changes in smoking in the home, and found no adverse effect of legislation (Akhtar *et al.*, 2007; Haw & Gruer, 2007; Edwards *et al.*, 2008; Hyland *et al.*, 2008b). In Norway, the proportion of households with a total ban on smoking in the home increased from 47%, a year prior to the 2004 comprehensive workplace legislation, to 59% one year later (Lund, 2006). Population data show no sign of "compensating" exposures to SHS resulting from restrictions in the workplace. In the USA, analysis of the long-running NHANES found that amongst individuals residing in counties with extensive smoking restrictions, the upper centiles of urinary cotinine were 80% lower than levels in counties with no restrictions (Arheart *et al.*, 2008). Another analysis of the NHANES data suggested that bans in US bars and restaurants were associated with higher cotinine levels among nonsmokers, possibly due to displacement of smoking to the home (Adda & Cornaglia, 2005). However, the latter study recorded only bans applied at the state level when most legislation in this time period was introduced at the municipality or county level.

In summary, research to date shows substantial reductions in exposure to SHS following legislation

to restrict smoking. The size of the effect depends on the nature of the restrictions and the context (including the extent of voluntary restrictions pre-legislation). SHS exposures are not prevented altogether, even with comprehensive legislation, but air quality and biomarker studies indicate that exposures of employees and patrons in what are typically the smokiest workplaces (bars and restaurants) can be cut by 80-90%.

Will these reductions in exposures to SHS be sustained in the long-term? The longest running evaluation studies come from California, and suggest that reductions can be maintained long-term. In California prior to 1995, there were many community level ordinances restricting smoking in public places and work settings, but in that year the California Assembly Bill 13 (AB-13) was implemented, banning smoking in most indoor workplaces. The law was extended in 1998 to cover bars and gaming venues. The proportion of indoor workers in California exposed to SHS fell from 29.1% in 1990 to 11.8% in 1996, and that figure has altered little in subsequent surveys (15.6% in 1999 and 12.0% in 2002) (Gilpin *et al.*, 2003). Elsewhere there have been few opportunities to examine long-term effects. Surveys in New Zealand show that reductions in perceived exposures to smoke in the workplace have remained two years post-legislation (Edwards *et al.*, 2008).

Effects of restrictions in settings other than the workplace

There are a number of residential settings, for example prisons, care homes, and hotel accommodations, which are workplaces for some and homes for others, and for this reason have often been exempted from statutory smoking restrictions.

SHS exposure in prisons is particularly elevated, as smoking rates amongst both inmates and prison guards are high. Indeed, it has been estimated that twice as many prisoners die each year in the USA from SHS as are executed (Butler et al., 2007). Prisons pose a particular challenge for enacting smoke-free policies, as inmates who smoke have few opportunities to do so without exposing others to SHS. By the end of 2007, however, 24 US states had enacted 100% smoke-free policies covering all indoor areas in correctional facilities (Proescholdbell et al., 2008). Though it has been claimed that prisoners commonly continue to smoke in jail, despite bans (Butler et al., 2007), there is evidence that smoking restrictions may be effective. A study of air quality in six North Carolina prisons found that levels of particles fell by 77% after a ban on smoking indoors was implemented (Proescholdbell et al., 2008). A similar study of facilities in Vermont and Massachusetts also reported evidence that bans in prisons substantially reduced levels of SHS in shared areas (Hammond & Emmons, 2005).

A Scottish study has examined levels of SHS exposure in care homes that were exempted from that country's 2006 smoke-free legislation. Data were collected from eight care home establishments in Aberdeen and Aberdeenshire, with a further eight static area measurements made in four designated smoking rooms within these establishments. Assessments were carried out during 2006 using a TSI Sidepak Personal Aerosol Monitor set to sample particulate matter of less than 2.5 microns in size ($PM_{2.5}$) (Semple et al., in press).

Measurements within the four smoking rooms showed very high SHS concentrations with $PM_{2.5}$ concentrations sometimes exceeding 5000 μg/m³. Time-weighted averages over periods extending to six hours revealed levels ranging between 81 and 910 μg/m³ (geometric mean value of 360 μg/m³ from all eight measurements), well in excess of the US Environmental Protection Agency (EPA) hazardous air quality index (250 μg/m³) for $PM_{2.5}$.

However, employees in the care homes studied did not appear to spend significant time in these environments; therefore, personal exposure levels to SHS were much lower with the geometric mean of the eight work-shift measurements being 24 μg/m³. Two of the eight (25%) time-weighted average exposures exceeded the US EPA 24 hour air quality index of 65 μg/m³ (rated as 'unhealthy' for outdoor air). Nevertheless, care home employees' exposures to SHS were on average nearly 10 times lower than those recorded in the hospitality sector in Scotland (before the introduction of smoke-free legislation), where full shift $PM_{2.5}$ levels had a geometric mean value of 202 μg/m³ (Semple et al., 2007a).

Salivary cotinine data from this group of workers also suggest exposure to SHS at work is much lower than for those in the hospitality trade. The geometric mean salivary cotinine level in nonsmoking care home workers (n=36) was 0.37 ng/ml prior to the smoke-free legislation in March 2006, compared to 2.94 ng/ml in bar employees (Semple et al., 2007b). Nonsmoking care home workers' levels reduced to 0.17 ng/ml after implementation of the legislation (Semple et al., in press). It seems likely that this decrease in salivary cotinine levels was from reduced exposure in social settings outside of work. This data is reflected from a population survey in Scotland, where levels in nonsmoking adults fell by 39% (from 0.43 ng/ml to 0.26 ng/ml) after introduction of the restrictions on smoking in enclosed public places in Scotland (Haw & Gruer, 2007).

Smoking in cars causes high levels of pollution, particularly in the absence of ventilation (average RSP levels of 271 μg/m³ were measured in driving trials by Rees & Connolly (2006)), and exposure to SHS in this setting is common. In a Canadian survey of youth in grades 5-9, just over a quarter reported they were exposed to smoking while riding in a car at least once in the previous week (Leatherdale et al., 2008). In a New Zealand study, smoking was observed in 4% (95% CI=3.8-4.4) of cars on city roads during the day (and the prevalence was three times higher in areas of high social deprivation) (Martin et al., 2006). In a phone survey in the same country, 71% of current smokers (n=272) reported smoking in their cars (Gillespie et al., 2005). In the United States, surveys have found similar levels of support for smoking bans in cars as in homes (70% and 62% respectively, in a 2005 study of African-American adults) (King et al., 2005). Studies in the USA have found that factors associated with smoking bans in homes, such as education, smoking histories, and ethnicity, tend to also apply to motor vehicles (King *et al.*, 2005; Gonzales *et al.*, 2006). However, those most seriously affected by SHS are often not protected. Exposure to SHS in cars has been reported to increase the rate of wheezing in young people (Sly *et al.*, 2007), but a US survey in 2005 found that only 64% of parents of children with asthma had household smoking bans that included the family car (Halterman *et al.*, 2006).

The only published data available so far on the impact of workplace legislation on smoking in cars comes from Scotland and Ireland. In Scotland, there was no change in reported exposures to SHS in cars, either amongst adults (Haw & Gruer, 2007) or primary school children (Akhtar *et al.*, 2007). The Irish results were similar: the prevalence of private smoke-free cars was reported to be 58% before comprehensive work-place legislation and 55% after (Fong *et al.*, 2006). Legislation that specifically bans smoking in cars with children has been introduced in two Australian states (Tasmania and South Australia) and in California, Arkansas, Louisiana, Maine, Puerto Rico, and Nova Scotia. No studies have yet been published on subsequent changes in exposures to SHS.

With the increasing prevalence of bans on smoking in enclosed public and workplaces, attention has moved to policies covering smoking in outdoor environments (e.g. sports arenas, parks, outdoor dining areas, and beaches) (Chapman, 2007), though there are few studies of exposure to SHS in outdoor settings. Airborne particles were measured

in 10 outdoor sites in California, and it was found that during periods of active smoking, peak levels nearby were similar to those observed indoors (Klepeis *et al.*, 2007). Outdoor levels were very sensitive to wind and proximity to smokers, and dropped almost instantly when smoking ceased. Declaration that the 2000 Sydney Olympic Games would be 100% smoke-free was an indication of growing willingness to extend smoking restrictions beyond indoors, however we know of no published studies that have examined the effect of outdoor bans on exposure to SHS.

Effects of smoke-free legislation on population exposure to SHS

Most SHS exposure studies have focused on employees, and, in the case of entertainment and hospitality venues, patrons. However, relatively few studies have examined the impact of legislation on population level exposure to SHS. Data were used from NHANES (1999-2002) to compare the proportion of adult nonsmokers exposed to SHS in counties classified as having extensive smoke-free laws, limited smoke-free laws, and no smoke-free laws (Pickett *et al.*, 2006). SHS exposure was defined as serum cotinine values of ≥0.05 ng/ml (the limit of detection for cotinine assays). The study found that 12.5% of nonsmoking adults living in counties with extensive smoke-free laws were exposed to SHS, compared with 35.1% from counties with limited coverage, and 45.9% from counties with no laws. Men and women from counties with extensive smoke-free laws had 0.1 (95% CI=0.06-0.16)

and 0.19 (95% CI=0.11-0.34) the odds, respectively, of SHS exposure, compared with men and women from counties without smoke-free laws.

In an analysis of data from the New York Adult Tobacco Survey (NYATS), it was found that as well as a large reduction in reported SHS exposure in restaurant and bar patrons, geometric mean cotinine fell by 47.4% from 0.078 ng/ml to 0.041 ng/ml (Centers for Disease Control and Prevention, 2007b). The proportion of adults who had no SHS exposure (cotinine <0.05 ng/ml) also increased from 32.5% to 52.4%. However, the very low response rates, both to the survey (22%) and amongst study participants to a request to provide a saliva sample (33%), suggests that the sample may not be representative of the New York population as a whole.

Two Scottish studies of the impact of smoke-free legislation on population exposure achieved more representative samples. The first, a repeat cross-sectional household survey of representative samples of adults aged 18-74 years (Haw & Gruer, 2007), found a 39% reduction in geometric mean cotinine in nonsmokers from 0.57 ng/ml at baseline to 0.26 ng/ml post-legislation, (p<0.001). However, only the reduction in mean cotinine concentrations for nonsmokers living in nonsmoking households was significant. For this sub-group, cotinine fell by 49%, from 0.35 ng/ml to 0.18 ng/ml (p<0.001). This compares with a non-significant reduction of 16%, from 0.92 ng/ml to 0.81 ng/ml in nonsmokers from smoking households. Reduction in SHS exposure was associated with a reduction in reported SHS exposure in public places (i.e. pubs, other workplaces, and public transport) post-legislation.

The second Scottish study was a repeat cross-sectional school survey of 11 year old children in their last year in primary school (Akhtar et al., 2007). Among nonsmokers, geometric mean salivary cotinine fell from 0.36 ng/ml to 0.22 ng/ml - again a 39% reduction. As in the adult study, significant reductions (51%) in SHS exposure were obtained for children living in households where neither parent smoked. There was also a significant reduction (44%) for children from households where only fathers smoked. For children living in households where either their mother or both parents smoked, mean cotinine fell by only 11%. In combination, the findings from both these studies suggest that the main beneficiaries of the Scottish smoking ban are nonsmokers from nonsmoking households. Indeed, Akhtar and colleagues (2007) conclude that after implementation of the Scottish legislation, nearly one in five Scottish school children are still exposed to SHS at levels (≥1.7 ng/ml) which have been shown to be damaging to arterial health in children (Kallio et al., 2007).

Health impacts of restrictions on smoking in the workplace

Studies of the health effects of smoking restrictions have focused almost exclusively on acute respiratory illness and cardiovascular disease. There is a short lag time between exposure to SHS and onset of symptoms, the evidence that SHS is causally related to these conditions

is strong, and the effects are thought to be largely reversible (Chapter 2). SHS also increases the risk of lung cancer, but the time period from exposure to evident disease may be 10-20 years, or longer, making it much more difficult to link changes in disease rates with introduction of smoking restrictions. Nevertheless, given the strength of the evidence linking SHS to increased risk of lung cancer, it is expected that the reduction in exposures following smoke-free legislation will ultimately be reflected in a fall in the incidence of this particular disease.

Studies of those most directly affected by smoke-free legislation have mainly focused on short-term changes in the respiratory health of workers in the hospitality sector. Most studies have measured changes in reported respiratory symptoms (e.g. wheeze and cough) and sensory symptoms (e.g. upper airway and eye irritation); a number have also assessed changes in lung function. The most common measures of lung function are forced expiratory volume in one second (FEV_1) and forced vital capacity (FVC). Some studies have also assessed peak expiratory flow rate (PEF), forced mid-expiratory flow rate (FEF_{25-75}), and total lung capacity (TLC).

A study of a cohort of San Francisco bar workers (Eisner et al., 1998) examined the impact of a smoke-free law on both sensory and respiratory symptoms and lung function. It found a large reduction in reported symptoms and a small, but significant, improvement in lung function following introduction of the smoke-free law. Mean FVC increased by 4.6% post-legislation and mean

FEV_1 by 1.2%. Complete elimination of workplace SHS exposure was associated with a 6.8% improvement in FVC and a 4.5% increase in FEV_1, after controlling for smoking status and recent upper and lower respiratory tract infection. A study of Dundee bar workers (Menzies et al., 2006) obtained very similar results to Eisner and colleagues, reporting a reduction in respiratory and sensory symptoms and a 5.1% increase in FEV_1 at two months post-legislation. Interestingly, this study also included measures of pulmonary and systemic inflammation. In asthmatics and rhinitis sufferers (n=23), there was a 20% reduction (p=0.04) in forced expired nitrous oxide (FE_{No}), a marker of pulmonary inflammation, at one and two months post-legislation. A significant reduction was not observed in otherwise healthy bar workers (n=54). For the sample as a whole, however, there was a reduction in markers of systemic inflammation with both total white blood cell (p=0.002) and neutrophil count (p=0.03) falling significantly at two months post-legislation.

In both the San Francisco and Dundee studies follow-up of respondents was two months after implementation. It is not clear what the impact of seasonal factors may be on the US results, but in the case of the Scottish study, temperature differences and differences in rates of respiratory infections between February and May provide an alternative explanation for the improvements in respiratory health. A similar issue arises in interpretation of a Norwegian study of 1525 hospitality workers, of whom 906 were contacted again five months later, following implementation of the national smoke-free legislation. Prevalence of five respiratory symptoms was lower after the legislation than before (Eagan *et al.*, 2006).

A study of staff from Norwegian pubs and restaurants adopted a different approach and assessed cross shift changes in lung function pre- and post-legislation (Skogstad *et al.*, 2006). For the whole sample, there was a reduction in cross shift changes in FEF_{25-75}, which fell from -199 ml/s to -64 ml/s (p=0.01). Significant reductions in cross shift changes in FEV_1 (p=0.03) and in FEF_{25-75} (p=0.01) were also observed in nonsmokers. In asthmatics, there were significant reductions in cross shift changes in FVC (p=0.04), FEV_1 (p=0.02), and FEF_{25-75} (p=0.01). In smokers, only a reduction in cross shift changes in PEF (p=0.02) was observed. Although cross shift changes in lung function fell after the legislation was introduced, with the exception of PEF, absolute values for the other lung function measures were also lower post-legislation. These findings may be explained by the lower mean outdoor temperature of 3°C during the follow-up period compared with 12°C at baseline.

Although there have been many studies on the respiratory health of bar workers, the sample sizes are often small, are drawn from a limited number of locations, and few attempt to eliminate seasonal influences on outcomes or have control groups. Even when studies have controlled for seasonal effects with follow-up at exactly one year after baseline, sample attrition rates have been high at over 40% (Hahn *et al.*, 2006). An exception is a study of the respiratory

health of bar workers in the Republic of Ireland (Allwright *et al.*, 2005) who were recruited from three areas in the Republic and one control location in Northern Ireland, where legislation had not yet been introduced. The follow-up rate at one year was 76%. In a sample of nonsmokers (n=158) from the Republic of Ireland, a significant fall in both respiratory (p<0.001) and sensory symptoms (p<0.001) were reported. The reduction in symptoms in this group was accompanied by an 80% reduction in salivary cotinine. By contrast, there was no change in reported symptoms in the control nonsmoking bar workers (n=20) from Northern Ireland, even though there was a 20% reduction in salivary cotinine. A subset of male bar workers from the Republic of Ireland (both smokers and nonsmokers) was tested for changes in lung function. Measurements were taken in a clinical setting. In never smokers, there were small, but significant, increases in predicted FVC, PEV, FEF, and TLC post-legislation. In ex-smokers, there were significant improvements in all measures, except PEF, but no significant changes in lung function measures were observed for smokers (Goodman *et al.*, 2007).

In summary, there is a growing body of evidence on the short-term impact of smoke-free legislation on respiratory health of employees (particularly bar workers). The majority of studies have found an improvement in reported respiratory and sensory symptoms irrespective of follow-up period.

Four studies have also reported small improvements in lung function. Three of the four (which

also demonstrated the largest improvements in lung function) did not, however, follow-up study participants a full 12 months after baseline data collection. Therefore, seasonal factors, such as ambient temperature, cannot be ruled out. The fourth study, a study of bar workers from the Republic of Ireland, found statistically significant improvements in lung function in nonsmokers at one year, but these changes were small in absolute terms and it is unclear if they have any immediate clinical significance for respiratory health.

Impact of smoke-free legislation on population health

Cardiovascular health

Most of the studies of the impact of smoke-free legislation on population health have examined the short-term effect of legislation on admissions for acute myocardial infarction and related cardiac conditions. These studies have relied largely on routine hospital data; as a result, they have encountered problems such as inconsistencies in case definition over time and between hospitals, and lack of information in patient level data on smoking status and exposure to SHS.

As previously noted, there is substantial scientific documentation on the acute and longer-term effects of SHS exposure on cardiovascular health, but particular interest in the effects of smoke-free legislation arose after admissions for acute myocardial infarction (AMI) to a single hospital that served Helena, Montana were reduced by 40% (Sargent *et al.*, 2004). This fall occurred in the six months after introduction of smoke-free ordinances and returned to the pre-restriction rate after the ordinances were repealed. Hospital admissions for AMI for a nearby comparison community, where no restrictions had been introduced, showed a slight increase in admissions for the same period. The size of the reduction was surprising and there have been a number of criticisms of the study. The total number of cases observed was small, the statistical approach to analysis did not account for the trend of increasing admissions over time, and the authors did not make any direct observations to confirm that exposure to SHS was reduced during the months when the law was in force.

Since the Montana investigation, another eight published studies have reported reductions in AMI after implementation of smoking bans (Table 6.2, Figure 6.1). Admissions for AMI in Pueblo, Colorado were examined for a three year period between 18 months before and 18 months after smoke-free legislation was introduced (Bartecchi et al., 2006). Hospitalisation rates for patients living within the city limits (where the ordinances applied) were compared with hospitalisation rates for patients residing outside the city limits (controls). Hospital admission rates were also compared with rates for a second external control: a geographically isolated community in El Paso County, Colorado. After smoke-free ordinances were introduced within the city limits, there was a 27% reduction (Rate Ratio (RR)=0.74; 95% CI=0.64-0.86) in AMI in residents residing within the

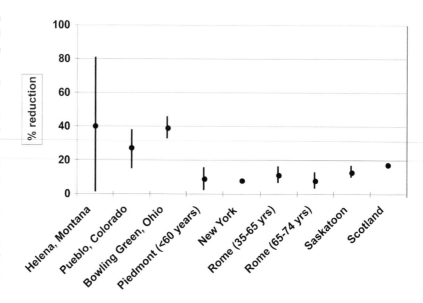

Figure 6.1 Summary of results from studies reporting reduction in hospital admissions for acute myocardial infarction/acute coronary syndrome following implementation of smoke-free legislation

One study has been published that did not detect evidence of a reduction in hospital admissions for acute heart disease (Edwards et al, 2008).

city boundary. A significant reduction was not observed for residents outside the city limits or in the external control.

A study in Bowling Green, Ohio examined a wider range of hospital admissions (ischaemic heart disease and heart failure) (Khuder et al., 2007). The post-legislation study period began six months after the ban was introduced in order to allow compliance to stabilise. Admissions with a diagnosis of ischaemic heart disease or heart failure fell by 39% (RR=0.61; 95% CI=0.55-0.67) after implementation of legislation. No change was observed in a matched control community from Kent, Ohio.

In a much larger study of admissions for AMI to all hospitals (number of hospitals=261 to 243

over the study period) in New York State, the impact of the 2003 comprehensive smoke-free legislation was examined (Juster et al., 2007). Prior to 2003, there was a patch work of different local laws that had been gradually introduced across the state beginning in 1989. A regression analysis of monthly hospital admissions for AMI against time, suggested an 8% decline attributable to the implementation of a statewide comprehensive ban following after local laws banning smoking. This is less than the effect reported in other US studies, and may be due to the relatively low levels of exposure to SHS in New York State as a consequence of the local ordinances implemented prior to the statewide law.

Table 6.2 Summary of studies on the impact of smoke-free legislation on cardiovascular health

Reference/ location	Control	Study period	Number of cases	Percent reduction (95% CI)	Rate ratio (95% CI)	Data source/end point/ comments
Sargent et al., 2004 Helena, Montana, USA	Patients residing outside Helena	Pre-ban: June-Nov1998 Ban: 5 June 2002 Post-ban: June-Nov 2002	Mean: 40 24	40 (1-79)	0.60 (0.21-0.99)	Hospital admission data/ Acute Myocardial Infarction (ICD9 code: 410)
Barone-Adesi et al., 2006 Piedmont Region, Italy	None	Pre-ban: Oct-Dec 2004 versus Oct-Dec 2003 Ban: 10 Jan 2005 Post-ban: Feb-June 2005 versus Feb-June 2004	3655 3581	< 60 yrs 11 ≥ 60 yrs NS	0.89* (0.81-0.98) 1.05* (1.00-1.11)	Hospital admission data/ Acute Myocardial Infarction (ICD9 code: 410)
Bartecchi et al., 2006 Pueblo, Colorado city limits USA	Pueblo (outside city limit) and El Paso County	Pre-ban: Jan 2002-June 2003 Ban: 1 July 2003 Post-ban: July 2003-Dec 2004	399 291	27 (15-37)	0.74** (0.64-0.86)	Hospital admission data/ Acute Myocardial Infarction (ICD9 code: 410) as primary diagnosis
Juster et al., 2007 New York State, USA	None	Pre-ban: Jan 1995-June 2003 Ban: 24 July 2003 Post-ban: July 2003-Dec 2004	44 000-48 000 per annum	Statewide after local bans: AMI: 8 Statewide without local bans: AMI:19 Stroke: No change		Hospital Admission data/ Acute Myocardial Infarction (ICD9 code: 410); Stroke (ICD9 codes: 430-438)
Khunder et al., 2007 Bowling Green, Ohio USA	Kent, Ohio	Pre-ban: Jan 1999-Jan 2002 Ban: March 2002; Post-ban: Jun 2002-Jun 2005	186	To 2003: 39 (33-45) To 2005: 47 (41-55)	To 2003: 0.61 (0.55-0.67); To 2005: 0.53 (0.45-0.59)	Hospitals admission data / Ischemic heart disease; Heart failure (ICD9 codes: 410-14, 428)
Seo & Torabi, 2007 Monroe County, Indiana, USA	Delaware County, Indiana	Pre-ban: Aug 2001-May 2003 Ban: Most workplaces 1 Aug 2003; Bars from 1 Jan 2005 Post-ban: Aug 2003-May 2005	Nonsmokers: 17 Smokers: 8 Nonsmokers: 5 Smokers: 7		Difference nonsmokers: -12 (-21.19 to -2.81) Difference smokers: -1 (-8.59 to -6.59)	Hospital admission data/ Acute Myocardial Infarction (ICD9 code: 410) patients without past cardiac history, hypertension, or high cholesterol

Table 6.2 Summary of studies on the impact of smoke-free legislation on cardiovascular health

Reference/location	Control	Study period	Number of cases	Percent reduction (95% CI)	Rate ratio (95% CI)	Data source/end point/comments
Cesaroni et al., 2008 Rome, Italy	None	*Pre-ban:* Jan 2000-Dec 2004 *Ban:* 10 Jan 2005 *Post-ban:* Jan-Dec 2005	11 939	35-64 yrs: 11.2 (6.9-15.3)	0.89† (0.85-0.93)	Values pre-ban used as reference Hospital admission data
			2136	65-74 yrs: 7.9 (3.4-12.2)	0.92† (0.88-0.97)	Acute Myocardial Infarction (ICD9 code: 410)
				75-84 yrs: NS	1.02† (0.98-1.07)	Acute and sub-acute ischaemic heart disease (ICD9 code: 411)
Edwards et al., 2008 Nationwide New Zealand	None	*Ban:* Dec 2004 Health data for the period 1996-2005 (including 12 months after introduction of ban)		Hospitalisation rates for acute asthma, acute stroke, unstable angina, and exacerbation of chronic obstructive pulmonary disease were lower in the 12 months after implementation of the legislation than in the 12 months before. However, no difference was apparent between these two periods when analysis adjusted for long term trends		Hospital admission data provided by the New Zealand Health Information Service
Lemstra et al., 2008 Saskatoon, Canada	None	*Pre-ban:* July 2000-June 2004 *Ban:* 1 July 2004 *Post-ban:* July 2004-June 2005	1377	All: 13 (10-16) reduction compared with mean for previous four years	176.1^ (165.3-186.3)	Hospital admission data for Acute Myocardial Infarction Note: Very small numbers; overlapping CIs for age adjusted admission rates
			312		152.4 (135.3-169.3)	
Pell et al., 2008 Nine Scottish Hospitals UK	None	*Pre-ban:* June 2005-March 2006 *Ban:* 26 March 2006 *Post-ban:* June 2006-March 2007	3235	All: 17 (16-18) Never smokers: 21 (18-24) Ex-smokers: 19 (17-21) Smokers: 14 (12-16)		Prospective study of all admissions to hospital with acute coronary syndrome (defined as chest pain with a detectable level of cardiac troponin in admission blood sample)
			2684			

* Age adjusted rate ratio
** Seasonally adjusted rate ratio
† Age adjusted rate ratio, controlling for outdoor PM_{10}, flu epidemic, holidays, and ambient temperature
NS=Statistically, not significant
^=Values reported are age-standardized incidence rates (cases per 100 000 population)

Indeed, the study authors estimate that implementation of the statewide ban without implementation of local laws would have been associated with a 19% reduction in AMI. As with the earlier studies, this one was limited by the absence of individual level data on variables such as occupation and smoking status, and the research design was unable to control for potential time-related confounders, such as long-term trends in smoking prevalence.

In spite of the limitations of these studies, the direction of the findings is consistent. In addition, there are now three large studies from Europe. The first is a study of the impact of the Italian smoking regulations on admission rates for AMI in Piedmont. Admission rates for October-December 2004 (pre-ban) and February-June 2005 (post-ban) were compared with admission rates in the corresponding periods one year earlier. Among men and women under age 60, the admissions for AMI for the period post-ban (February-June 2005) fell by 11% compared with February-June 2004 (RR=0.89; 95% CI=0.81-0.98). The rates of admissions decreased for both men (RR=0.91; 95% CI=0.82-1.01) and women (RR=0.75; 95% CI=0.58–0.96), but notably, no decrease was seen before the ban (comparison of October-December 2004 with October-December 2003). In addition, no decrease was observed in people over 60 years of age (RR=1.05; 95% CI=1.00-1.11). An analysis of hospital data 18 months post-legislation, found there was a cumulative reduction of 9% in hospital admissions for AMI in individuals under age 60 (Barone-Adesi et al., 2006).

A study in Rome also reported a fall in admissions for AMI and acute and sub-acute ischemic heart disease (IHD) in the year following implementation of the Italian smoking ban (Cesaroni et al., 2008). After controlling for outdoor air pollution (PM_{10}), flu epidemic, holidays, and ambient temperature, admissions in 35-64 year old patients fell by 11.2% (RR=0.89; 95% CI=0.85-0.93) and by 7.9% in 65-74 year olds (RR=0.92; 95% CI =0.88-0.97). There was no change in admissions in the oldest group aged 75-84 years. When further terms were included in the analysis for time trends and rates of hospitalisation, the reduction for 35-64 year olds was only marginally significant (RR=0.94; 95% CI =0.89-1.01), with a slightly stronger effect for 65-74 year olds (RR=0.90; 95% CI=0.84-0.94).

The only published study that has so far reported no evidence of effect comes from New Zealand. As part of a national evaluation of the 2004 smoke-free legislation, admission rates for AMI and unstable angina were tracked between 1997 and 2005 for the whole country (Edwards et al., 2008). A comprehensive ban on smoking in the workplace came into force in December 2004. Rates of admission due to AMI increased throughout the study period, counter to the trends in all coronary risk factors (with the exception of obesity), suggesting the increase was more likely due to changes in clinical practice (affecting re-admission rates and recording of diagnoses) than to a change in the underlying incidence of disease. Rates of admission for unstable angina decreased throughout the study period. After adjusting for underlying trends, there was no discernible change in admissions for AMI, unstable angina, or AMI and unstable angina combined, associated with the smoke-free legislation (Edwards et al., 2008). The New Zealand evaluation also analysed hospital admissions for acute asthma, acute stroke, and chronic obstructive pulmonary disease, but again, after adjusting for underlying trends and other potential influences on hospitalisation rates, there was no sign that rates were reduced in the 12 months after implementation of the smoke-free law (Edwards et al., 2008).

Because of the limitations of routine datasets, it is not possible without going back to case notes (as Seo & Torabi, 2007 did in a very small study) to ascertain individuals' smoking status, and thus any observed reductions in AMI admissions could be due to changes in smoking behaviour among smokers, or a reduction in exposure to SHS, or both. To some extent, this was overcome by modelling the impact of the observed reduction in smoking following the introduction of the Italian ban on AMI admissions (Barone-Adesi et al., 2006). It was estimated that the observed reduction in active smoking, after the introduction of the ban, could account for no more than a 0.7% reduction (0.6% among men, 0.9% among women) in admissions for AMI during the study period. Nevertheless, inability to ascertain smoking status (and level of SHS exposure) remains a major problem in interpreting study results in this, and other, time-series analyses.

To surmount the methodological problems associated with post-hoc analysis of routinely collected data, researchers in Scotland carried out a large prospective study of admissions for acute coronary syndrome (ACS) (Pell *et al.*, 2008) as part of a national evaluation of Scotland's smoke-free legislation (Haw *et al.*, 2006). Data on ACS admissions were collected prospectively on all patients admitted with ACS to nine Scottish hospitals over a ten month period prior to the smoke-free legislation (June 2005-March 2006 inclusive) and over the same ten month period following the ban (June 2006-March 2007 inclusive). ACS was defined as chest pain and raised I or T troponins in the admission blood sample. Participating hospitals accounted for 63% of all ACS admissions in Scotland during the pre-legislation period, and 64% post-legislation. Dedicated research nurses identified all eligible patients and completed structured interviews to confirm the diagnosis of ACS, to obtain information on demographic and socioeconomic status, self-reported smoking status, and information on SHS exposure. Blood samples taken on admission were tested for cotinine.

The number of ACS admissions in Scotland fell from 3235 pre-legislation to 2684, a 17% (95% CI=16-18%) reduction. The number of admissions per month fell across the whole period, and the monthly reduction increased with time from implementation of the legislation (chi-square trend, p=0.02). Amongst those admitted with ACS, the number of current smokers fell by 14% (95% CI=12-16%) from 1176 to 1016. There was a 19% (95% CI=17-22%) reduction in ACS admissions among ex-smokers from 953 to 769, and a 21% (95% CI=18-24%) reduction among never smokers from 677 to 537 (Table 6.2). The authors concluded that 56% of the admissions avoided post-legislation were in nonsmokers and never smokers, with a greater reduction among women (28%; 95% CI=23-33%) than men (13%; 95% CI=9-17%).

Following implementation of legislation, the observed drop in admissions was much greater than expected based solely on the underlying trend in ACS admissions. During the preceding 10 years, the fall each year in ACS admissions averaged 3% (95% CI=3-4%) with a maximum reduction of 9% in 2000. The post-legislation fall in admissions was not due to an increase in pre-hospital deaths from ACS. Death certificate data showed there was a 6% decline in pre-hospital deaths due to ACS, from 2202 in 2005/2006 to 2080 in 2006/2007. In England, where legislation had not yet been introduced, there was a 4% reduction in ACS admissions over a similar period.

In summary, the introduction of smoke-free legislation may influence cardiovascular disease by consequent reduction in active smoking (see Chapter 7), or by reduction in exposures to SHS (Dinno & Glantz, 2007). There is strong epidemiological evidence that exposure to SHS is associated with the development of coronary heart disease, and is backed up by experimental and clinical studies of the physiological effects of SHS (Samet, 2006). In smokers, it is estimated that the risk of coronary heart disease is halved one year after quitting smoking. Little research has been conducted to assess the reduction in risk after exposure to SHS has stopped, but current exposure to SHS appears to be more harmful than past exposures. At least one study found that the risk declines as more time elapses since the last exposure (Rosenlund *et al.*, 2001). This finding is consistent with the assumption that the acute effects of SHS exposure on platelet aggregation and epithelial function will be quickly reversed (U.S. Department of Health and Human Services, 2006) and that there is a rapid reversal of epithelial dysfunction when exposure to SHS ceases.

On the basis of what is known about the acute effects of SHS, it follows with a high degree of confidence that a substantial reduction in SHS will cause heart disease rates to fall, assuming there is no change in other risk factors. The magnitude of the reduction in disease due to comprehensive workplace smoking restrictions is less certain. A total of ten studies have now been published, nine reporting reductions in hospital admissions for AMI (six studies), acute coronary syndrome (one study), ischaemic heart disease and heart failure (one study), and AMI and ACS (one study) following implementation of smoke-free legislation. We know of no study reporting negative results (i.e. an absence of an effect of legislation) apart from the New Zealand evaluation. The research reported so far includes only a small fraction of all populations that have implemented state, municipal, or national restrictions on smoking (Chapter 3), raising the possibility that publication and reporting bias may be active. The four studies which found the largest reductions in hospital admissions (along the order of 30%) were based on relatively small populations and included only a small number of admission events. The bigger studies, which covered large geographical areas and included thousands of cases (i.e. Italy, Scotland, and New York State), but did not include control areas, found smaller reductions of between 8% and 17%. This effect size is closer to what one would expect from first epidemiologic principles, based on the change in prevalence of exposure and the strength of the association between SHS and CHD, according to the standard formula for Population Attributable Risk (Population Attributable Risk = Pe (RR-1)/ [Pe (RR-1) + 1], where Pe is prevalence of exposure, RR is relative risk). Applying this formula, if the legislation caused a 40% reduction in population exposure to SHS (as reported in Scotland), and that exposure to SHS increases the risk of CHD by 30% (Chapter 2), then the risk of CHD would be projected to fall by 10.7%.

The Scottish study (Pell *et al.*, 2008) contains the strongest evidence so far of cause and effect. The researchers ascertained the smoking status of patients admitted to the hospital, applied a common diagnostic standard throughout the study period, and found a reduction in rate of hospital admission for ACS in both nonsmokers and smokers alike (although the reduction in admission rates for smokers was smaller). It was possible to relate the change in admission rates

to a reduction of nearly 40% in exposure to SHS at a population level in Scotland, all of which adds weight to the argument that the before/after reduction in ACS admissions in nonsmokers can be attributed at least in part to the smoke-free legislation. Since the Scottish legislation was recently introduced (2006), the evaluation thus far includes data for only a short time post-smoking ban, and further follow-up is needed to confirm the reduction in disease burden is sustained.

Epidemiological studies have also established associations between SHS exposure and other conditions, such as chronic respiratory disease and stroke, but to date no study has yet reported a reduction in these conditions following implementation of smoke-free legislation. It will be 10-20 years before the impact of smoke-free laws on lung cancer morbidity and mortality can be assessed.

Summary

In the past, voluntary restrictions on smoking in the workplace have been an important vehicle for reducing exposure to SHS in many countries. However, such restrictions have uneven coverage, and are generally not applied in some of the highest exposure settings (such as bars and gaming venues). Further, they have typically offered little protection for groups in the working population with the poorest health status, and therefore increase the likelihood of widening health inequalities. Comprehensive, mandatory restrictions do not have these shortcomings.

Studies of smoke-free legislation, that prohibits smoking in virtually

all indoor workplaces, consistently demonstrate reduced exposure to SHS in high-risk settings by 80-90%. The residual exposures are likely caused by seepage of SHS from smoking around the boundaries of venues, including designated smoking areas on patios and verandas. As a result, indoor smoke-free workplace laws greatly reduce, but do not remove altogether, the potential for harm to health caused by SHS around bars, restaurants, and similar settings.

The most comprehensive study to date indicates that legislation may reduce exposure to SHS population-wide by up to 40%. Several large, well-designed studies have found that comprehensive smoke-free policies do not lead to increased exposure to SHS in the home. Another important feature of comprehensive legislation is its impact on inequalities; the largest absolute reductions in exposure to SHS in the workplace tend to occur among those groups that had the highest pre-legislation exposures.

Given the relatively recent introduction of comprehensive bans, there is only one study reporting on sustained changes in SHS exposure. More than 10 years of follow-up data from California show that the early, large reductions in SHS exposure have been maintained.

There are short-term improvements in health linked to these restrictions on smoking. Workforce studies have reported reductions in acute respiratory illnesses after smoking bans, and early findings of substantial declines in hospital admissions for acute myocardial infarction have been replicated in numerous studies. The literature also indicates that wide-ranging bans on smoking in the workplace are followed by as much as a 10-20% reduction in hospital admissions for acute coronary events in the general population in the first year post-ban. At present, it is not possible to distinguish the contributions to the decline in hospital admissions from changes in smoking behaviour and those of reduced exposures to SHS. The precise magnitude of the reduction in admissions is uncertain, but will vary with the background incidence of heart disease, the prevalence of exposure to SHS preceding the ban, and the extent of the legislation and its implementation.

SHS increases the risk of lung cancer, but the time period from exposure to evident disease may be 10-20 years or longer, making it difficult to link changes in disease rates with introduction of smoking restrictions. However, given the strength of the evidence linking SHS to increased risk of lung cancer, the reduction in exposure following smoke-free legislation is expected to ultimately be reflected in a decrease in the incidence of this particular disease.

Chapter 7
The effect of mandated smoking restrictions on smoking behaviour

Introduction

The primary reason for smoking restrictions is to protect nonsmokers from secondhand tobacco smoke (SHS). Restrictions on smoking also help make tobacco use less socially acceptable and reduce opportunities to smoke. Therefore, it would be expected that besides protecting nonsmokers, smoking restrictions would also tend to reduce smoking prevalence and consumption in smokers. The purpose of this chapter is to further explore if and how mandated restrictions in various settings (e.g. public places, workplaces) might act in this manner, and to present results from a number of studies that have investigated this issue. Smoking restrictions in the home are by agreement among household members, and are considered separately in Chapter 8.

Methodological issues

Identification of relevant literature

A preliminary search of the Web of Science, covering the publication period from January 1, 1990 to March 30, 2008, including the title subjects (TS) ('Smoke Free' SAME ban*) OR TS=('Smoke Free' SAME polic*) OR

TS=('Smoke Free' SAME legislation) OR TS=('Smoke Free' SAME Law*), generated a preliminary, extensive list of articles. Papers identified from this search were reviewed for relevance to the topic of the effect of smoking restrictions on smoking behaviour. Additional searches of PubMed paired various permutations of smoke-free (e.g. smoking restrictions, smoking rules, etc.) with words describing venues (e.g. workplaces, worksites, homes (Chapter 8), schools, etc.) and words related to smoking behaviour (e.g. smoking prevalence, smoking initiation, cigarette consumption, smoking cessation, etc.). Several studies that were particularly appropriate were used as templates to extract "related articles." These lists of related articles were then scanned for additional relevant studies. More pertinent articles were found in the references cited by the studies already identified. These were obtained and examined for further citations until no further studies were identified. While this procedure does not ensure that all relevant studies were captured, it goes well beyond a single set of search criteria.

Typical study designs

There are several typical study designs found in the body of research summarised in this chapter. These are commented on throughout, but a few general characteristics of such studies are mentioned briefly here.

Some studies compare smoking behaviour before and following the implementation of new smoking restrictions. Unless a comparable group of people, not subject to the new restrictions, is available for comparison purposes, it cannot be decided whether any changes observed in the group subject to the new restrictions resulted from the restrictions or were simply following a population secular trend. Using multiple observation points before the new restrictions were implemented would help establish any existing secular trend. In some cases, changes are studied using data from large, cross-sectional population surveys, conducted before and after the new restrictions. This approach assumes that no changes in the composition of the population have occurred that might be related to smoking behaviour. In population studies, changes in population composition could be from immigration or emigration, and in surveys of worksites, those who quit or take a job in a given workplace might self select according to workplace smoking policy. Advantages of the cross-sectional approach are that the surveys are usually large and representative of the population.

Single cross-sectional population survey samples cannot establish causality, but only identify associations. For instance, while people subject to smoking restrictions might smoke less, it may be because of the restrictions, or because of some other characteristic (e.g. higher socioeconomic status or health consciousness) that is related both to their likelihood of smoking and to their being in a situation where smoking is or is not restricted. These cross-sectional studies examined the correlation between the presence of smoking restrictions and such outcomes as smoking status, consumption, making a recent quit attempt, or intention to quit smoking. These measures are described in Appendix 2.

In other studies, a cohort of subjects interviewed before the new smoking restrictions were implemented is followed-up again months or years later and re-interviewed. The cohort (or longitudinal) approach usually involves fewer subjects, and while this design is particularly appropriate for studying changes in individuals' smoking behaviour over time (e.g. cessation), typically a significant percentage of the subjects is lost to follow-up. If the group lost differs in some important respect (e.g. propensity to quit smoking or

switched to a job where smoking is not restricted) to the group successfully followed, the results can be compromised. Behavioural outcomes typically examined in these longitudinal studies were changes in consumption and in smoking status.

Conventions for reporting results

Many of the studies reviewed used some form of multivariate logistic regression analysis to relate smoking restrictions to various aspects of smoking behaviour. Unless otherwise specified, the results cited in this chapter are adjusted odds ratios (OR) together with their 95% confidence intervals (CI). Typically, such analyses adjusted for a number of demographic and other factors. Generally, if the odds ratio fails to include 1.0, it is statistically significant. In a few cases, rounding leads to a value of 1.0 as the upper or lower 95% confidence limit, but if the author indicated that the odds ratio was significant, it is reported as significant here. Most of theses studies do not report p-values for the odds ratios if they give 95% confidence intervals. Report of actual p-values or p-value thresholds were more common in studies employing multiple linear regression models. In this chapter, results are reported as the authors presented them.

Scope of chapter

The prevalence of workplace smoking restrictions and who is subject to them is described in Chapters 5 and 6, and issues related to economic impact are presented in Chapter 4.

Here the focus in on how smoking restrictions in the workplace and in other settings might affect both adult and youth smoking behaviour.

The first section below looks at changes in smoking behaviour following the implementation of new laws restricting smoking. It also reviews studies that correlate the strength and breadth of smoking restrictions in specific localities to the smoking behaviour of the residents there, both adults and youth. The second section is concerned with the effect of workplace smoking policies on workers' smoking behaviour, and the last section examines the evidence for an effect of smoke-free school campuses for everyone, not just students, on youth smoking behaviour.

Mandated restrictions on smoking and population level smoking behaviour

There are two types of studies that address the impact of mandated restrictions on smoking behaviour: those that compare pre-law and post-law smoking behaviour within a specific population subject to a new law, and those that correlate variable strength and extent of local laws restricting smoking with smoking behaviour in the same localities. This section reviews both types of studies.

Pre- versus post-law studies

Most studies of the assessment of changes after the implementation of local, regional, or national anti-smoking laws (such as those implemented in Ireland, Italy or

Norway) or comprehensive tobacco control programmes (such as those implemented in the USA: California, Massachusetts or New York City) have used data collected on a periodic basis in health interview surveys or in more specific tobacco surveys. These studies select representative samples of the adult population (mostly ≥18 years), with comparable methods and measures across time.

In some studies, the analysis is limited to simple before and after comparisons of adult smoking prevalence, but a number of studies analysed trends over time, including estimates from several surveys before and after the law or programme was implemented. A few studies have combined data from different surveys to reconstruct birth and age-cohorts for the analysis of smoking prevalence and cessation over longer periods of time. Some studies have modeled the effect of the law or the total programme by means of indicator variables for when the intervention commenced in the regression models used for the statistical analysis. Also, a few evaluations have used 'control groups' (comparison populations not exposed to the law or programme), or other designs such as prospective cohort studies. The studies in each section below are discussed in order according to the time the new law was implemented.

Before/after law implementation comparisons

Two articles have evaluated the effects of smoking restrictions using two independent cross-sectional surveys: one before and one after the implementation of a new law restricting smoking. These were in Madrid Region, Spain (Galàn *et al.*, 2007), and Scotland, UK (Table 7.1), and assessed the entire population (Haw & Gruer, 2007). Another study (Braverman *et al.*, 2008) used a longitudinal sample to look for changes in smoking behaviour in hospitality workers following law implementation.

In Spain, a comprehensive law on smoking prevention and control implemented in 2006 included a prohibition on smoking in all enclosed workplaces, with the exception of the hospitality sector. The law called for only partial restrictions in the hospitality sector with venues larger than 100m^2 mandated to be smoke-free, but owners could decide to have separated, ventilated smoking areas of less than 30% of the total floor area. In venues <100m^2, however, smoke-free environments were not compulsory and depended on the owner's decision. An early evaluation of the impact of the law on secondhand smoke (SHS) exposure at the population level in the Region of Madrid (including the city of Madrid) included information on the prevalence of smoking (Galàn *et al.*, 2007). Using the continuous Behavioural Risk Factors Survey System, two independent telephone surveys were carried out among the adult (18-64 years) population before the law (October-November 2005; n=1750) and after the law (January-July 2006; n=1252). The surveys collected information on active and involuntary smoking. The prevalence of smoking was similar both before (31.7%) and after the law (32.7%) was implemented.

In Scotland, a law to prohibit smoking in virtually all enclosed places and workplaces including bars, restaurants, and cafes was implemented by March 2006. The comprehensive evaluation of the impact of the law (Haw *et al.*, 2006) has included the assessment of changes of the exposure to SHS of the adult population (Haw & Gruer, 2007). From this study, the short-term effect of the law on smoking prevalence in the adult population can be derived, although the study was designed to assess SHS exposure (self-reported in a questionnaire and measured by means of saliva cotinine concentrations). Two independent cross-sectional surveys among representative samples of the adult (18-74 years) population were conducted before (September-November 2005 and January-March 2006; n=1815) and after (September-December 2006 and January-April 2007; n=1834) the law was implemented. No apparent short-term changes in the adult tobacco use prevalence among Scottish adults was found: the prevalence of smoking (cigarettes, pipes, or cigars) was 35.6% in the pre-law survey and 35.1% in the post-law survey.

These two studies (Galàn *et al.*, 2007; Haw & Gruer, 2007) were designed to assess changes in SHS exposure, and from questions used to characterise smoking status, smoking prevalence rates can be derived. However, the articles did not include a specific analysis of smoking prevalence beyond presenting the prevalence rates within a descriptive table (Galàn *et al.*, 2007) or within a descriptive paragraph in the results section (Haw & Gruer, 2007).

Table 7.1 Studies comparing smoking behaviour pre- and post-implementation of new laws restricting smoking

Reference Location	Population and design	Year of assessment	Type of intervention (law)	Outcomes assessed	Covariates and analysis	Results	Comments
Single cross-sectional pre- versus post- new law comparisons of population smoking prevalence							
Galán et al., 2007 Madrid Region, Spain	Adults (18-64 years). BRFSS surveys before/after law. 2 surveys; n0=1750; n1=1252	Pre-law Oct-Nov 2005 Post-law June-July 2006	Comprehensive law covering all enclosed places, with partial restrictions in hospitality venues, effective Jan 2006	Smoking prevalence	Simple, no adjustment for covariates (see comments)	Smoking prevalence pre-law (31.7%) and post-law (32.7%) were not statistically different.	Response rates: 77% pre- and 66% post-law. The paper is aimed at evaluating changes in SHS exposure in different settings, but it also presents smoking prevalence.
Haw & Gruer, 2007 Scotland, UK	Adults (18-74 years). Face-to-face at-home interviews. 2 surveys: n0=1815; n1=1834	Pre-law Sept 2005-Mar 2006 Post-law Sept 2006-April 2007	Comprehensive law including smoking prohibition in hospitality venues, effective March 2006	Prevalence of tobacco use (cigarettes, pipes, or cigars)	Simple, no adjustment for covariates (see comments)	Tobacco use prevalence pre-law (35.6%) and post-law (35.2%) were not statistically different.	Response rates around 70%. The paper is aimed at evaluating changes in SHS exposure, but it also presents tobacco use prevalence.
Longitudinal study pre- versus post- new law comparisons of hospitality workers							
Braverman et al., 2008* Norway	Longitudinal study of 1525 restaurant and bar employees.	Pre-law and 4 and 11 months post-law	Comprehensive smoke-free policy, June 2004	Smoking prevalence and daily cigarette consumption	No covariates	Significant declines in prevalence and consumption were identified from baseline to 4 months, with behaviour stable between 4 and 11 months. Prevalence of daily smoking declined 3.6%, daily smoking at work declined by 6.2%, the number of cigarettes smoked by continuing smokers declined 1.55 CPD, and the number of cigarettes smoked at work by 1.63 CPD. Occasional smoking was stable across all three survey waves.	Analysis of sample attrition suggested results unaffected. Attrition mostly due to job changing. The authors suggested that the stable rates between 4 and 11 months indicate that the initial drop was because of the law, and not a result of a secular trend for decreased smoking

Multiple cross-sectional population surveys or other data pre- and post- new law

Reference Location	Population and design	Year of assessment	Type of intervention (law)	Outcomes assessed	Covariates and analysis	Results	Comments
Heloma et al., 2001; Heloma & Jaakkola, 2003. Helsinki metropolitan area, Finland	Adult employees. Trends. Sample of workplaces (n=8). Self-administered questionnaire. Before/after law. 3 surveys: n0=880; n1=940; n2=659	1994-5; 1995-6; 1998. Law passed on March 1995	Smoking prevalence. Mean number cigarettes smoked	Simple analysis, by sex. No adjustment for potential confounders		Prevalence smoking 1994-5: 29.8% 1995-6: 24.6% 1998: 25.2%; p trend <0.05. Mean cigarettes smoked 1994-5: 19 CPD 1995-6: 16 CPD 1998: 16 CPD. Smoking at work 1994-5: 83.1% 1995-6: 47.4% 1998: 31.1%; p trend <0.05	2 papers (2001 & 2003) with results 1 year after and 3 years after the law. Response rates: 69%; 74%; not known 3rd survey. Reduction significant only among men (33.1%; 26.9%; 24.8%), whilst increase among women (22.0%, 18.4%; 21.1%)
Galeone et al., 2006. Italy (country-wide)	Changes in indicators of tobacco consumption and NRT use. Trends. Pre/post law.	Monthly sales Jan 2005 through Nov 2005	Comprehensive smoke-free policy, Jan 2005	Cigarettes sales (in Kg), per capita sales (packs per capita) and sales of NRT products	No covariates, differences not statistically analysed	Decline cig sales: -5.7%. Decline per capita consumption: -6.6% (previous declines before law were 2.8% between 2003 and 2004, and 1.3% between 2002 and 2003). Increase in sales of NRT products: 10.5%.	
Gallus et al., 2007. Italy (country-wide)	>15 years. Face-to-face interview. Before/after law. 3 surveys: n0=6534; n1=6585; n2=6153	2001-2; 2003-4; 2005-6. Law effective Jan 2005	National law prohibiting smoking in all enclosed workplaces (smoking areas allowed in hospitality sector under strict conditions)	Adult smoking prevalence. Mean CPD	Simple analysis, by sex and age. No adjustment for potential confounders	Prevalence smoking 2001-02: 27.8% 2003-04: 27.0% 2005-06: 25.0%; p<0.05 versus 2003-4. Mean cigarettes smoked 2004: 15.4 CPD 2006: 13.9 CPD Not statistically tested	Response rate: quota sample. Reduction significant in men (2003-04 versus 2005-06: 31.7% versus 29.0%), but not in women (22.5% versus 21.2%), and in <45 years (32.4% versus 30.0%), but not ≥45 years (20.5% versus 20.2%).

Table 7.1 Studies comparing smoking behaviour pre- and post-implementation of new laws restricting smoking

Multiple cross-sectional population surveys or other data pre- and post- new law

Reference Location	Population and design	Year of assessment	Type of intervention (law)	Outcomes assessed	Covariates and analysis	Results	Comments
Edwards et al., 2008 New Zealand (country-wide)	Overview evaluation NZ Smoke-free Environments Amendment Act (SEAA) 2003. Annual cross-sectional population surveys conducted as part of the evaluation.	1997-2005	SEAA 2003	Adult and youth prevalence and cigarette consumption (sales)	Only qualitative comments regarding smoking behaviour presented	There did not appear to be any discernable effect of SEAA on adult smoking prevalence or overall cigarette consumption. Youth prevalence declined, but not differrently than what would be expected from on-going trend.	
Office of Tobacco Control, 2007 Ireland	Monthly surveys (n=1000) of persons aged 15+ years	June 2003 to Dec 2007	Comprehensive smoke-free law March 2004	Running average of smoking prevalence	No statistical analysis presented	Prevalence: March 2004: 25.5% March 2005: 23.8% April 2006: 24.5%	Short-term decline appeared to be partially reversed.

Studies where laws restricting smoking were part of multiple tobacco control measures implemented. Generally, studies involved multiple, representative cross-sectional population surveys

Reference Location	Population and design	Year of assessment	Type of intervention (law)	Outcomes assessed	Covariates and analysis	Results	Comments
Emmanuel et al., 1988 Singapore	Pre-post cross-sectional surveys of persons aged 15 years and older, n=92 500 in 1984 n=78 600 in 1987	1984-1987	National Smoking Control Programme of 1986	Adult and youth smoking prevalence, per capita tobacco consumption	Simple comparisons pre versus post new law	**Adult** (15+ years) prevalence 1984: 19.0% 1987: 13.6%, $p<0.01$ **Youth** (15-19 years) prevalence 1984: 5.1% 1987: 2.9%, no p-value reported Per capita consumption 1984: 3.21 kg/person 1987: 2.38 kg/person, no p-value reported	
Pierce et al., 1998b; Gilpin et al., 2001 California versus rest of USA	18+ years. Different health and tobacco interview surveys: NHIS, CTS, BRFS/CATS,	1982-1999 (tobacco sales) 1978-1999 (adult smoking prevalence)	California Tobacco Control Programme (1989). Includes new taxes on cigarettes, laws restricting	Per capita cig consumption (1983-1999) Adult (≥18 y) smoking prevalence (1978-1999)	Prevalence standardised for age, race, and education level. Piecewise linear regression	Pre-programme annual rate of decline in per capita consumption was -0.46/ packs in CA, and -.35 in the rest	

Studies where laws restricting smoking were part of multiple tobacco control measures implemented. Generally, studies involved multiple, representative cross-sectional population surveys

Reference Location	Population and design	Year of assessment	Type of intervention (law)	Outcomes assessed	Covariates and analysis	Results	Comments
Pierce et al., 1998b; Gilpin et al., 2001 California versus rest of USA	and CPS. Tobacco sales from the Tobacco Institute		smoking, mass media, local media, local agency actions, research, and school education programmes.	Several periods: pre-programme 1978-1989; early period 1989-1993; middle period 1994-1996, late period; 1996-1999		of the USA. In the early period these rates were significantly different at -0.58 versus -.40. In the middle period the rates of -.16 and -0.7 were not significantly different, but in the later period, they were: -1.56 versus -0.78.

Only in the early period was the rate of annual decline in prevalence different from that in the rest of the USA (-1.01 versus -0.51). | |
| Laugesen & Swinburn, 2000 New Zealand | Annual cross-sectional surveys of 10 000+ persons aged 15+ years each year | 1985-1998 | Tobacco Control Programme of 1985-1998 | Adult and youth smoking prevalence, per capita tobacco consumption | Simple comparisons and comparisons of trends in New Zealand and other countries with comparable data over this period | **Adult** (15+ years) prevalence 1985: 30% 1998: 26% **Youth** (15-24 years) prevalence 1985: 35% 1998: 29% Per capita consumption 1985: 2493 1995: 1472 | New Zealand ranked 8th in the extent of decline in adult prevalence among 21 countries. It ranked 3rd in the decline of youth prevalence among 17 countries with comparable data. In 1995 New Zealand was second lowest in per capita consumption. |
| Biener et al., 2000. Massachusetts (MA), USA; with comparison to rest of states, excluding California | Adult population (18-64 years) Trends. Telephone interview. BRFSS survey. Sample size around 1500 subjects (between | Adult smoking prevalence: 1989-1999 | MA Tobacco Control Programme: 1: mass media campaign; 2: services (treatments, youth programmes, telephone | Adult (≥18 years) cigarette per capita consumption Adult smoking prevalence | Simple trend analysis Simple linear regression with splines | Before 1993 (tax operating), the decline was similar in MA (-15%) and the comparison states (-14%) (annual decline of 3-4%). In 1993, MA decline was 12%, | |

Table 7.1 Studies comparing smoking behaviour pre- and post-implementation of new laws restricting smoking

Studies where laws restricting smoking were part of multiple tobacco control measures implemented. Generally, studies involved multiple, representative cross-sectional population surveys

Reference Location	Population and design	Year of assessment	Type of intervention (law)	Outcomes assessed	Covariates and analysis	Results	Comments
Biener *et al.*, 2000. Massachusetts (MA), USA; with comparison to rest of states, excluding California	1221 in 1989 to almost 1800 in 1997; with 4944 subjects in 1999). Data tobacco sales from the Tobacco Institute		counseling educational materials); 3: promotion of local policies The MA TC programme funding comes from a surcharge of 25 cents per dollar implemented in January 1993			compared to 4% in the comparison states, followed by a continuous 4% year decline in MA versus just 1%/year in the rest of the states. Decline in smoking prevalence in MA from 24% in 1989 to 19% in 1999, with a significant slope of -0.43%/year (-0.66 to -0.21%/year) after 1992. Decline in rest of the USA from 25% to 23.5% in 1992, and no significant changes thereafter (slope after 1992 of -0.03).	
Helakorpi *et al.*, 2004, 2008 Finland (country-wide)	15-64 years. Trends. Self-administered postal questionnaire. Pool of surveys (~5000 subjects per year, 33 080 men and 34 991 women)	1979 to 2002	Tobacco Act (1976)	Smoking prevalence by birth cohorts by sex	Age, period, and cohort analysis, by sex, and by SES (second paper) Logistic regression to assess the effect of age, cohort, and the 1976 Tobacco Act	**Paper 1.** Prevalence declined concurrent to 1976 Tobacco Act in men and women OR men=0.74 (p<0.05) OR women* cohort=0.45, 0.34, and 0.26 (p<0.05). **Paper 2.** Men, declining cohort trend in all SES groups. Women, increasing in early cohort and declining thereafter.	Average response rate 70% men and 79% women. Second paper adds socioeconomic status by means of record linkage (health interview-census): entrepreneur, farmer, upper white collar, lower white collar, blue collar. * Values correspond to birth cohorts: 1961-1965, 1966-1970, 1971-1975 respectively

Studies where laws restricting smoking were part of multiple tobacco control measures implemented. Generally, studies involved multiple, representative cross-sectional population surveys

Reference Location	Population and design	Year of assessment	Type of intervention (law)	Outcomes assessed	Covariates and analysis	Results	Comments
Frieden et al., 2005 Centers for Disease Control and Prevention, 2007c New York City	Adult (≥18 years). BRFSS surveys and ad hoc surveys. Telephone questionnaire. Multi-language Approximately 10 000 subject per survey.	"Background" prevalence from 1993-2001 surveys. Pre-law survey: 2002; post-law 2003. Centers for Disease Control and Prevention paper adds surveys for 2005 and 2006	Tobacco Control strategy, including: 1: Increased tax; 2: Smoke-free Air Act 2002 (March 2003) for all indoor workplaces; 3: guidelines to physicians + NRT; 4: education through broadcast and print media; 5: systematic evaluation (surveys)	Adult smoking prevalence % heavy smokers (>10 CPD) Average CPD	Analysis by age groups, race/ethnicity, sex, district, income, education, place of birth. Changes in % from rate ratios, derived from ORs calculated by means of age-adjusted logistic regression models.	No changes in smoking prevalence during the 10 years preceding the 2002 programme (21.5%) Smoking prevalence: 2002: 21.6% (23.4% men; 19.8% women); 2003: 19.2% (21.6% men; 17.2% women); 11.3% decrease (p<0.05) Significant decrease in men and women, all age groups except ≥65 years (larger at 18-24 years), all race groups (significant only among non-Hispanic blacks and Hispanics), all education groups (larger and significant only for "some college"). Decrease in heavy smoking from 8.0% (2002) to 6.2% (p<0.05). Decrease from 11.2 CPD (2002) to 10.6 CPD (2003).	Response rates 2002-2003: around 60%. The groups that experienced the largest declines in smoking prevalence were young people, women, people in lowest and highest income brackets, people with higher educational levels, and heavy smokers. Centers for Disease Control and Prevention paper with 2005 and 2006 data confirms previous findings 2002: 21.6% 2005: 18.9% 2006: 17.5% Decrease in men and women, all age groups (2002-2006), and all educational groups (larger among more educated).

Table 7.1 Studies comparing smoking behaviour pre- and post-implementation of new laws restricting smoking

Incidence of smoking cessation, no direct evaluation of new laws restricting smoking

Reference Location	Population and design	Year of assessment	Type of intervention (law)	Outcomes assessed	Covariates and analysis	Results	Comments
Gilpin & Pierce, 2002a USA	20-50 years. Trends. (7 surveys from 1965 to 1992). Face-to-face at-home questionnaire. Pool of surveys yielded 140 199 subjects.	1950-1990	Partial restrictions in 1978, 1986, and 1988	Incidence of quitting smoking	Analysis by age, sex, ethnicity, and educational level	Increase in quitting from <1% to 5%. Gender differences occurred following the beginning of public health campaigns (danger to the fetus). Quitting increased among younger smokers in the 1970s, around nonsmokers' rights movement. Quitting incidence was larger among more educated subjects (some college).	Effect of smoking restrictions or campaigns not directly assessed with statistical models.
Schiaffino et al., 2007 Spain	≥20 years. Trends. 5 surveys (1993, 1995, 1997, 2001, and 2003). Face-to-face at-home. Pool of surveys yielded 33 532 subjects.	1965-2000	Partial restrictions in 1978, 1986, and 1988	Incidence of quitting smoking	Analysis by age, sex, and educational level	Increase in quitting incidence 20-50 years: men (0.5% to 4.9%) women (1.1% to 5.0%) Larger increases ≥50 years, 8% by 2000. Differences according to education: level-off in men and women with primary or less than primary education, while cessation incidence among more educated continued to increase.	Effect of restrictions not assessed in models. No clear pattern according to laws and decrees passed. None of them prohibited smoking in workplaces or promoted NRT treatments.

Respondent report/perceptions regarding changes in smoking due to law

Reference Location	Population and design	Year of assessment	Type of intervention (law)	Outcomes assessed	Covariates and analysis	Results	Comments
Hammond et al., 2004 Ontario, Canada	191 former smokers who quit before and after new law	2001	Before and after law (January 2000) restricting smoking and requiring new warning labels on cigarette packages	Cite restrictions as motivation to quit Cite warning labels as motivation to quit	Logistic regression adjusted for age, sex, CPD prior to quitting, and number of years smoked. Indicator variable included for quit pre- and post-law	Increase in those citing smoking restrictions as motivation OR=3.06; 95% CI=1.02-9.19 Increase in those citing warning labels as motivation OR=2.78; 95% CI=1.20-5.94	
Fong et al., 2006 Ireland	Representative longitudinal sample of the adult ≥18 years) smoking population (n=1679) before law and followed-up after law (n=769)	Dec/Jan 2003-04 and Dec/Jan 2004/05	Before and after new law (implemented March 2004)	In smokers (n=640): Had the law made them more likely to quit? Had the law made them cut CPD? In quitters (n=119): Had the law made them more likely to quit? Helped them to stay quit?	Report of simple percentages and 95% CIs	46% (41-50%) 60% (55-65%) 80% (71-88%) 88% (81-95%)	

*Braverman study not cross-sectional
BRFS/CATS = Behavioral Risk Factor Survey/California Adult Tobacco Survey
BRFSS = Behavioral Risk Factor Surveillance System
CPD = Cigarettes per day
CPS = Current Population Survey
CTS = California Tobacco Survey
NHIS = National Health Interview Surveys
SES = Socioeconomic status
SHS = Secondhand smoke

If the studies were designed to assess changes in SHS exposure, they might not have been adequately powered (sample size too small) to detect changes in prevalence. In both studies, moreover, the post-law survey was conducted within a year after law implementation (six months in Spain and within the first year in Scotland) so that there was limited likelihood of observing any potential effect of the restrictions on smoking prevalence.

The short-term effects of Norway's comprehensive clean air policy, that took effect in June 2004, were evaluated (Braverman et al., 2008). A longitudinal sample of randomly selected restaurant and bar employees was used; subjects were interviewed at baseline immediately before the policy and at four and 11 months afterwards. Sample attrition was considerable, but extensive analyses of those followed and not followed led the researchers to conclude that it was unlikely that attrition would affect the study results. Restaurant and bar employees were chosen for study, because they are relatively younger (changes in smoking would have long-term health benefits), they have historically experienced high levels of exposure to SHS in the workplace, and they have relatively higher smoking rates than the general population (52.9% daily versus 26.3% in a similarly aged group from the general population). Significant declines in prevalence and consumption were identified from baseline to four months, with behaviour stable between four and 11 months. Prevalence of daily smoking declined 3.6 percentage points, daily smoking at work

declined by 6.2 percentage points, the number of cigarettes smoked by continuing smokers declined 1.55 cigarettes per day (CPD), and the number of cigarettes smoked at work by 1.63 CPD. Occasional smoking was stable across all three survey waves. The authors concluded that the stable rates between four and 11 months mean that the initial drop was real and not just a result of a secular trend for decreased smoking.

While the longitudinal study (Braverman et al., 2008) found a short-term effect, the repeated cross-sectional studies did not. In the cross-sectional approach, cessation would have to offset initiation and relapse of former smokers to current smoking to show an effect, but the longitudinal study involved only smokers at baseline, so a change in prevalence in the same subjects would be due to cessation, assuming no bias due to sample attrition.

Trends from multiple cross-sectional surveys before/after new laws

A number of studies have evaluated pre-post legislation changes in the prevalence of smoking using trends across time by means of repeated representative population cross-sectional surveys (Table 7.1). Two of these papers present Finnish data with reference to smoking in workers in Metropolitan Helsinki (Heloma et al., 2001; Heloma & Jaakkola, 2003). Other papers are from New Zealand (Edwards et al., 2008) and Italy (Galeone et al., 2006; Gallus et al., 2007). Online data are available for Ireland (Office of Tobacco Control, 2007).

In March 1995, an amendment to the previous 1976 Tobacco Act took effect in Finland. The 1995 Act prohibited smoking in all workplaces; however, the employer could implement it by means of a total prohibition or by allowing designated smoking rooms with separate ventilation systems and lower air pressure. The 1976 law prohibited smoking in most public places, along with a number of other tobacco control measures.

Studies to evaluate the short-term (one year) (Heloma et al., 2001) and long-term (three years) (Heloma & Jaakkola, 2003) impact of the new law implemented in 1995 were conducted among representative samples of the working population in the Helsinki Metropolitan area. Repeated in-dependent cross-sectional surveys were conducted among employees in a sample of nine medium-sized and large workplaces (eight participating in the three surveys), including 880 workers at baseline before the law in 1994-95, 940 workers in 1995-96 one year after the law, and 659 workers three years after the law. Information on smoking status, including mean CPD and whether smokers smoked at work were collected using a self-administered questionnaire. The main results indicate a significant trend for a reduction in smoking prevalence, from 29.8% at baseline to 24.6% and 25.2% at short- and long-term post legislation. However, this reduction was only present among men (33.1% at baseline, 26.9% at one year later, 24.8% at three years, *p for trend* =0.026), but not among women (22.0% at baseline, 18.4% at one year, 26.1% at three years, *p for trend* =0.128). Cigarette consumption declined from 19 CPD at baseline to 16 CPD at three years after the law (difference not statistically tested). With regard to smoking during work shifts, a substantial reduction was observed; while 83.1% of smokers said they smoked at work before the law, this percentage was reduced to 47.4% and 31.1% at the short- and long-term evaluations (*p for trend* <0.05).

A recent paper provides an overview of evaluations of the implementation of the New Zealand 2003 Smoke-free Environments Amendment Act (SEAA) (Edwards *et al.*, 2008). SEAA introduced a range of tobacco control measures, including smoke-free schools and early childhood centers beginning in January 2004, and it extended smoke-free status to nearly all other indoor workplaces, including bars, casinos, members' clubs, and restaurants in December 2004. As part of the evaluation, the effects on smoking behaviour were mentioned briefly. Based on a series of annual cross-sectional smoking surveys in random samples of the population, the authors stated:

"Youth smoking rates decreased significantly between 2004 and 2005, but in line with long-term trends with no discernable effect of the SEAA. There was also a small reduction in reported parental smoking in the year 10 survey between 2004 and 2005. The per capita release of tobacco onto the New Zealand market (a marker for overall consumption) was fairly constant from 2003-5, with no evidence of any change in 2005 following implementation of the SEAA."

These comments do not suggest a notable impact of SEAA on smoking behaviour. Other effects reported included reductions in socially-cued smoking in hospitality settings, increased calls to the national quitline, and the dispensing of vouchers for nicotine replacement therapy (NRT) via the quitline service.

Ireland implemented its smoke-free law in March 2004. The Office of Tobacco Control conducts monthly quota telephone surveys of 1000 persons aged 15 years or older. Results are weighted to standard demographics and a 12-month running average is computed to smooth the data (Office of Tobacco Control, 2005). After June 2003, the first month depicted in the smoothed trend plot, smoking prevalence increased to 25.5% in March 2004. It then declined fairly steadily to 23.8% in March 2005, but increased again to 24.5% in April 2006. Between then and July 2007, it remained fairly steady at between 24.5% and 24.8%. Another decline was apparent beginning in August 2007 that brought prevalence down to 24.0% by December 2007, the latest point plotted (Office of Tobacco Control, 2007). Thus, there appeared to be a short-term effect by one year post-law implementation (decline by 6.7%) that was partially reversed by two years. No statistical testing was reported.

Beginning in January 2005, smoking in Italy was prohibited in all indoor public places including cafes, restaurants (except for a few separate and regulated smoking areas), airports, railway stations, and all public and private indoor workplaces. An early evaluation of the Italian anti-smoking law (Galeone *et al.*, 2006) included a short-term trend analysis of indicators of tobacco consumption and sales of nicotine replacement therapies. During the 11 months following implementation of the law (January-November 2005), total sales of cigarettes decreased in Italy by 5.7%, in comparison with the same period in 2004 before the law. Accordingly, the adult per capita sales of cigarettes packs decreased by 6.6% between 2004 and 2006, while declines before 2004 were lower (1.3% between 2002 and 2003, and 2.8% between 2003 and 2004). Finally, total sales of nicotine replacement products was 10.8% higher between January and September 2005 compared to the same period in 2004 before the law took effect.

For the initial evaluation of the impact of the new comprehensive legislation, data were examined from three independent cross-sectional surveys conducted in 2004, 2005, and 2006, and for comparative purposes, earlier data from 1990 and 2001-2003 surveys (Gallus *et al.*, 2007). These surveys were conducted among representative samples of the adult (>15 years) Italian population by means of face-to-face at-home interviews. Data were combined to compute prevalence estimates for the periods 2001-2002 (6534 subjects), 2003-2004 (6585 subjects), and 2005-2006 (6153 subjects). A simple analysis by sex and age showed that smoking declined from 26.2% (30.0% in men and 22.5% in women) in 2004 to 25.6% (29.3% in men and 22.2% in women) in 2005, and to 24.3% (28.6% in men and 20.3% in women) in 2006, with an acceleration in the decreasing rate from 2004 onward. Using the earlier 1990 data, up until the law came into force in 2004, smoking prevalence declined by 0.40% per year (0.53% in men and 0.25% in women), and thereafter, smoking prevalence declined by 1.08% per year (1.11% in men and 1.03% in women). When three subsequent two-year calendar periods were considered, a significant difference between 2003-04 and 2005-06 was present in men (31.7% versus 29.0%), but not in women (22.5% versus 21.2%), and also in subjects aged <45 years (32.4% versus 30.0%), but not ≥45 years (20.5% versus 20.2%). While no significant differences were found between smoking prevalence in 2001-02 versus 2003-04, mean CPD decreased from 15.4 (16.7 in men and 13.7 in women) in 2004 to 13.9 (15.1 in men and 12.4 in women); however, statistical tests were not reported. It appears that the new law may have led to an acceleration of an existing downward trend, at least for some demographic groups.

Changes in smoking behaviour in programmes where smoking restrictions were only one strategy used to reduce health effects from tobacco use

A number of localities have included restrictions on smoking in public and private places as one component of a multi-component effort to reduce tobacco use. While in some cases the introduction of the laws restricting smoking occurred during a period when other tobacco control strategies were more or less at a relatively steady state, in other cases, implementation

of new laws occurred at the same time as other new tobacco control measures, such as cigarette excise tax increases or new anti-tobacco media campaigns. Thus, it is not generally possible to attribute any changes in population smoking behaviour to the new laws restricting smoking. The studies described below also appear in Table 7.1.

Two studies examined the effect of the 1976 Tobacco Control Act in the patterns of ever smoking among Finnish adults by sex and birth cohort (Helakorpi *et al.*, 2004) and by sex, birth cohort and socioeconomic groups (Helakorpi *et al.*, 2008). The 1976 Act prohibited smoking in most public places (including public transport), prohibited the sale of tobacco products to those aged 16 years and younger, required health warnings on tobacco packages, and funded tobacco-related health education and research. The researchers pooled annual nationwide postal cross-sectional surveys (from 1978 to 2001/2002) with random samples of about 5000 subjects, totaling 33 080 men and 34 991 women for analysis. From respondents' smoking histories, they constructed age-cohort ever smoking prevalence rates for men and women. In the first article (Helakorpi *et al.*, 2004) the authors assessed the independent contribution of age, cohort, and the 1976 Tobacco Control Act by means of logistic regression models. A significant decline in the prevalence of ever smokers concurrent with the 1976 Tobacco Act was present in men (OR=0.74; 95% CI=0.68-0.81) for the Tobacco Act term after adjusting for cohort and age profile, indicating reduced

ever smoking after compared to before the law was implemented. In women, an interaction term between the Tobacco Act and the cohort trend was included in the model, and a decline in the prevalence of ever smokers concurrent with the Tobacco Act was clear (OR=0.45; 95% CI=0.35-0.57, OR=0.34; 95% CI=0.26-0.45, and OR=0.26; 95% CI=0.19-0.36 for the three birth cohorts studied). These effects were for the entire programme, not just the new smoking restrictions.

In the second paper (Helakorpi *et al.*, 2008) the authors extended the previous analysis by stratifying by socioeconomic status (from Census data) according to a person's life cycle stage (family member, student, pensioner, economically active, etc.), occupational status (self-employed, employee, unpaid family worker), and nature of occupation (upper white collar workers-upper level employees, lower white collar workers-lower level employees, blue collar workers-manual workers, farmers, and entrepreneurs-otherself-employed). In all socioeconomic groups a declining cohort trend was observed among men, with significant reduced odds ratios for the pre-post 1976 Tobacco Control Act effect in all socioeconomic groups (OR=0.52; 95% CI=0.40-0.66 in upper white collar workers, OR=0.55; 95% CI=0.44-0.68 in lower white collar workers, OR=0.76; 95% CI=0.65-0.88 in blue collar workers, and OR=0.66; 95% CI=0.45-0.97 in entrepreneurs), except farmers (OR=0.89; 95% CI=0.60-1.33). In women, however, an increasing trend in prevalence was present in the earliest cohort, but a declining trend was observed thereafter.

From 1985 to 1998, New Zealand undertook an extensive tobacco control programme that included increased, but not total restrictions, on smoking in enclosed public and workplaces, restrictions on tobacco advertising and sponsorships, increased taxation of tobacco products, regulation of nicotine and tar yields in manufactured cigarette brands, stronger warnings on cigarette packaging, school-based education programmes, a prohibition on the sale of tobacco products to those under age 16 years, and public education through both paid advertising campaigns and news items (Laugesen & Swinburn, 2000). However, the paid advertisements were limited because of cost. The campaign effect was evaluated by annual cross-sectional population surveys (1985 through 1995) of 10 000+ persons age 15 years and older, and data were compared to available published data from other Organization for Economic Cooperation and Development (mostly European) countries. Adult smoking prevalence fell from 30% in 1985 to 26% in 1998, and was then the eighth lowest among 21 comparison countries. Youth (15-24 years) prevalence decreased from 35% to 28% over this period. Among the 17 comparison countries with data for this age group, New Zealand ranked third in the rate of decline. The decline was also observed among the Maori population, which was an important programme goal, but, in general, the declines were greater among the higher educated. Between 1975 and 1985 adult per capita tobacco consumption fell 23%, and nearly doubled to a 45% decline from 1985 to 1995. The adult

per capita consumption level in 1995 was second lowest behind Sweden among the comparison countries.

In 1986, Singapore introduced a coordinated tobacco control programme that sought to denormalise tobacco use with its theme, "Towards a Nation of Non-Smokers" (Emmanuel et al., 1988). The programme aimed both to prevent youth smoking, encourage smokers to quit, and protect the rights of nonsmokers. Tobacco control measures included restriction of smoking in public and workplaces, restriction of tobacco advertising, increased excise duties on imported cigarettes, and provision of cessation assistance. Educational programmes in schools, clubs, worksites, and within the community also were undertaken. Cross-sectional population-based surveys (1984: n=92 500; 1987: n=78 600) indicated that smoking prevalence (age 15 years and older) fell from 19.0% in 1984 to 13.6% in 1987, or 28% (p<0.01). Per capita tobacco consumption also fell 26% over this period from 3.21 Kg/person in 1984 to 2.38 Kg/person in 1987. Youth (15 to 19 years) smoking prevalence fell from 5.1% to 2.9% over this period. No statistical tests were reported for youth prevalence or per capita consumption. Declines in prevalence were observed for all age groups, genders, and ethnic groups. Smoking prevalence had already been declining in Singapore prior to this tobacco control effort; the rate of decline increased during the campaign.

Repeated cross-sectional surveys and trends in per capita cigarette sales in California, and the rest of the USA, were used to evaluate California's

Tobacco Control Programme (Pierce et al., 1998b; Gilpin et al., 2001). Both smoking prevalence (standardised to account for changes in the population composition) and per capita cigarette consumption declined faster in California compared to the rest of the USA following programme implementation, which included a new excise tax ($0.25/pack), a media campaign, and funding for local level (county) efforts to reduce smoking. Pre-programme (1983-1988), the annual rate of decline in per capita consumption was 0.46/packs in California, and 0.35 in the rest of the USA. In the early period (1990-1993) these rates were significantly different at 0.58 versus 0.40/packs/year. The decline appeared to halt from 1994 to 1998 when funding for the media and local efforts was substantially reduced. Then in 1995, California implemented its smoke-free workplace policy (that exempted bars and clubs until January, 1998), and lawsuits initiated and won by non-profit organisations (e.g. American Heart Association, American Cancer Society, American Lung Association) against the state restored programme funding in late 1996. From 1998 to 1999, per capita cigarette consumption resumed its decline at 1.56 packs/year, significantly different from the 0.78 packs/year decline in the rest of the USA. Annual pre-programme prevalence declines were nearly the same for California and the rest of the USA (0.77% and 0.78%, respectively). From 1989 to 1993, prevalence declined significantly faster in California than in the rest of USA (by 1.01% and 0.51% annually, respectively). However, thereafter the annual rates of decline did not differ significantly. Nevertheless, compared to pre-programme levels, prevalence by 1993 declined by 24% in California compared to 17% in the rest of the USA. It cannot be determined whether the new smoke-free workplace law, or other factors such as the restoration of programme funding, was responsible for the new downturn in cigarette consumption. However, if smoking restrictions tend to decrease consumption more than they do prevalence, the results described above are consistent with that hypothesis.

Massachusetts implemented its own tobacco control programme in 1994, using funds from a new $0.25/pack cigarette tax. The Massachusetts programme was media led, but included efforts to prevent youth initiation and promote adult smoking cessation. A statewide law prohibiting smoking in indoor workplaces was not implemented until July 2004. However, there was an increase in the number of local laws restricting smoking in public places from programme inception through passage of the state law. Analyses of per capita cigarette consumption from tobacco sales data showed downward trends in Massachusetts (3-4%/year) and the rest of the USA, omitting California (4%/year) (Biener et al., 2000). In 1993, the decline was 12% in Massachusetts compared to 4% in the comparison states. Thereafter (to 1999), the decline was 4% in Massachusetts compared to 1% in the comparison states. Repeated cross-sectional surveys indicated that smoking prevalence declined in Massachusetts from 24% in 1989 to 19% in 1999, with

a significant decline of 0.43%/year (95% CI=-0.66, -0.21%/year) with no significant downward slope in the comparison states.

Between 2002 and 2003, New York City undertook a number of tobacco control activities: a large increase ($1.42/pack) in the excise tax on cigarettes; implementation of a new law that restricted smoking in all indoor workplaces, including restaurants and bars; an emphasis on the treatment of nicotine dependence; and a complementary media campaign that focused heavily on the health risks of SHS and the health benefits of smoking cessation. Using repeated cross-sectional surveys, the impact of these measures on smoking prevalence was evaluated (Frieden et al., 2005). After nearly a decade of stable adult smoking prevalence, between 2002 and 2003 (pre- to post-programme implementation), prevalence dropped from 21.6% to 19.2%, or by 11%. A subsequent analysis of later survey data (Centers for Disease Control and Prevention, 2007c) showed a further decline in prevalence to 18.9% in 2005 and to 17.5% in 2006. Another study conducted in New York City monitored sales of nicotine replacement products (gum and patches) weekly from July 2001 to February 2004 (Metzger et al., 2005). Trend analyses indicated a significant increase in sales of these products during the weeks of the cigarette tax increase and of the smoke-free workplace law implementation. These immediate increases tended to taper off in the following weeks, but the increases were larger and remained higher longer for higher-resource areas of the city.

Several other US states (e.g. Oregon and Arizona) have implemented comprehensive tobacco control programmes that included laws restricting smoking, and again significant declines in smoking behaviour were observed pre- to post-programme implementation (Center of Disease Control and Prevention, 1999; Porter et al., 2001).

Incidence of smoking cessation in countries with tobacco control measures including smoking restrictions

Two studies (Table 7.1), one in the USA (Gilpin & Pierce, 2002a) and the other in Spain (Schiaffino et al., 2007), analysed time trends in the incidence of successful quitting (i.e. the ratio of those newly successfully quit each year to those eligible to quit at the beginning of the year). This approach, using incidence quit rates for short periods (annual or bi-annual), allows rapid shifts in successful cessation to be identified in population subgroups (by sex, age, race, and educational level) potentially resulting from varied intervention strategies.

In the USA, annual cessation incidence rates were computed from 1950 to 1990 using pooled data from seven National Health Interview Surveys conducted between 1965 and 1992 (Gilpin & Pierce, 2002a). The age when regular smoking began and when cessation occurred, together with the survey year, allowed the year of these events to be determined. Each survey considered between 10 000 and 80 000 respondents; 140 199 ever smokers aged 20-50 years old were included in the analyses. Overall, incidence increased from

<1% in 1950 to 5% in 1990. Gender differences were seen following the beginning of public health campaigns of the mid 1960s (e.g. emphasising the dangers of smoking to the fetus). Younger adult smokers appeared to show increased quitting in the 1970s, around the beginning of the nonsmokers' rights movement in the USA, where proponents lobbied for smoke-free public and workplaces with local success in many cases. The pattern of quitting in middle-aged African Americans was similar to whites, although at reduced levels. Cessation incidence rates were higher among more educated subjects, regardless of age, during the 1970s and 1980s.

In Spain, biannual quitting incidence rates were computed from 1965 to 2000 according to sex, age, and educational level, using pooled data from five National Health Interview Surveys conducted between 1993 and 2003 (Schiaffino *et al.*, 2007). Altogether the analyses included 33 532 ever smokers aged >20 years with complete information on smoking history and educational level. The incidence of quitting smoking, for those age 20 to 50 years, increased from 0.5% in 1965-1966 to 4.9% in 1999-2000 in men, and from 1.1% in 1965-1966 to 5.0% in 1999-2000 in women. For those aged >50 years, larger increases in the incidence of quitting were observed (from 0.4% to 8.7% in men and from 7.9% to 8.8% in women). Educational disparities were present: by the last decade, a levelling off of cessation rates was apparent in both men and women aged 20 to 50 years with lower educational levels, while cessation rates among those with higher

educational attainment continued to increase. No clear changes in cessation incidence rates were observed surrounding the tobacco control laws passed between 1978 and 1997. However, none of these laws included prohibition of smoking in enclosed public or workplaces.

In both studies above (Gilpin & Pierce, 2002a; Schiaffino *et al.*, 2007), no direct analysis of the effect of public health campaigns, comprehensive programmes or mandated smoking restrictions were included in any statistical models.

Report/perceptions about changes in smoking behaviour due to law

Two studies (Table 7.1) asked smokers how new laws affected their smoking behaviour (Hammond *et al.*, 2004; Fong *et al.*, 2006). Researchers contacted 191 former smokers in southwestern Ontario, Canada in October 2001 and compared former smokers who had quit before the new law (restricting smoking and requiring warning labels on cigarette packages) to those who had quit following the new law, which was implemented January 2001 (Hammond *et al.*, 2004). From logistic regression analyses, that adjusted for age, sex, CPD prior to quitting, and number of years smoked, those who quit following the new law were 3.06 (95% CI=1.02-9.19) times more likely to cite the law as a motivation for quitting than those who quit earlier, and were 2.78 (95% CI=1.20-5.94) times more likely to cite the warning labels as a motivation.

The self-reported behavioural changes among Irish smokers were investigated (Fong *et al.*, 2006). A

representative sample of the adult (≥18 years) smoking population was identified in Ireland (n=1679) before the comprehensive law restricting smoking became effective (December 2003-January 2004); subjects (n=769) were re-contacted from December 2004 to January 2005 after the law was implemented in March 2004. Relevant questions asked of Irish smokers at follow-up (n=640) included whether the law had made them more likely to quit smoking (46% (95% CI=41-50%)), or made them cut down on the number of cigarettes they smoke (60% (95% CI=55-64%)). Former smokers were asked whether the law made them more likely to quit (80% (95% CI=71-88%)), and helped them stay quit (88% (95% CI=81-95%)). Numbers in parentheses are percentages of the relevant subgroup and 95% confidence intervals.

These two studies indicate that smokers notice new laws and perceive that they motivate them to change their smoking behaviour. However, these studies are not direct measures of current population smoking behaviour before and after the law took effect, and possibly overstate the affect of the new laws on smoking behaviour.

Summary

The studies that assessed smoking behaviour before and after the implementation of a new law restricting smoking can at least identify that any change in smoking behaviour observed occurred following implementation of the law. Multiple surveys before the law can establish that the changes observed following the law were not just a continuation of an ongoing secular trend. However, if other interventions occurred simultaneously with the introduction of the new law, any changes cannot be definitely attributed to it. The results from two cross-sectional studies concerning changes in smoking behaviour pre- to post- new laws failed to find a significant decline in smoking prevalence early after the law took effect. However, these studies were designed to assess changes in exposure to SHS and may not have been appropriately powered to detect differences in smoking prevalence. The study using a longitudinal sample of hospitality workers did find an early and significant decrease in smoking prevalence and cigarette consumption.

Results from the five studies with multiple pre- and/or post-law surveys were mixed. Of the four that reported changes in adult smoking prevalence, two found a significant overall difference and one study did not provide a statistical test. Two of these studies examined prevalence changes by sex and found greater changes in men than in women, and one also showed greater changes in younger compared to older smokers. While changes in consumption were examined in four studies, no significant change was reported in one study, and the declines were not tested in the others, although they appeared to be meaningful. One study reported a decline in youth prevalence, but indicated that the decline was not different from the secular trend. Increases in nicotine replacement sales were noted in two studies, but again no statistical test was performed.

However, in locations with multiple tobacco control efforts that included smoking restrictions, significant declines in prevalence and consumption for both the short- and long-term were consistently observed following programme implementation compared to earlier. Two studies also reported declines in youth smoking prevalence, but no statistical tests were performed. Sales of nicotine replacement products increased significantly in the one study that reported this outcome.

Correlative studies

A number of articles were identified that related the strength and extent of local laws regarding smoking in public places to the smoking behaviour of adults or youth. About half of these articles are econometric analyses, and several of these studies published in 1990 or later utilised data collected in the USA earlier than 1990 (Wasserman et al., 1991; Chaloupka, 1992; Chaloupka & Saffer, 1992). In the 1970s, 1980s, and into the 1990s, laws governing smoking in public places in the USA were not widespread and tended to be weak compared to present day standards. Typically they covered specific public places such as buses or trains, elevators, health care facilities, student smoking in schools, government workplaces, restaurants, or private workplaces. Also, restrictions generally did not imply a total prohibition. For instance, restrictions in restaurants might dictate separate sections for smokers and nonsmokers, but without separate ventilation.

The econometric studies employed specialised multivariate regression techniques and generally considered many different model formulations that omitted or included certain sets of variables. These studies were mainly concerned with estimating the price-elasticity of demand for cigarettes; the percent decrease in cigarette consumption that would result from a 10% increase in cigarette prices. However, these studies also included variables for the strength or extent of laws restricting smoking, and some also included other tobacco-control-related factors. The econometric studies generally report regression coefficients together with t-statistics and their corresponding p-values at the <0.10, <0.05, or <0.01 levels of statistical significance. All dollar ($) amounts included in the models were adjusted for inflation.

Other studies relating the extent and strength of clean air laws to smoking behaviour tended to use standard logistic regression analyses (categorical outcomes such as smoking status) or multiple linear regression (continuous variables such as daily cigarette consumption) and considered fewer model formulations. In the subsections below and in Appendices 3 and 4, the word "analysis" is used in a very general sense, and only if the study used a different (usually simpler) method than outlined above is a description provided. The studies reviewed below are presented under two headings, econometric and other studies, in roughly chronological order of data collection. Most of the studies controlled for demographic factors and other types of policies, such as taxation, that might affect smoking behaviour.

Econometric studies

Table 7.2 summarises the results of the econometric studies reviewed which are described in detail in Appendix 3. These studies, all from the USA, matched data on smoking restrictions at the local level to survey data that included information about where the respondent resided. These studies employed a number of strategies to capture the scope and strength of local ordinances restricting smoking in public and workplaces. In some studies, a set of indicator variables was included, one for each possible venue such as private worksites, restaurants, government worksites, healthcare facilities, grocery stores, schools, and other public places. Some used multilevel indicators for strength of the ordinance in each venue considered. In other cases, the set of indicator variables was reduced to three or four (e.g. workplaces, restaurants, other places). Other studies constructed an ordered categorical variable where the highest level was reserved for workplaces, the next highest for localities with no workplace restrictions but many restrictions in other public places, the next lower level for those with no workplace restrictions and only a few restrictions in other public places, and the lowest level for localities with no restrictions at all on smoking. Still others analysed a 'continuous' index to capture both the scope and strength of the local laws.

The indicator variables tended to be correlated with one another; for example, localities with workplace restrictions tended to have smoking restrictions in other venues as well. Thus, an ordered categorical or index variable probably gives a better representation of both law scope and/or strength. However, the quality of these index schemes for grading local ordinances might depend on the decision rules used for scoring the individual local laws.

The summary (Table 7.2) shows that all of the studies found at least some relationship between the variables for smoking restrictions and the smoking behaviour considered. When a set of variable was used, it may have only been for one or two of them that were significantly related (see Appendix 3). Most of the studies evaluated some measure of cigarette consumption and seven of eight found some association of smoking restrictions with this outcome. Only one study examined smoking cessation (Tauras & Chaloupka, 1999b), and it only found an effect for females working in workplaces with smoking restrictions. All but one of the six studies that examined smoking prevalence concerned youth. While all of the youth studies found an association, the one adult-only study did not.

Data were examined on self-reported smoking status and cigarette consumption among current smokers from the National Health Interview Surveys (NHIS) of 1970, 1974, 1976, 1979,1980, 1983, and 1985 for adults (n=207 647), and from the National Health and Nutrition Examination Survey (NHANES) II conduced from 1976 to 1980 for adolescents (n=1960) (Wasserman *et al.*, 1991). Information on smoking restrictions

was merged into the survey datasets by location and was formulated as an index: 1=restricted smoking in private workplaces; 0.75=restricted smoking in restaurants, but not private worksites; 0.50=restrictions in at least four public places, other than private workplaces or restaurants; 0.25=restrictions in one to three of these public places; 0=no restrictions. The adult regression model included year, log cigarette price by year, income by year, family size, log family size, education, and education by year, sex, age, birth cohort, sex by age, birth cohort by age, non-white race/ethnicity, and marital status, as well as the regulation index, which was significantly ($p < 0.05$) related to lower reported cigarette consumption among current smokers, but not to being a current smoker. The teen model included year, log cigarette price by year, family size, log family size, family income, household head education level, sex, age, non-white race/ethnicity, and a variable about restrictions on sales of cigarettes to minors, as well as the regulation index. In this analysis, the index was significantly ($p < 0.01$) related to being a current smoker but not to cigarette consumption.

The effect of regulations regarding smoking in public places on average self-reported cigarette consumption for adult males and females, separately, using NHANES II data collected from 1976 to 1980, was studied (Chaloupka, 1992). In this analysis the smoking restrictions were coded separately (binary variables) as nominal (restrictions in one to three public places not including restaurants or private workplaces), basic (restrictions in four or more

Table 7.2 Summary of econometric studies relating scope and strength of smoking restrictions to smoking behaviour

Reference	Population	Type of ordinance variable	Prevalence	Consumption	Cessation	Other
					Outcomes	
Wasserman et al., 1991	Adults	Ordered categorical	NS	SIG		
Wasserman et al., 1991	Youth	Ordered categorical	SIG	NS		
Chaloupka,1992	Total*	Four indicator variables		SIG		
Chaloupka & Saffer, 1992	Total*	Two indicator variables		SIG		
Keeler et al., 1993	Adults	Index		SIG		
Chaloupka & Grossman, 1996	Youth	Five multi-level variables	SIG	SIG		
Chaloupka & Wechsler, 1997	College students	Three binary Ordered categorical	SIG NS	SIG NS		
Lewit et al., 1997	Youth	Index	SIG			NS-intent to smoke among nonsmokers
Tauras & Chaloupka, 1999a	Youth	Ordered categorical	SIG	SIG		
Tauras & Chaloupka, 1999b	Young Adults	Three binary Ordered categorical			NS-quit at follow-up NS-males; SIG-females	
Tauras, 2005	Youth	Five indicator variables				NS-transition from non-daily to daily smoking SIG-transition from light to heavy daily smoking NS-transition from mode-rate to heavy daily smoking

*Total = when per capita consumption is analysed, it is for the entire population
SIG = significant difference in smoking behaviour indicated between workers with and without workplaces smoking restrictions. All significant differences were in the direction of reduced smoking (i.e. less consumption, more quitting) in workplaces with restrictions. NS = no significant difference. No entry means that the outcome was not considered.

public places not including restaurants or private workplaces), moderate (restrictions in restaurants but not private workplaces), or extensive (restrictions in private workplaces). Variables for current, past, and next year cigarette prices, and past and next year consumption were also included in the regression analysis. Whether or not all respondents or just ever smokers (zero cigarettes per day) were analysed, the variable for basic regulations was significantly related to reduced consumption overall ($p < 0.01$). When male and female ever smokers were analysed separately, the basic restrictions variable was only significant for males. The authors concluded that stronger than basic restrictions are unlikely to impede smoking further.

Data were analysed from 1970 to 1985 on a state level (50 US states as data points) basis (Chaloupka & Saffer, 1992). They were gathered from various sources and included cigarette prices, tobacco production, three variables related to export and import of cigarettes (smuggling), income, percent of the population who were Mormons or Southern Baptists, the percentage of the population who voted, the percent divorced, and the percent unemployed. The dependent variable in the regression analysis was cigarette sales per capita, and restrictions were handled as two separate binary variables. One variable was coded one if the state restricted smoking in at least four public places (including restaurants but not private workplaces) and zero otherwise, and the other was coded one if smoking was restricted in private workplaces and zero otherwise. Both restriction variables were significantly

($p < 0.01$) related to lower per capita cigarette sales. Another analysis involved simultaneous equations with sales as the dependent variable in one equation, and each restriction variable as the dependent variable in the other two equations. All other variables including sales or restrictions, as appropriate, were included as independent variables. These simultaneous equations also adjusted for the other factors mentioned above. Public place laws were significantly ($p < 0.01$) related to reduced sales, while higher cigarette prices were related to private place laws. The authors concluded that laws restricting smoking are more likely to be passed in states with higher cigarette prices, and that passing more smoking restrictions may not decrease cigarette sales.

Another time series analysis examined monthly per capita cigarette consumption in California from 1980 to 1990 (Keeler *et al.*, 1993). This study used a regulation index that accounted for the percent of the state's population affected by smoking restrictions and the strength of the restrictions for the population covered. The index was computed on a monthly basis from data in an NHIS report and from a telephone survey of local health departments. The regression models included the average of Arizona and Oregon taxes divided by the California tax, federal tax, per capita income, cigarette price, state tax, and a time trend. The results, without the time trend included, showed a strong effect for the regulation index on lower per capita consumption ($p < 0.001$). However, when the time trend was included in the model, the regulation index

was no longer significant, and other terms in the model (e.g. cigarette tax) also became less significant. Most of the tax increase occurred in 1989, following Proposition 99. However, models based on the period up to two months before the new tax produced very similar results. The authors suggest that while including a time trend to account for secular changes in smoking behaviour is standard, its effect is questionable. The time trend appears to capture the long-term effects inherent in regulation, price, and other factors.

The relation of young adult smoking behaviour to cigarette prices and clean indoor air laws was the subject of several analyses, which involved longitudinal samples of high school seniors followed periodically as part of the Monitoring the Future project (Tauras & Chaloupka, 1999a,b; Tauras 2005). The data analysed were collected from 1976 to 1993. All of these studies considered venues possibly subject to smoking restrictions: private worksites, restaurants, government worksites, healthcare facilities, grocery stores, and other public places. Each subject was matched to the restriction indicators by locality and time of response to the Monitoring the Future surveys. The studies also included a number of variables from the survey and at the locality level such as age, sex, income, college (attending less than half time, attending half time, attending full time), religiosity, marital status, household composition, region, cigarette prices, etc.

One of the studies (Tauras, 2005) examined transition from non-daily to daily smoking, from light smoking (1-5 CPD) to moderate (6-10 CPD), or transition from an average of 10 CPD to heavy smoking (20+ CPD). In regression models, the smoking restriction variables (private workplace, restaurants and other public places) were significantly (p<0.01) associated with reduced transition from light to moderate smoking, but not to the other transitions examined.

Smoking status and consumption among current smokers was examined in another of the studies (Tauras & Chaloupka, 1999a). Here, the authors formed an index from the individual venue restrictions variables; 0=no restrictions, 1=nominal restrictions (other public places), 2=basic restrictions (health care facilities, grocery stores, government worksites), 3=moderate restrictions (restaurants but not private worksites), and 4=extensive restrictions (private worksites). The index variables were preferred because of multiple collinearities among the separate binary indicator variables. In all the regression models considered, the clean air index variable was significantly (p<0.01) related to both less current smoking and reduced daily cigarette consumption. The authors also discussed that many previous researchers may have computed price elasticities of demand for cigarettes that were inflated, because they did not control for clean indoor air laws. There is a correlation between these factors, and variance attributable to the clean indoor air laws was confounded with that for cigarette prices.

The third paper examined smoking cessation among young adults by sex (Tauras & Chaloupka, 1999b). In this study, the clean indoor indicators were used in a

different manner: in one model the index was considered; in another analysis three indicators were used (private workplace, restaurants, all other venues); and in the third analysis the index without the workplace indicator was used, along with a second variable computed as the interaction between work status of the respondent and private workplace restrictions. For males, none of the clean indoor air variables significantly predicted cessation in their respective models. For females, the interaction variable was significant (p<0.01); indicating that employed females working in worksites where smoking was restricted were more likely to quit.

Another study using a different data source, the 1993 Harvard College Alcohol Study, also examined smoking behaviour among 16 570 college students in 140 four-year colleges in the USA (Chaloupka & Wechsler, 1997). The authors analysed any smoking in the past 30 days, and an ordered variable for amount smoked per day: 0=none, 1=light (1-9 CPD), 2=moderate (10-19 CPD), and 3=heavy (20+ CPD). A set of binary indicator variables for restrictions on smoking in various venues and a composite index were analysed as in the Wasserman et al. (1991) study. Other variables analysed included local cigarette prices, age, sex, race/ethnicity, marital status, religiosity, parental education, on-campus residence, fraternity or sorority membership, and employment. Several additional variables characterised the college: co-ed, private, commuter, rural, with a fraternity or sorority, and region. In probit regression models, including

only the individual venue binary variables, restrictions in restaurants were fairly consistently (p<0.10) related to both less current smoking and lower amount smoked. School smoking restrictions were significant (p<0.10) for lower consumption. The index variable was not significant in any of the models analysed. The authors suggested that the restaurant variable might reflect restrictiveness of smoking in general within the communities.

Investigators analysed data on 15 432 ninth graders gathered in 1990 and 1992, as part of the Community Intervention Trial for Smoking Cessation (COMMIT) in 21 communities in the USA and Canada (Lewit et al., 1997). This study included a broad set of variables related to tobacco control policy: price, clean indoor air policy, school smoking policy, school anti-tobacco classes, minimum age of purchase requirements, vending machine restrictions, limits on free cigarette sample distributions, anti-tobacco media exposure, and pro-tobacco media exposure. Analyses also controlled for sex, age, race/ethnicity, whether the community was part of the COMMIT intervention, and year. The clean indoor air variable was a composite score of three separate indices related to workplaces, restaurants, and other public places, with the individual indices capturing both the relative frequency of venue type, the extent (number of public places), and the restrictiveness (allowed or prohibited areas) of the laws in each community. The composite index ranged from 2 to 46, with a mean of 28.8 and standard deviation (SD) of 10.6. The dependent variables analysed were any smoking in the past 30 days, and among nonsmokers, in the past 30 days their intention to smoke in the future. In the multiple logistic models including all the variables, the school smoking policy variable ($p < 0.10$), but not the clean indoor air policy variable showed some relation to lower current smoking; however, neither the school nor the clean indoor policy variables appeared related to intention to smoke. Minimum age of purchase and cigarette prices were related to reduced smoking, while pro-tobacco media and paradoxically anti-tobacco media were related to increased smoking.

Eight, tenth and twelfth graders (n=110 717), from Monitoring the Future surveys conducted in 1992, 1993, and 1994, were the subject of another study (Chaloupka & Grossman, 1996). The authors analysed any smoking in the past 30 days, and a self-reported measure of daily cigarette consumption. A set of five variables captured the fraction of the population in each adolescent's place of residence subject to restrictions on smoking in private workplaces, restaurants, retail stores, schools, or other public places. Other locality variables analysed included a set related to cigarette prices, a set related to restrictions on youth purchase of cigarettes, whether a portion of cigarette tax revenue is devoted to tobacco control activities, and whether a locality has any laws protecting smokers. Individual level variables included age, sex, weekly income (work and/or allowance), race/ethnicity, marital status of youth, parental education, family structure, work status of mother, whether youth had siblings, average hours of work weekly, rural residence, and religiosity. When each restriction variable was analysed separately along with all the other variables listed above, limitations on smoking in private workplaces, restaurants, and retail stores were negatively associated with lower current smoking ($p < 0.01$). Restrictions in private workplaces and restaurants were also related to reduced cigarette consumption ($p < 0.01$). However, when all five of the restriction variables were included together, only restrictions in workplaces ($p < 0.05$) was significantly related to lower current smoking, but restaurant restrictions, school smoking restrictions, and other public place restrictions were still related to reduced consumption ($p < 0.01$).

Other studies

A number of other studies have also investigated the relationship between smoking restrictions and smoking behaviour. These studies differ from the econometric data in that they generally involved more recent data and used somewhat different analytical approaches. These studies are summarised in Table 7.3 and described in detail below and in Appendix 4. As for the econometric studies, data on laws and individuals were matched by locality and most studies used an index of some sort to rate the scope and strength of the local laws restricting smoking. All four of the studies that examined smoking prevalence found a significant effect, as did the three studies that studied consumption. The studies that looked at cessation were mixed. Three studies examined transitions in the smoking uptake process, and at least for some transitions, each study found a significant effect.

Aggregate state level adult smoking prevalence and quit ratio estimates from the 1989 Current Population Survey and Tobacco Institute tax reporting sales data (to estimate per capita cigarette consumption), were linked to cigarette prices and strength of clean indoor air legislation (Emont et al., 1993). Fifty one data points were analysed; the 50 US states and the District of Columbia. State clean air laws were classified as in Chaloupka (1992). The hypotheses of lower adult smoking prevalence, higher quit ratio, and lower per capita cigarette consumption were tested using a Jonckhere test for ordered data; in this case, the increasing restrictiveness of the clean air laws. This bivariate test was significant for prevalence ($p < 0.001$), for per capita consumption ($p < 0.005$), and for the quit ratio ($p < 0.00005$). Mean prevalence ranged from 28% for the states with no restrictions to 24.5% for those with extensive restrictions. Analogous ranges for per capita consumption and the quit ratios were 118.6 packs/person/year to 105.3/ packs/person/year, and 43.5% to 49.6%. The bivariate Pearsons's correlations of cigarette prices to the three outcome variables were also significant ($p < 0.001$). No state or individual level control variables were included in this study.

In contrast, data were compiled for a multitude of variables on all 50 US states and the District of Columbia covering the period from 1970 to 1995 (Yurekli & Zhang, 2000).

Table 7.3 Summary of other studies relating scope and strength of smoking restrictions to smoking behaviour

Reference	Type of variable	Outcomes				
		Prevalence	Consumption	Cessation	Initiation	Other
Emont et al., 1993	Four indicator variables as for Chaloupka (1992)	SIG	SIG	SIG-quit ratio		
Yurekli & Zhang, 2000	Index		SIG			
Moskowitz et al., 2000	Ordered categorical			SIG-recent cessation		SIG-report of workplace policy
Wakefield et al., 2000a	Index	SIG			SIG-transitions on uptake continuum	
Stephens et al., 2001	Index	SIG-males and females	SIG-females not males			
Viehbeck & McDonald, 2004	Index			NS		
McMullen et al., 2005	Index	SIG-youth NS-adults				
Siegel et al., 2005	Ordered categorical				SIG-becoming an established smoker	
Albers et al., 2007	Ordered categorical			SIG-attempt NS-quit at follow-up		
Siegel et al., 2008	Ordered categorical				SIG-transition from experimentation to established	

SIG = significant difference in smoking behaviour indicated between workers with and without workplaces smoking restrictions. All significant differences were in the direction of reduced smoking (i.e. less consumption, more quitting) in workplaces with restrictions. NS = no significant difference. No entry means that the outcome was not considered.

The main purpose of this study was to gauge the impact of cigarette smuggling on excise tax revenue. However, also included in the analyses of per capita cigarette consumption was a variable for clean indoor air laws. A state level index was constructed that considered both the time people spent in venues subject to regulations and the strength of such regulations. The value of the variable changed over time in states as they adopted broader or strict regulations. Other variables compiled and analysed included per capita disposable income, price of cigarettes, cigarette tax, percent of the state population with at least a bachelor's degree, percent of the state that is Native American, African-America, Asian, of Mormon religion and unemployed, per capita expenditures on tourism, and a set of variables related to smuggling. They constructed a number of linear regression models including and omitting various sets of variables, but the variable for the clean indoor air laws was included in all the models and significant ($p<0.05$) in them all for reduced per capita consumption. From the final model, the researchers estimated that without such laws, total demand for cigarettes would have been 4.5% greater in 1995.

A study in California related the strength of community ordinances regulating smoking in the workplace to both report of a workplace smoking restriction and recent smoking cessation (Moskowitz et al., 2000). Data from 4680 employed current and recent former smokers from the 1990 California Tobacco Survey were linked by workplace zip code (postal code) to a database with rankings of the strength of local ordinances (none, weak, moderate, strong). In a multivariate analysis adjusting for age, sex, race/ethnicity, education, type of work area, and workplace size, those working in a community with a strong ordinance were 1.61 (95% CI=1.20-2.15) times more likely to report that their workplace had a smoking policy than those in communities with no ordinance. Even those working in communities with moderate ordinances tended to be more likely to report a workplace policy. Further, a strong ordinance was associated with cessation in the past six months; the adjusted odds ratio was 1.52 (95% CI=1.14-1.71) compared to those working in a community with no ordinance. Moderate or weak ordinances had smaller odds ratios with lower 95% confidence intervals of about 0.95-2.00.

Researchers appended data on cigarette prices and price increases, and the percentage of provincial populations covered by no-smoking bylaws to data records from a nationwide survey of 11 652 Canadians conducted in 1991 (Stephens et al., 1997). In a logistic regression of current smoker (coded 0) versus nonsmoker (coded 1) that adjusted for demographics (age, sex, marital status, and education) and the price variables along with significant interactions, the odds ratio of being a nonsmoker for the no-smoking bylaw variable was 1.21 (95% CI=1.08-1.36); for price it was 1.26 (95% CI=1.11-1.43), but changes in price were not significant. The authors repeated their analyses with data from the 1990 survey and attained essentially the same results.

Another analysis was conducted by the same group using data from another population survey conducted in 1995 and 1996 (Stephens et al. 2001). Data from 14 355 persons aged 25 years and older were analysed. This time they used a somewhat broader set of policy variables, analysed men and women separately, and constructed models for smoking status and for reported daily cigarette consumption by current smokers. The policy variables included were a dummy for a tax cut enacted in some localities (for analysis of consumption), current cigarette prices, expenditures for tobacco control in the previous year, a rating of strength of municipal no-smoking bylaws, signage requirements (no smoking signs), and strength of provisions for enforcement. The bylaw strength, enforcement and signage requirements were scored separately for 12 venues and the results summed. Strength codes were: 0=no limits on smoking, 1=designated smoking areas required or allowed, and 3=area smoke-free. Signage received a point for using both words and symbols and a point for requirements at doorways and entrances. Points for enforcement were given as 1 for specifying a designated enforcement official and 1 for fines that escalate with repeated offences. For both men and women in a logistic regression, cigarette price was positively related to being a nonsmoker (men OR=1.02; 95% CI=1.00-1.03; women OR=1.01; 95% CI=1.00-1.02). For women, the variable for the clean air bylaw was also significant, 1.02 (95% CI=1.00-1.04). For men, the clean indoor air variable was not significant, but the provisions for signage (OR=1.25; 95% CI=1.01-1.55) and enforcement (OR=1.21; 95% CI=1.00-1.46) were.

The public education expenditure variable was also significant for men. In a multiple linear regression analysis of daily cigarette consumption, the tax cut indicator, but not current cigarette prices, was significant for both men (p<0.01) and women (p<0.05), although an interaction term for these two variables was significant (p<0.001 for men and p<0.07 for women). Those subject to the tax cut smoked more. Again, the clean air bylaw variable was significant for women (p<0.05) but not for men, with women who were subject to these laws smoking less.

A Canadian study, using data from 2001, failed to demonstrate a significant association between municipal smoke-free laws and being a former smoker (Viehbeck & McDonald, 2004). In this study, the strength of ordinances regarding smoking in all public places (e.g. bars, restaurants, public auditoriums, etc.) was linked by postal code of residence. Law strength was actually an indication of extensiveness (number of public places covered). Enforcement and signage scoring was also added into the scale and was determined similar to the earlier study (Stephens et al., 1997). Communities with strong laws (top tertile of law strength scale) were matched to communities of similar socioeconomic status with weak or no bylaws (bottom tertile). Data from 9249 current and former smokers were analysed in a multivariate logistic regression analysis; the adjusted odds of being a former smoker were 0.95 (95% CI=0.82-1.11) if the communities had strong ordinances versus if they had no or weak ordinances.

A smoking regulation index, based on state laws effective in 1996 from records maintained by the Centers for Disease Control and Prevention, was merged into survey data from 17 287 US high school students in 202 schools by the location of the school (Wakefield et al., 2000a). Successive stages of a smoking uptake continuum and any smoking in the past 30 days was looked at. The smoking uptake continuum included stages for non susceptible never smokers (strong intentions not to smoke in the future), susceptible never smokers (weak intentions not to smoke in the future, or had taken a puff on a cigarette), early experimenters (had puffed on a cigarette, but not in the past 30 days and had weak intentions not to smoke in the future, or had smoked a whole cigarette but not in last 30 days and had strong intentions not to smoke in the future), advanced experimenters (had smoked a whole cigarette, but not in the past 30 days and had weak intentions not to smoke in the future, or had smoked in the past 30 days, but not 100 cigarettes in their lifetime), and established smokers (had smoked at least 100 cigarettes in their lifetime irrespective of future intentions). The models included grade, sex, race/ethnicity, adult smokers in the home, sibling smokers, living in a smoke-free home, attending a smoke-free school, and strength of enforcement of such a policy. The regulation index was significantly associated with reduced advanced experimentation versus early experimentation, and with less established smoking versus advanced experimentation. It also was associated with less smoking

in the past 30 days. Similar trends were also present in the analysis of the first two and second two stages on the smoking uptake continuum, but they failed to reach statistical significance.

A study of US states examined multiple population surveys conducted between 1996 and 1999, and related adult and youth (12-17 years) smoking prevalence, to an index of the strength of clean indoor air laws in each state (McMullen et al., 2005). The index was complex and summed scores for nine venues according to whether the venue was unrestricted to being completely smoke-free (0-4 points). Some categories (e.g. worksites, childcare facilities) could receive a bonus point if the surrounding area was also smoke-free. The maximum score could be 42, and averaged 8.7 in 1993 to 10.98 in 1999. These analyses used multiple linear regression models that adjusted for state poverty rates and cigarette excise taxes. It was found that the index was significantly related to the percentage of indoor workers reporting a smoke-free workplace (p<0.01), and to reduced youth (p<0.01), but not adult smoking prevalence (p<0.07) in linear regression models. Their analysis included 51 data points; one for each US state and the District of Columbia.

Massachusetts investigators used longitudinal population data to examine the association between baseline local laws restricting smoking in restaurants to both adult and youth smoking behaviour (Siegel et al., 2005, 2008; Albers et al., 2007). At the time of the baseline survey in 2001-2002, such restrictions varied widely among Massachusetts towns. Data on regulations from 351 cities and towns were categorised as strong (no smoking allowed in restaurants and no variances allowed), medium (smoking restricted to separately ventilated area or variances allowed), and weak (smoking in designated areas without separate ventilation or not restricted). The survey included a cohort of 2623 youth aged 12-17 years, who were not already established smokers at baseline; data from the smoking restrictions were appended to the survey data by zip code (Siegel *el al.*, 2005). The main outcome variable was progression to being an established smoker during the two-year follow-up period. An established smoker is defined as someone who has smoked at least 100 cigarettes in his or her lifetime. Using a generalised estimating equations logistic regression model, the researchers controlled for a number of individual and town level characteristics. Individual characteristics included age, sex, race/ethnicity, smoking experience at baseline (non-susceptible never smoker, susceptible never smoker, puffer, experimenter, smoked in last 30 days), having close friends who smoke, exposure to anti-smoking messages at school, having smokers in the household, the education level of the adult informant (gave permission for adolescent to be interviewed), and household income. Besides strength of smoking restrictions in restaurants, town level variables included percentage of residents who are college graduates, percentage of voters voting in favor of a voter initiative to increase cigarette taxes and expand state

tobacco control efforts, percentage of residents who are white, percentage of residents who are youth, number of restaurants in town (<5, ≥5), and population size (<20 000, 20 000-50 000, >50 000). After adjusting for all these factors, compared to adolescents living in towns with weak regulations, those living in towns with strong ordinances were 0.39 (95% CI=0.24-0.66) less likely to progress to being an established smoker. A medium strength ordinance was not protective.

Further analyses of a subsequent follow-up of these same adolescents after another two years (n=2217) used the same control variables, and again found the association of strong regulations to impeded progression (OR=0.60; 95% CI=0.42-0.85) to established smoking. It was determined that the transition interrupted was the one from being an experimenter to becoming an established smoker (Siegel *et al.*, 2008). Strong, but not weak, regulations were related to reduced transition from experimenting to established smoking (OR=0.53; 95% CI=0.33-0.86), but there was no significant relation regarding the transition from never smoking to any experimentation (OR=1.18; 95% CI=0.94-1.49). The findings suggest that reduced exposure to smokers in communities might reduce adolescents' perceptions of smoking prevalence, and affect their perceptions of the social acceptability of smoking. Both of these factors lead to reduced smoking initiation.

Adult smokers (n=1712) in these same households were also followed-up two years after the baseline survey (Albers *et al.*, 2007). They were

asked about their perceived social acceptability of smoking in restaurants and bars and quitting behaviour (making a quit attempt or being quit at follow-up). Analyses controlled for age, sex, race/ethnicity, education, household income, marital status, children <18 years in the household, and baseline level of addiction. This time, using hierarchical linear models to adjust for individual and town level characteristics, a strong restaurant regulation was predictive of making a quit attempt (OR=3.12; 95% CI=1.51-6.44), but not of being quit when interviewed again. There was a marginal effect with respect to perceptions about the social acceptability of smoking.

While these three longitudinal studies have the advantage of knowing the status of a community before observing future smoking behaviour, it is likely that the restaurant restriction variable is a proxy for an overall community sentiment unfavorable to smoking. Thus, it may not be just the restrictions themselves that are influencing smoking behaviour, but the norms inherent in these communities.

Summary

While not every correlative study (econometric and others) found an association between the strength and/or extent of laws prohibiting smoking in public places and smoking behaviour, most (17 of 19) of them did, at least in a particular subgroup or for a specific behaviour. The measures of law strength and extent differed among the studies reviewed, as did the smoking behaviours considered. Nevertheless, these studies cannot determine whether it is localities with strong anti-smoking norms, and thus less smoking, that are more likely to adopt laws restricting smoking, or whether such laws lead to reduced smoking. Even the longitudinal data from Massachusetts cannot definitively attribute the effects noted to the laws, as other normative influences may have been associated with the existence of the laws.

Workplace smoking restrictions

Workplace smoking restrictions might be implemented either to conform with a law mandating them, or because of a policy voluntarily adopted by individual worksites. Most of the studies reviewed later in this section took place during a time when local or state-wide mandated restrictions were not widespread.

Why workplace restrictions might affect smoking behaviour

It would be expected that smokers not being able to smoke whenever they want during the workday would have some affect on their smoking behaviour. At the least, they would have to plan ahead for when they would be able to smoke. They might think about having a last cigarette in their cars or even on their way from the parking lot or transportation center to the workplace before entering. They would also have to leave their work area and make their way to an area where smoking was allowed or go outside to smoke during breaks. A total prohibition on smoking indoors would probably have a greater impact on choice of when and where to smoke, than a lesser restriction that

allowed smoking in certain common or designated areas.

With their limited options for smoking, they also might be inclined to smoke fewer cigarettes during the workday. Also, if they do not witness others smoking, they may experience fewer cues to smoke. If they do not compensate by smoking more otherwise, their daily consumption might decline.

Some smokers may quit rather than put up with the inconvenience that smoking restrictions would impose. Further, if consumption is reduced, some smokers might find it easier to eventually successfully quit (Farkas *et al.*, 1996; Pierce *et al.*, 1998c). More subtle factors may also encourage cessation. A smoker might never think about quitting if smoking was considered acceptable everywhere in the workplace. Restrictions communicate the idea that it is not acceptable to smoke in the presence of nonsmokers, and perhaps not at all, which might stimulate thoughts about quitting. Also, the image of addicts huddled outside by the building entrance getting their nicotine fixes might not fit some smokers' self images, leading them to consider quitting. Once quit, the smoker might find it easier to remain abstinent in a smoke-free environment; cues to smoke from smokers smoking would be less (Payne *et al.*, 1996; Shiffman *et al.*, 1996).

Smoking restrictions might also affect the transition from experimental or intermittent smoking to daily smoking among young adults (Hill & Borland, 1991; Pierce *et al.*, 1991; Trotter *et al.*, 2002). There is evidence that some smoking initiation during

young adulthood occurs in the workplace (Hill & Borland, 1991). While they are now of legal age to smoke, if smoking was not perceived as a normative behaviour, or no smoking was observed in the workplace or on college campuses, fewer young adult never smokers might initiate, and those who have already initiated and who smoke intermittently might be less likely to transition to daily smoking (Pierce *et al.*, 1991). Also, those already smoking daily may adapt to a lower consumption level (lower tolerance level) if they could not smoke anytime they wished. By providing fewer cues to smoke, smoking restrictions in bars and clubs might also hinder both initiation and transition to heavier levels of smoking (Trotter *et al.*, 2002).

Previous reviews of the effects of workplace restrictions on smoking behaviour

Seven published reviews of the effects of workplace smoking restrictions on smoking behaviour were located (Brownson *et al.*, 1997; Eriksen & Gottlieb, 1998; Chapman *et al.*, 1999; Hopkins *et al.*, 2001; Fichtenberg & Glantz, 2002; Levy & Friend, 2003; Moher *et al.*, 2005). These reviews considered basically two types of studies: analyses of workers employed in specific individual worksites, or analyses of workers from population surveys who were asked about smoking restrictions in their workplaces. Altogether 36 separate studies of the first type were reviewed, only one was considered by all seven previous reviewers, three by six of the reviews, 10 by five, three by four,

four by three, eight by two and eight by only one.

The literature databases searched and study selection criteria varied among the reviews. Sample sizes for the studies reviewed tended to be modest (in general, <300 workers), and most concerned the relatively short-term (<12 months). The most recent data reported in any of these reviewed papers were collected in 1995. For these reasons, rather than re-reviewing all 36 of these relatively old, small studies, the results and conclusions of the reviewers regarding this general type of study are summarised below. Current smoking prevalence and cessation are related outcomes, and some studies examined one but not the other. Cross-sectional evaluations pre- and post- or just post-implementation of restrictions were more common to evaluate prevalence, and longitudinal studies tended to evaluate quitting, but studies based on retrospective recall were inclined to evaluate both.

Nineteen such studies were reviewed and indicated that most (17 of 18 that evaluated this outcome) showed a significant decrease in cigarette consumption following implementation of the smoking restrictions (Brownson *et al.*, 1997). Also, most showed a decline in smoking prevalence or an increase in quitting (17 of 19 that evaluated this outcome); little is known about the longer-term effect. Eriksen & Gottlieb (1998) evaluated 23 studies and their table appeared more complete and comprehensive than any of the other reviews, although the discussion in the text was more limited. Results were similar to the

Brownson *et al.* (1997) review; 16 of 17 found reduced consumption after implementation of workplace smoking restrictions, and 9 of 17 found some evidence for reduced prevalence or increased quitting (by 5% or more). Both these reviews endeavored to be as comprehensive as possible, and did not exclude studies based on study design criteria. A number of the studies were single surveys of respondents' perceptions of changes in their behaviour in response to the workplace smoking restrictions.

The review by Chapman *et al.* (1999) considered only studies (n=15) with information on completely smoke-free workplaces. They categorised the studies into three sub-types: prospective cohort studies (n=9), studies with cross-sectional pre- and post-evaluations (n=2), and studies where workers recalled their smoking behaviour before the workplace smoke-free policy took effect, and provided current information after working under the smoke-free policy (n=4). The authors noted that all of these studies showed declines in daily cigarette consumption rates, but fewer than half (5/14) showed declines in smoking prevalence or increases in quitting. Based on these observations, the authors concluded that smoke-free workplace policies reduced smoking. The authors then used six of the nine prospective cohort studies to estimate a mean change in daily cigarette consumption. The other three did not report these data sufficiently for inclusion in the calculation. The result was decrease of 3.5 CPD or a 20.7% decrease in daily cigarette consumption; the percentage decline

ranged from 5% to 52.6%. If heavier smokers quit their jobs because of the smoke-free policies and were not surveyed again, this estimate may be high. Not enough data were reported in the nine cohort studies to estimate a mean decline in prevalence.

One review included just eight studies of this type, out of about 50 that they identified, due to stringent inclusion criteria ("least suitable study design" – did not include a control group or a pre-post comparison), but a perusal of the excluded article titles suggested that many did not evaluate smoking behaviour (Hopkins *et al.*, 2001). All eight of the studies reviewed showed a significant decline in cigarette consumption following implementation of restrictions. In the four studies that examined quitting, three showed a significant effect, but in the six studies that examined prevalence, only three detected a significant decline. The reviewers concluded that smoking restrictions appear to reduce cigarette consumption and increase cessation, but the effect on prevalence is less consistent.

Another review considered the same three study subtypes as the Chapman *et al.* (1999) review, and considered eight prospective cohort studies, seven sequential cross-sectional, and six retrospective cross-sectional (Fichtenberg & Glantz, 2002). Two papers included more than one type of study. Of the 14 studies that evaluated consumption, 12 showed a reduction, but only 3 of 16 showed a significant reduction in prevalence. They included all the studies that reported on declines or differences in consumption or prevalence to compute their estimate of an aggregated decline of 3.1 CPD and of 3.8 percentage points in prevalence with a smoke-free workplace. They concluded that smoke-free workplaces do influence smoking behaviour.

In another review, all of the previous reviews were investigated, but only those studies (n=19) that had been conducted in the USA were selected for summary (Levy & Friend, 2003). The rationale was to minimise possible cultural differences in response to workplace smoking restrictions by focusing on one country. As for the other reviews, they express more confidence in the effect of smoking restrictions on reduced cigarette consumption (12 of 14 studies) than on increased quitting or reduced smoking prevalence (12 of 19). Some interesting points are made about such studies. By comparing results by length of follow-up, it was observed that reductions in quantity smoked appeared greatest relatively early (within 6 months) following implementation of smoking restrictions, while the effects on quit rates were more apparent over the longer-term, either from studies with repeated follow-ups or with follow-ups after one year from imposition of the restrictions. They comment regarding the considerable variation in study results that likely stems from differences in sample size, time of follow-up, type of industry, differences in how behaviour is measured, and differences in extent of restrictions and the presence of other ongoing interventions. In particular, they note that the type of workplace or industry (typically hospitals or government agencies) where the studies were conducted might limit the ability

to generalise from the results. Such industries may attract mainly nonsmokers so that restrictions might be more enforceable, and the smokers in these settings might be more susceptible to pressure to change their behaviour.

In the most recent article, multiple strategies for reducing smoking in the workplace were reviewed, including a section on the imposition of smoking restrictions (Moher et al., 2005). The inclusion criteria were more strict than in the other reviews; to be included, the study must have used pre- and post-measures of smoking behaviour (n=14). Two studies included a control group, but in both cases this consisted of only one workplace. Thus, any change over time in the control could either be from a secular trend or to some characteristic of the worksite. Three of the studies reviewed used cross-sectional pre- and post-measures and the others all used a prospective cohort design. Several of the studies also included other strategies for encouraging smokers to quit smoking; some included policies that were less than a completely smoke-free policy regarding smoking indoors. Declines in cigarette consumption during working hours after restrictions were implemented were noted in 9 of 11 of the studies that evaluated this outcome; smaller decreases were seen in overall daily consumption in eight studies, and three studies reported no change or a slight increase in daily consumption. Of the 10 studies that considered prevalence, five showed a decline and five showed no change. One study found higher quit rates during the evaluation period in those working

under a smoke-free policy compared to a control group without smoking restrictions. A number of the studies reviewed did not statistically test the changes observed. The authors concluded that the evidence was 'not consistent' for decreased cigarette consumption, and 'conflicting' for decreased prevalence with smoking restrictions.

Both the Chapman et al. (1999) and Fichtenberg & Glantz (2002) reviews used their estimates to gauge the economic impact to the tobacco industry of smoking restrictions. Chapman et al. (1999) calculated the revenue currently lost to the tobacco industry because of current smoking restrictions and if all workplaces became smoke-free. With the level of implementation of smoke-free policies introduced in Australia in 1995, the retail value lost sales total $90 (95% CI: 77.4, 100.7) millions of which 18.5% represented lossess to the industry. If all workplaces became smoke-free, the annual loss would be $171 (95% CI=147-191) million US$ in the USA and A$274 million in Australia. There would be a reduction in tax revenue as well (Chapman et al., 1999). According to Fichtenberg & Glantz (2002), if all workplaces became smoke-free, per capita consumption would drop by 4.5% in the USA and by 7.6% in the UK. These reductions would cost the tobacco industry $1.7 billion and £310 million annually in lost sales, equivalent to increasing the tax on cigarettes by $1.11 and £4.26 per pack, respectively.

Only the review by Chapman et al. (1999) mentioned the possibility that smokers working in smoke-free workplaces may be able to smoke their cigarettes sufficiently 'harder' so that they can maintain their accustomed nicotine levels by smoking fewer cigarettes. This is often called compensatory smoking (Scherer, 1999). Smoking a cigarette 'harder' can be accomplished by taking more puffs, taking deeper puffs, or smoking more of the cigarette. Several studies evaluated smokers' reported consumption on work days and non-work days with mixed results; a few found an increase in consumption on non-workdays, a few found no change, and a few found a decrease. It is likely that for some smokers, the 3.5 or 3.1 CPD less for workers in smoke-free worksites that was estimated from the Chapman *et al.* (1999) review, and the one by Fichtenberg & Glantz (2002), is within the realm of possible compensatory smoking (smoking 'harder').

Another issue not addressed in any of these reviews was workers leaving a smoke-free workplace to smoke. Such behaviour would both reduce the effect of smoke-free policies on cigarette consumption, and perhaps cost the employer in terms of unauthorised breaks. A survey of smokers working in smoke-free workplaces assessed this behaviour (Borland *et al.*, 1997). Of those who smoked during working hours (88%), consumption averaged 5.4 (SD=4.21) cigarettes during work breaks each day. Overall, 39% of workers said they left workplace premises to smoke. This occurred at least once a day during tea/coffee breaks for 25% of smokers, at lunch for 40% of smokers, and during work time for 13%. Factors related to this behaviour mainly related to level of addiction. The authors concluded

that smoke-free workplace policies would be more effective in reducing smoking if "exiled smoking" could be reduced.

Population surveys

All but the review by Moher *et al.* (2005) also included a few studies based on population survey data. Employed respondents were asked about their workplace situation, and those working in a smoke-free environment were compared to those working under partial or no smoking restrictions. Altogether, 11 population studies were reviewed previously (Brenner & Mielck, 1992; Wakefield *et al.*, 1992; Kinne *et al.*, 1993; Woodruff *et al.*, 1993; Patten *et al.*, 1995; Glasglow *et al.*, 1997; Biener & Nyman 1999; Evans *et al.*, 1999; Farkas *et al.*, 1999; Farrelly *et al.*, 1999; Longo *et al.*, 2001). Of these, two were reviewed in four of the previous reviews, two by three, three by two, and four in only one, likely due to later publication date. Other population studies (n=13) have been published subsequently (Pierce *et al.*, 1998c, 2009; Gilpin *et al.*, 2000, 2002a; Bauer *et al.*, 2005; Shields, 2005, 2007; Shavers *et al.*, 2006; Shopland *et al.*, 2006; Morozumi & li, 2006; Burns *et al.*, 2007; Lee & Kahende, 2007; Messer *et al.*, 2008).

Table 7.4 briefly summarises the results of all the population studies, which are described in detail in Appendix 5. All but three (Biener & Nyman, 1999; Shields 2005; Messer *et al.*, 2008) of these 24 population studies found a significant association between workplace smoking restrictions and some facet of smoking behaviour. The negative

studies only examined cessation. Of the 17 studies that compared cigarette consumption according to the presence or level of smoking restrictions, all but one (Brenner & Mielck, 1992) found significantly lower consumption among smoking workers in workplaces with restrictions. Smoking prevalence in the sample of workers was examined by eight of the studies, and two failed to find a significant association (Patten *et al.*, 1995; Shavers *et al.*, 2006). Making a recent quit attempt was examined in six studies, and three of these failed to find a higher rate among smokers working under restrictions (Bauer *et al.*, 2005; Shavers *et al.*, 2006; Messer *et al.*, 2008). Twelve studies reported on recent quitting (continuous abstinence of varying length when interviewed), and three of these (Biener & Nyman, 1999; Shields *et al.*, 2005; Messer *et al.*, 2008) failed to find significantly higher rates among workers with smoking restrictions. Several studies examined other outcomes: duration of smoking (Burns *et al.*, 2007), progress toward cessation (Pierce *et al.*, 1998c), and intent-to-quit (Woodruff *et al.*, 1993), and found significant pro-health associations of these outcomes with workplace smoking restrictions.

However, cross-sectional population studies cannot determine whether it is the type of workplace or worker characteristics (e.g. employing predominately white or blue collar workers) that are responsible for any observed association, or whether smokers in these environments do indeed alter their smoking behaviour because of the restrictions.

Table 7.4 Summary of results of 24 longitudinal and cross-sectional population studies examining associations between (all) worksite smoking policies and smoking behaviour

Reference	Locale	Occupation analysed	Outcome				
			Cigarette consumption	Smoking prevalence	Quit attempt	Cessation	Other
Longitudinal studies							
Patten et al., 1995	California, USA		SIG	NS			
Glasglow et al., 1997	USA		SIG		SIG	SIG	
Pierce et al., 1998a	California, USA						SIG-progress toward cessation
Biener & Nyman, 1999	Massachusetts, USA					NS	
Longo et. al., 2001	USA	yes				SIG	
Bauer et al., 2005	USA and Canada	yes	SIG		NS	SIG	
Shields et al., 2005	Canada					NS	
Shields et al., 2007	Canada	yes	SIG			SIG	
Cross-sectional studies							
Brenner & Mielck, 1992	Germany		NS		SIG	SIG	
Wakefield et al., 1992	Australia	yes	SIG				
Kinne et al., 1993	Washington, USA	yes	SIG-males only	SIG			
Woodruff et al., 1993	California, USA		SIG	NS			SIG-intent to quit
Farkas et al.,1996, 1999	California, USA	yes	SIG		SIG	SIG	
Farrelly et al., 1999	USA	yes	SIG	SIG			
Evans et al., 1999	USA	yes	SIG	SIG			
Gilpin et al., 2000	California, USA		SIG	SIG			
Gilpin & Pierce, 2002b	California, USA		SIG				
Shavers et al., 2006	USA	yes	SIG	NS	NS		
Shopland et al., 2006	USA	yes	SIG			SIG	
Morozumi et al., 2006	Japan		SIG	SIG		SIG	
Lee et al., 2007	USA					SIG	
Burns et al., 2007	Colorado, USA						SIG-smoking duration
Messer et al., 2008a	USA				NS	NS	
Pierce et al., 2009	USA		SIG				

SIG = significant difference in smoking behaviour indicated between workers with and without workplaces smoking restrictions. All significant differences were in the direction of reduced smoking (i.e. less consumption, more quitting) in workplaces with restrictions. NS = no significant difference. No entry means that the outcome was not considered.

More educated individuals generally smoke less and are more inclined to quit than those less educated (Pierce et al., 1989; Escobedo & Peddicord, 1996; Centers for Disease Control and Prevention, 1999; Gilpin & Pierce, 2002b; Schulze & Mons, 2005; Federico et al., 2007); thus, technical and professional businesses would be expected to employ more nonsmokers, and the smokers they do employ might smoke less and be more motivated to quit than would workers employed in factories or warehouses. Also, in the absence of a law requiring indoor workplaces to be smoke-free, workplaces that are smoke-free may be so because their highly educated workforce comprised mainly of non-smokers demanded it. All of the population studies included education and/or income as covariates, which could account to some extent for this possible source of confounding, and a number of the studies explicitly included a variable for occupation (see Table 7.4).

Rather than review all of the population studies in detail, the next sections describe results from the few published longitudinal surveys (Patten et al., 1995; Glasglow et al., 1997; Biener & Nyman, 1999; Bauer et al., 2005), including one that is not, strictly speaking, a population survey, but was nevertheless a survey of workers (Longo et al., 2001). Also described are a couple of cross-sectional studies that employed novel analytical strategies in an attempt to account for possible industry or work-er effects that might possibly explain the observed results of less smoking in workplaces with restrictions (Evans et al., 1999; Farrelly et al., 1999). The longitudinal design can compare changes in smoking behaviour over time between smokers working in an environment where smoking is restricted or not. The other cross-sectional surveys are described in detail in Appendix 5.

Longitudinal studies

One of the studies investigated in several of the previous review articles, conducted a cross-sectional comparison of smoking cessation among 1469 current and former smokers who worked in hospitals, to 920 who worked in other employment settings (Longo et al., 1996). Hospitals in the USA were mandated to be smoke-free by 1993, but many went smoke-free earlier. The post-smoke-free policy quit ratios (quit since policy imposed / all ever smokers) were higher among the hospital workers and tended to increase with time since the policy took effect. The subjects of this cross-sectional study became the basis for a cohort interviewed one or two times later up to 1996 (Longo et al., 2001; Appendix 5). Using the last follow-up data available, the time post-policy differed for each subject, so a Cox proportional hazard model was constructed for time to quit post-policy with censored observations as appropriate. The adjusted hazard ratio for quitting was 2.29 (95% CI=1.56-3.37) for the hospital compared to other workers, after adjusting for employee group (blue collar, clerical, white collar), education, age, sex, and education. Unadjusted quit ratios computed for groups with data at increasing time points post-policy showed increased quitting for both the hospital and other workers, and up through 84 months, these differed significantly, with the hospital workers showing consistently ever higher quit ratios. After that, sample sizes were small. Simple relapse rates at the follow-up surveys were compared for those not smoking at baseline, but were not found to be significantly different. At the first follow-up, nearly the same percentages of those in the hospital and other group were smoking again, 19.3% and 20.4%. At the second follow-up, these rates were 19.3% and 24.5%, respectively. Thus, these data suggest that while a smoke-free workplace might prompt quitting, it may not help prevent relapse among those initially quit.

A longitudinal sample of 1844 adult indoor workers (follow-up rate 50%) were asked about the smoking restrictions in their workplaces in both 1990 and 1992 (Patten et al., 1995). A smoke-free work area (not a completely smoke-free workplace) was reported by 57% of the sample in 1990 and by 67% in 1992. California did not mandate that all indoor workplaces be smoke-free until 1995. This study assessed changes in smoking status and cigarette consumption among four groups: work area under no restrictions both years, work area smoke-free in 1992 but not 1990, work area smoke-free in both years, work area smoke-free in 1990 but not in 1992. Besides smoking prevalence, the study assessed change in smoking status (smoker to nonsmoker or nonsmoker to smoker) from 1990 to 1992, and changes in daily consumption among those smoking in either year, with zero imputed if they were not smoking in a given year. Two multivariate analyses, adjusting for age, sex, education, and race/ethnicity, were conducted for consumption with increases or decrease (by 5 CPD or not smoking) from 1990 to 1992 as the dependent variable.

Smoking prevalence changed over time with work area restriction category (overall chi-square, p<0.06), but separate analyses of changes within category showed no significant difference because of small samples sizes. The group working in a smoke-free work area both years showed a decline in prevalence from 18.3% to 16.3%. Where the work area was smoke-free in 1992 but not 1990, prevalence changed from 20.3% to 19.1%. The group working in unrestricted work areas showed no change (~26.6% in both years). The group that worked in a smoke-free area in 1990 but not 1992, actually showed an increase in prevalence from 15.3% to 23.1%.

The groups that included those with smoke-free work areas in 1992 showed about double the rates of change in status from smoker to nonsmoker (about 18%) than the other groups (about 8%). Change in status from nonsmoker to smoker was highest (38%) in the group with a smoke-free work area in 1990 but not 1992. Some of this change may be relapse among former smokers and some may be initiation. This percentage ranged from 9% to 11% in the other groups. The overall chi-square for the analysis of change in status was p<0.05.

There was a small but significant decline in consumption (0.90 CPD) for the group with smoke-free work areas in both years. The group with a smoke-free work area in 1990 but not in 1992 showed a non-significant increase of 4.25 CPD. These changes

may be due to changes in prevalence and not to changes in consumption among continuing smokers. The multivariate analysis indicated that working in a smoke-free work area in 1990 but not 1992 was inversely associated with a decrease in consumption compared to having restrictions in both years. Overall, the results of this analysis suggest that moving from a job where smoking is not allowed in the work area to one where it is may increase smoking. The evidence for the opposite effect was less consistent.

The above study prompted investigators in Massachusetts to analyse their longitudinal population survey data in a similar fashion (Biener & Nyman, 1999), although they had even a smaller sample size (n=369). Two-thirds of smokers who were workers at baseline in 1993 were able to be contacted again in 1996. The outcome of interest was smoking cessation (a report of smoking "not at all" when interviewed again). Smoke-free workplaces were contrasted to all others (including those with partial restrictions), and categorised as continuously smoke-free, became smoke-free, or not smoke-free. Analyses adjusted for sex, age, education, smoking level at baseline (<15 versus 15+ CPD), and intent to quit within 30 days. Although the odds ratio for the group continuously working in a smoke-free environment was 2.0 (95% CI=0.7-6.0), it was not statistically significant compared to cessation in the group working continuously under no restrictions. For a new smoke-free workplace, the odds ratio was 1.4 (95% CI=0.3-6.1). Only being a light smoker or intending to quit were significantly

associated with cessation at follow-up. An additional analysis substituted exposure to SHS (exposure variable codes as: continuously low, became low, became high, continuously high) for workplace smoking policy. If exposure was continuously low or became low, cessation was higher, 6.99 (95% CI=1.79-27.3) and 6.44 (95% CI=1.04-28), respectively, compared to continuously high. The authors concluded that problems with enforcement of smoke-free policies may be partly responsible for the lack of a cessation effect.

A secondary analysis of longitudinal data from the Community Intervention Trial for Smoking Cessation (COMMIT) examined employed smokers (n=8271) interviewed in 1988 and again in 1993 (Glasglow et al., 1997). Worksite smoking policy was categorised as prohibiting smoking, allowing it only in designated areas, and allowing it everywhere. This study analysed cessation by follow-up, quit attempts, and cigarette consumption in continuing smokers and smokeless tobacco use. Multivariate analyses adjusted for sex, age, race/ethnicity, education, income, cigarette consumption in 1988, desire to quit, and number of past quit attempts. Compared to those working where smoking was allowed everywhere, those working where it was prohibited were 1.27 times more likely to be quit at follow-up (p<0.05). Designated areas were not significantly associated with increased quitting. However, both a designated area (1.16 times higher) and a smoke-free workplace (1.27 times higher) were significant when compared to where it was allowed everywhere (p<0.05). Both conditions were also associated with reduced cigarette consumption, by 1.17 (designated area), and by 2.78 (smoke-free) CPD. Smokeless tobacco use at follow-up was unrelated to smoking policy at baseline.

Another analysis of cohort data from COMMIT assessed the longer-term effects of working under a smoke-free workplace policy (Bauer *et al.*, 2005). A subset (n=1967) of smokers was identified who were initially interviewed in 1988, re-interviewed in 1993 and 2001, and who worked indoors in both years. These participants provided information about their employer's smoking policy in both 1993 and 2001. The proportion of these smokers working in a completely smoke-free environment increased markedly, from 27% in 1993 to 76% in 2001. Two different classifications taking account of worksite policy in both years were constructed. One was a three-level variable: maintained no restrictions or regressed from partial to none, maintained partial restrictions or regressed from smoke-free to partial, and maintained smoke-free status or changed to smoke-free. The other variable had nine levels, ranging from worked under no restrictions in both years to worked in a smoke-free workplace in both years. The study analysed several outcomes: quit for at least six months at follow-up, making a serious attempt to quit between surveys (including all those quit at follow-up), daily cigarette consumption and smokeless tobacco use, and adjusted for age, sex, race/ethnicity, education in 2001, desire to quit in 1988, number of previous quit attempts in 1993, amount smoked in 1993, and occupation in 2001.

For the three-level outcome, compared to the first category, the likelihood of quitting for six months was 1.73 (95% CI=0.96-3.11) higher for the second level, and for those working under smoke-free conditions at follow-up, it was 1.92 (95% CI=1.11-3.32) higher. Workplace smoking restrictions did not predict making a quit attempt. However, those in the third category, but not the second, showed a significant decline in daily consumption of 2.57 CPD (p<0.05) compared to those in the first category. For the nine-level categorisation, those working in a smoke-free workplace at both surveys were 2.29 (95% CI=1.08-4.45) more likely to be quit, and smoked 3.85 (p<0.05) fewer cigarettes than those working under no restrictions at both times. Lower levels of the categorisation were not associated with being quit for at least six months. Again, for the nine-level variable there was no significant relation of worksite restrictions to making a serious quit attempt. For daily consumption, the beta coefficients for the intermediate categories of worksite restrictions were less than for full restrictions, and were significant for the categories where the workplace was smoke-free at follow-up or for partial restrictions at both times. These results suggest that there may be a longer-term effect of smoke-free workplaces on successful cessation and consumption, and that smoke-free workplaces might help someone remain abstinent rather than prompt a quit attempt. Very few smokers (n=6 or 0.3%) indicated that they had switched jobs to avoid smoking restrictions in their workplace. Also, in 2001 only about 1% of the workers reported using smokeless tobacco at least three times per week, indicating no significant shift to this tobacco type as a result of working where smoking was not allowed.

Cross-sectional studies

An example of a study that went to considerable length to account for a possible "type-of-industry" effect is the one that analysed 1992-93 Current Population Survey data (Farrelly *et al.*, 1999). Smoking prevalence was examined in nearly 100 000 non-self-employed adult (18+ years) indoor workers, and daily cigarette consumption in a subset of nearly 25 000 current smokers according to the level of restrictions on smoking in their workplaces. These were categorised into four levels: no restrictions, partial work area/ common area restrictions, work area prohibition and partial common area restrictions, and completely smoke-free. Besides being asked about workplace restrictions on smoking, respondents provided information on their sex, age, race/ethnicity, educational attainment, marital status, number of persons in their households, urban/rural status, state, income, hours worked per week, and type of industry where they worked (seven categories: wholesale/retail trade; manufacturing; transportation; common utilities, including communications; medical services; finance, insurance, and real estate; and other professions, including law, education, architecture, etc.).

In an analysis that included all these variables, a smoke-free work area was only about half as strongly related (coefficients in model) to smoking prevalence as a fully smoke-free workplace. Model coefficients indicated that a smoke-free work area was associated with lower smoking prevalence by 2.6 (95% CI=1.7-3.5) percentage points, and a fully smoke-free workplace policy by 5.7 (95% CI=4.9-6.5) percentage points compared to no restrictions. Lesser restrictions were unrelated. For daily consumption among current smokers, the pattern was similar. For a completely smoke-free workplace policy, cigarette consumption was 2.7 (95% CI=2.3-3.1) CPD lower, for a smoke-free work area it was 1.5 (95% CI=1.1-1.9) CPD lower, and for partial restrictions it was 0.6 (95% CI=0.1-1.1) CPD lower compared to no restrictions. These results suggest a dose-response relationship between level of smoking restrictions and smoking behaviour.

The large sample sizes afforded by national surveys allow for sub-group analyses. Separate multivariate analyses were conduced within subgroups (e.g. sex, age group, race/ethnicity group, education group, industry group, etc.) and included all other factors as covariates. The difference in prevalence and consumption for workplaces that were completely smoke-free versus those with no restrictions were reported. Although the magnitude of the difference (smoke-free versus no restrictions) in prevalence or consumption varied among the subgroups analysed, in each one those working in smoke-free work-places showed a significantly lower

smoking prevalence, and smoking workers showed significantly lower daily cigarette consumption than those in workplaces with no restrictions. The differences tended to be greater in specific education (e.g. those without a high school diploma) or industry groups (e.g. wholesale retail trade), with higher relative prevalence or consumption rates overall. It is possible that smoke-free workplaces have a greater impact on smokers who smoke more.

In the second study, a standard analysis was performed of both adult smoking prevalence and smoker's cigarette consumption that adjusted for age, age squared, family size, log income, region, education, race/ethnicity, city size, marital status, cigarette tax, occupation, and year (Evans et al., 1999). Worksites were categorised as smoke-free work areas, having restrictions in other indoor areas, or no restrictions. The primary data source was the 1991 and 1993 NHIS that included 18 090 indoor workers. Results indicated that smoking prevalence among indoor workers in smoke-free work areas was 5.7 percentage points less than among indoor workers working under no smoking restrictions, and smokers in smoke-free work areas smoked 2.5 CPD less. The remainder of the paper presents a multitude of analyses trying to dispute this result. The highlights are summarised below.

First, the findings were replicated using the 1992/1993 CPS (n>97 000 indoor workers). Then additional analyses were conducted to explore whether this result was due to excluded variable bias; that is, if a worker's unobserved propensity to smoke is related to having a smoke-

free workplace, the results reported above are biased. The NHIS includes a comprehensive set of variables about respondent health and lifestyle, and if healthier workers or those with healthy lifestyles (including not smoking) tend to congregate in smoke-free workplaces. Including these variables and interactions with worksite policy should diminish the effect, but the original estimates proved robust. Other models included such factors as duration of employment at the current worksite (perhaps newer employees sought out worksites that were either smoke-free or not), or whether the worksite had unions, and again the results were unchanged. Next, it was determined that worksite size was the factor that was most related to whether or not the worksite was smoke-free; workplaces with more than 50 workers (22%) were more likely to be smoke-free. All possible worker characteristics were explored in small versus larger worksites. The differences were minimal, even for smoking prevalence, and when they included worksite size in the model, again it did not alter the effect. Another analysis included the number of hours worked; cigarette consumption was inversely related to number of hours worked if the workplace was smoke-free. Taken together, these results are fairly convincing for a causal effect: smoke-free workplaces have led workers to smoke less. A final analysis of data from other sources correlated the prevalence of worksite smoking policies, which increased from 25% in 1985 to 70% in 1993, to smoking prevalence trends among workers and non-workers. If indeed smoke-free workplaces reduce smoking prevalence by 5.7%, the observed widening discrepancy in the downward trend in smoking prevalence between workers and non-workers is completely explained by the rise in workplace smoking restrictions.

The detailed analyses employed by the above two studies suggest that declines in smoking behaviour occur in all types of workplaces, regardless of size, type of occupation or industry, and health consciousness. Thus, the generally consistent findings from all the other cross-sectional surveys likely identify real differences in smoking behaviour between those employed in smoke-free workplaces compared to those working in workplaces with lesser or no restrictions.

Shifts from cigarettes to other forms of tobacco as a result of workplace smoking restrictions

The analyses of the COMMIT longitudinal sample described above, failed to find any noticeable shift to smokeless tobacco use among smokers at baseline who became subject to smoke-free workplaces (Glasgow *et al.*, 1997; Bauer *et al.*, 2005). However, if smokeless tobacco, particularly Snus, is successfully marketed as a way for smokers to maintain access to nicotine during the workday without having to go outside or leave the premises to smoke, aggregated tobacco use may not decline as a result of smoke-free workplace policies. Smokers who might have quit because of the smoke-free policies, might choose to use smokeless products when they cannot smoke, but continue to smoke cigarettes when they can.

Summary

There appeared to be a fairly strong consensus among the previous reviews of worksite-based studies that workplace smoking restrictions lead to smokers reducing their daily cigarette consumption. These reviews were not as ready to claim an effect on smoking prevalence or cessation, because of very mixed results from the individual studies. Again, there were different study designs, smoking behaviour definitions, and categorisations of workplace smoking policy. The more inclusive the review, the more likely it was to conclude that the policy affected behaviour.

It would be expected that if partial restrictions are associated with reduced smoking, including this group with those having no restrictions in an analysis of smoke-free workplaces, versus all others, might limit the ability of the analysis to detect an association. There was some evidence that smoke-free work areas or completely smoke-free worksites might reduce daily cigarette consumption in the shorter-term with a cessation effect more likely to be observed in the longer-term. In general, smokers who have lower daily cigarette consumption find it easier to successfully quit.

The results from the population surveys of smokers working and not working under smoking restrictions were generally consistent with the worksite-based studies concerning the finding of reduced daily cigarette consumption. Further, among the population studies, there was a more consistent trend for lower smoking prevalence or higher rates of cessation among workers in workplaces with restrictions. While these mostly cross-sectional studies cannot prove that workplace smoking restrictions reduce smoking, two such studies provided additional evidence for a causal effect: one by examining smoking behaviour differences within industries which should employ similar workers, and the other by convincingly ruling out an effect for other worker or worksite characteristics that might have produced the observed results.

Smoking restrictions in schools

Besides the home, children and adolescents spend a good portion of their time at school. Therefore, this section focuses on the potential effect on student smoking of a complete prohibition on smoking for everyone, including adults, on school campuses compared to lesser or no restrictions.

Why school smoking restrictions might affect youth smoking behaviour

The traditional rationale for instituting a prohibition on smoking for students on school campuses is related to smoking prevention. If society thinks it is harmful for adolescents to smoke, and anti-tobacco curricula are used in its schools, then adolescents should not be given the conflicting message that it is permissible to smoke on school property. Furthermore, if such rules are well enforced, the availability of cigarettes and the opportunity for students to smoke is diminished, and even if they experiment outside of school, their progression to regular smoking might be impeded or at least delayed. Finally, if students do not see other students smoking on campus, they may perceive a relatively lower adolescent smoking prevalence, and such perceptions are associated with reduced smoking uptake. There is a large body of research on the effect of smoking prohibitions for students in secondary schools. The results have been mixed, with the extent and type of enforcement (punitive or cessation focused) or the combination (or not) of smoking policies with anti-tobacco curriculum the subject of most investigations.

More recently, the school has also been seen as a workplace, and especially in indoor areas, there is the rationale to prohibit smoking for everyone, including teachers, staff, and visitors to protect the health of nonsmokers. However, if smoking is prohibited indoors and not outdoors on campus, the effect might be that students would see many more adults smoking on campus. A study of seven European countries indicated that national and school policies restricting teacher smoking are negatively associated with students' seeing teachers smoking indoors, but positively associated with seeing them smoke outdoors (Wold et al., 2004b). Four countries had no policies regarding teacher smoking. Only one of the countries studied (Finland) prohibited smoking by teachers outside buildings on campus; it restricted it indoors (presumably to rooms to which students had no access). This study did not examine student smoking behaviour.

Teachers are important role models for students (Bewley et al., 1979; Poulsen et al., 2002), and students are well aware of the

hypocrisy of forbidding students to smoke, but allowing teachers or other adults to smoke on campus. In California, students who smoked were less likely to support smoke-free school policies if they perceived that teachers smoked on campus (adjusted OR=0.40; 95% CI=0.20-0.82) (Trinidad et al., 2005).

The review presented in the next section is confined to the relatively few studies to date that address the issue of the effect on student smoking of completely smoke-free schools, where no one including teachers, staff, or visitors is allowed to smoke on campus (Table 7.5).

Results for studies examining the association of smoke-free schools with youth smoking behaviour

The prevalence of student smoking in secondary schools is related to a multitude of factors and varies widely depending both on the characteristics of the students and of the school (Aveyard et al., 2004; Sellström & Bremberg, 2006). School level factors associated with student smoking prevalence include urban location, a school health policy, an anti-smoking policy, a good school climate, and a high average socioeconomic status (Sellström & Bremberg, 2006). Because of such differences, recent studies of school smoking policies have tended to use hierarchal statistical models that account for both school and student level characteristics. Studies that did not use a hierarchical analytic approach will be discussed in the text and in Table 7.5 before the studies that did. To date, all of the studies

related to this topic have been cross-sectional.

Data for 2464 students aged 16-17 years in 74 secondary schools and colleges in England and Wales were analysed (Charlton & While, 1994). In 1990, school directors filled out questionnaires concerning their school's smoking policies, and these were related to student smoking (at least weekly) and daily cigarette consumption separately in the secondary schools and colleges. Although some sample sizes were small, prevalence was 16% for students in smoke-free schools, 24% if staff but not students could smoke, 27% if staff not permitted to smoke but students are, and 34% if both staff and students could smoke. After adjusting for age, whether a best friend smokes, and whether a sibling smokes, it appeared that removal of staff smoking was associated with reduced current smoking in colleges, but not in schools. Because there was no suggestion from bivariate analyses that total daily consumption (school and non-school hours) was related to smoking policy, the authors did not perform a multivariate analysis.

Variables for student smoking policy, staff smoking policy, visitor smoking policy, and the presence of no-smoking signs were evaluated in a study of 26 429 students from 347 secondary schools in Australia (Clarke et al., 1994).

Table 7.5 Studies examining the association of school smoke-free policies for everyone with youth smoking behaviour

No hierarchical analyses

Reference Location	Population	Year	Definitions of smoking	School level characteristics other than smoking policy	Individual level characteristics	School policy	Analysis	Results	Comments
Charlton & White, 1994 England and Wales UK	2467 students 16-19 years in 74 schools and colleges	1990	At least weekly. Daily cigarette consumption also analysed	None in multivariate analysis	Age, best friend smokes, sibling smokes	Allowed for students and staff; not allowed for students, but allowed for staff; allowed for students but not for staff; not allowed for anyone.	Separate logistic regression analyses were conducted for secondary and college students.	Prohibition for staff, but not students significantly associated with reduced smoking for college students (p=0.034), but not for secondary school students.	The smoking policy was unrelated to cigarette consumption for both secondary and college students.
Clarke et al., 1994 Australia	26 429 students 12-17 years from 347 schools	1990	1 or more cigarettes in last week	Gender and age composition of school, school type, urban versus rural, staff smoking prevalence, and others related to school organisation	None	Three variables: staff smoking policy (not allowed, some areas, no restrictions), visitor policy (same categories as above), no smoking signs around school (none, few, most parts).	Bivariate analysis of variance of school level characteristics. Separate analyses by grade level (7-8, 9-10, 11-12).	None of the smoking policy variables considered were significantly related to student smoking.	Smoking was prohibited for students in nearly all schools.
Wakefield et al., 2000a USA	17 287 students 14-17 years from 202 schools	1996	Continuum: non susceptible, susceptible, early experimenter, advanced experimenter, established smoker. Any smoking in past 30 days	Restrictions on smoking in public places from other sources was merged into the dataset	Adult smokers in home, living siblings smoking, living in a smoke-free home, gender, race/ethnicity, and grade in school	Smoke-free for everyone versus lesser restrictions, level of enforcement of complete ban	Multivariate logistic regressions of each smoking stage level compared to lower level and of any smoking in the past 30 days.	A smoke-free school was not significant for the various transitions. However, an enforced smoke-free policy was. It was also significant for lower likelihood of being a current smoker OR=0.86; 95% CI=0.77-0.94	

Table 7.5 Studies examining the association of school smoke-free policies for everyone with youth smoking behaviour

Reference Location	Population	Year	Definitions of smoking	School level characteristics other than smoking policy	Individual level characteristics	School policy	Analysis	Results	Comments
No hierarchical analyses									
Osthus et al., 2007 Norway	16-20 years. 2400 current and former senior high students	2004	Daily smoking	School type (preparation for manual work, preparation for university)	Sex, age, work status	Smoke-free for everyone versus some restrictions versus no restrictions. Prevalence was 16%, 45%, and 40% for the policy types.	Separate multivariate logistic regression analyses for current and former students	Current students: OR=0.3;95% CI=0.1-0.5 smoke-free versus no restrictions. Former students OR=0.2; 95% CI=0.1-0.8 smoke-free versus no restrictions. Lesser restrictions not significant.	No interaction effect between policy type and school type was examined, so it is unknown whether the policy effect was present to the same extend in each school type.
Hierarchical analyses									
Moore et al., 2001 Wales, UK	15-16 years. 1246 students in 55 schools	1998	Weekly smoking Daily smoking	None	Mother's smoking, parents' expectations of school achievement, gender, socioeconomic status, school performance, alienation from school, best friend smokes	Strong: written policy about prohibition for everyone; Average: prohibition for everyone but not written for at least one group; Weak: no policy, or only policy for students. Also, whether policy strongly enforced or not for students and for teachers	Individual level characteristics associated with smoking in multivariate logistic regression were then included in the hierarchical models.	Average (OR=2.04; 95% CI=1.04-4.00) or weak (OR=2.77; 95% CI=1.25-6.12) policies were significantly associated with increased daily smoking, but not for weekly smoking. Strong enforcement for students was significantly related to both daily (OR=1.52; 95% CI=1.03-2.243) and weekly (OR=1.49; 95% CI=1.01-2.20) smoking. Strong enforcement for teachers was not significantly	Policy strength and enforcement were highly correlated, so they were not analysed in the same models.

Hierarchical analyses

Reference Location	Year	Definitions of smoking	School level characteristics other than smoking policy	Individual level characteristics	School policy	Analysis	Results	Comments
Moore et al., 2001 Wales, UK							related to either daily or weekly student smoking.	
Kumar et al., 2005 USA	1999 and 2000	Daily smoking, and attitude toward adult daily smoking	Public versus private, urbanicity, school size, aggregated parental education attainment. Year also included in full models	Grade in model for high school students, parental education, student race/ethnicity, and sex	3 variables: good monitoring of school policy prohibiting student smoking; strict consequences for student violation of smoking rule; teachers not permitted to smoke anywhere on school premises	Separate analyses for middle and high school students. Each policy variable analysed separately, then all three together, and finally with all other school and individual-level variables in hierarchical analyses.	For middle schoolers, monitoring was significantly related ($p<0.01$) to reduced daily smoking at all levels of analysis. For high schoolers, staff policy was significantly related ($p<0.05$) to reduced smoking in the final model with all factors included. Severity of consequences was significantly related to reduced smoking in individual and multiple policy models ($p<0.05$), but not in the full model.	There were no variables included for smoking among parents, siblings or friends.
Barnett et al., 2007 Quebec, Canada	1999	Daily smoking, not daily but in last 30 days, no smoking in past 30 days	Urban or rural, private or public, income in area of school	Sex, parents smoke daily, siblings smoke daily, live with both parents	3 variables: students can smoke outdoors, staff can smoke indoors, staff can smoke outdoors	Preliminary analyses identified individual, policy and other school level characteristics to include in final separate hierarchical models for age and sex groups.	Staff allowed to smoke outdoors was significantly related ($p<0.05$) to increased daily smoking in 13-year-old girls.	Sample sizes were relatively small for the age-sex subgroup analyses (<406 students). Student smoking policy was not significant in preliminary analyses.

Smoking cigarettes in the past week was bivariately (analysis of variance) related to these policy variables, as were other school level characteristics (sex composition; urban versus rural location; school type (government, Catholic or independent); proportion of students in level 7-10; proportion of students in level 11-12; school uniform compulsory; prefects selected by principal, staff or students; student representative on school council, etc.). None of the smoking policy variables was related to student smoking in any of the grade levels analysed (7-8, 9-10, or 11-12). No factor analysed was consistently related across all three grade level groups, but type of school (government, Catholic, or independent) showed the largest F-ratios in the analyses of variance for the 7th and 8th graders and for the 9th and 10th graders.

In 1996, a study conducted in the USA contrasted a completely smoke-free policy for everyone on campus to lesser or no restrictions for different levels of adolescent (14-17 years) smoking (Wakefield et al., 2000a). The 17 287 adolescents were either nonsusceptible never smokers, susceptible never smokers, early experimenters (puff in the past but not in last 30 days and weak intentions regarding future smoking, or a whole cigarette in past 30 days but strong intentions about not smoking again), advanced experimenters (a whole cigarette but less than 100 in lifetime and weak intentions not to smoke in future), or established smokers (had smoked at least 100 cigarettes in lifetime). Any smoking in the past 30 days was also analysed. Besides the smoke-free school variable, there was a school level variable for

strength of policy enforcement and for smoking restrictions in public places in the town were the school was located, obtained from external sources. Individual characteristics analysed included grade, sex, race/ethnicity, adult smoker in the home, sibling smoker, and home smoking restrictions. Multiple logistic regression analyses compared each smoking level to the one previous to it. Only for the transition to established smoking from advanced experimentation was a smoke-free school policy significant and it was positively associated with this transition (OR=1.22; 95% CI=1.07-1.37). However, a strongly enforced smoke-free policy was significantly related to reduced transition in every analysis, including the one of smoking in the past 30 days (OR=0.86; 95% CI=0.77-0.94). Thus, it is not sufficient for there to be a smoke-free policy for everyone; the policy must be consistently enforced.

Daily smoking in 2400 current and former students (aged 16-20 years) from Norwegian schools, with three levels of smoking policies in 2004, was evaluated (Osthus et al., 2007). Schools were classified as having smoke-free campuses, lesser smoking restrictions, or no smoking restrictions. For the three policy types, overall (current and former students) smoking prevalence was 16%, 45%, and 40% respectively. Separate multivariate analyses for current and former students adjusted for sex, age, work status, and school type (preparation for manual labour or for attending a university). For the current students, a smoke-free policy compared to no restrictions was associated with reduced daily

smoking (OR=0.3; 95% CI=0.1-0.5). A similar relationship was present for former students (OR=0.2; 95% CI=0.1-0.8). The odds ratios for a less than smoke-free policy were not significant. The authors did not examine an interaction between school and policy type, so it is unknown whether the policy affect was present equally for both school types.

The remainder of the studies used a hierarchical analysis. A survey of 11th graders in 55 randomly selected schools in Wales, classified school smoking policy as strong, average, or weak based on separate questionnaires completed by the head teacher and the teacher responsible for health education (Moore et al., 2001). A strong school policy was defined as a clearly written policy prohibiting smoking by students and staff anywhere on the school premises. An average policy also required the campus to be smoke-free, but the written policy was not clear and/or did not specifically mention all groups. A weak policy was defined as one that only covered students or where there was no policy at all. Whether or not the policy was consistently enforced for students and for teachers was analysed as two separate variables. In schools where there was a strong policy, mean daily smoking prevalence was 9.5% (95% CI: 6.1-12.9%). For those with an average policy it was 21.0% (17.8-24.2%), and for those with a weak policy it was 30.1% (23.6-36.6%). Weekly smoking prevalences for these policy categories were 17.1% (14.1-20.0%), 25.5% (21.7-29.2%), and 34.7% (24.7-44.7%), respectively. For daily smoking, students in schools with high enforcement for students showed a prevalence of daily smoking of 17.7% (13.4-22.0%) compared to 23.7% (20.2-27.2%) in schools with low enforcement. The comparable data for weekly smoking were 22.7% (18.3-27.0%) and 28.6% (24.0-33.2%), respectively. The student smoking prevalence for low and high enforcement of teacher smoking was not very different (Moore *et al.*,2001).

In the above study, preliminary logistic regression analyses identified student level characteristics that were related to report of daily or weekly smoking. These included sex, mother's smoking, parents' expectations about school performance, best friend's smoking, and alienation from school. Preliminary analyses also examined the school smoking policy variables. For daily smoking, an average or weak policy was related to increased smoking, and strong student enforcement marginally related to reduced smoking. Enforcement for teachers was not significantly related. For weekly smoking, the policy level and student enforcement variables were significant. Because the enforcement and policy level variables were highly related, separate hierarchical models analysed each. Compared to a strong policy, an average (OR=2.04; 95% CI=1.04-4.00) or weak (OR=2.77; 95% CI=1.25-6.12) school policy was still significantly related to increased daily smoking. In the separate model, low enforcement for students was also related to increased daily smoking (OR=1.52; 95% CI=1.03-2.24). For weekly smoking, policy level was unrelated, but low enforcement for pupils was marginally related (OR=1.49; 95% CI=1.01-2.20). Based

on their findings, the authors suggest that wider introduction of smoke-free school policies might help reduce teenage smoking.

Monitoring the Future school survey data were used to examine the relationship of school smoking policies to student daily smoking in middle (8th grade) and high school students (10th and 12th grades) in over 37 000 students from 342 schools in the USA (Kumar *et al.*, 2005). The study also analysed students' attitudes toward adult daily smoking. Separate variables accounted for three facets of school smoking policy: strength of monitoring for violations of school policy against student smoking, severity of consequences for student violations, and whether staff were permitted to smoke anywhere on school property. These and other school level factors were determined from questionnaires answered by an administrator at each participating school. Student level variables were demographics (gender, race/ethnicity, parental education), and other school level factors besides smoking policy were school type (public or private), school size, urbanicity, year of survey, and aggregated (from student's report) parental education attainment.

In the above study, models first considered only each separate smoking policy variable, then all three simultaneously, and finally hierarchically all school level and individual level factors. For middle-school students, strong monitoring of student smoking was the only significant policy variable related to daily smoking (p<0.001 in the individual model, p<0.01 in the policy and full models). However, in the

full model, the beta coefficient for staff smoking (0.22) was actually larger than for this same variable (0.19) in the analysis of high school students. In the high school students, staff smoking was significant in the full model (p<0.05), but not in the individual or combined policy analyses. Severity of consequences was significant individually (p<0.01) and in the policy model (p<0.01), but not in the full model. In the analyses of attitudes toward adult smoking, for the middle school students, the staff smoking variable was significant individually (p<0.05) and in the policy model (p<0.05), but lost significance in the full model. The opposite was true for the high school students: staff smoking was not significant in the individual or policy models, but was significant in the full model (p<0.05). Neither of the other two school policy variables was significant in any of the analyses of attitudes for either middle or high school students. The authors conclude that staff who smoke are likely poor monitors and should be provided with smoking cessation programmes.

In separate school samples of 763 13-year-old and 768 16-year-old Quebec students, school smoking policies were related to student smoking (Barnett *et al.*, 2007). The study assessed smoking policy for staff indoors, for staff outdoors, and for students indoors. Among 13-year-olds, daily smoking prevalence was 6.1% if students were permitted to smoke, versus 3.4% if they were not permitted to smoke. Related to staff smoking indoors, these prevalences were 4.3% versus 5.8%, and to staff smoking outdoors they were 6.5% versus 2.3%. The prevalences for less than daily smoking were similar regardless of policy. For the 16-year-olds, daily smoking prevalence was 23.6% if students could smoke outside, versus 20.8% if they could not. For staff smoking indoors these percentages were 28.1% versus 20.9%, and for staff smoking outdoors they were 23.3% and 22.8%. Again, the prevalence of less than daily smoking did not vary much according to policy.

Because there were some interactions by sex for individual level characteristics, the final hierarchical models in the above study analysed daily smoking in each sex-age group separately, resulting in fairly small sample sizes (n=357-405). Individual level variables included in the final models were daily smoking by parents and daily smoking by siblings, but neither of these variables was significant in any analyses. Other school level factors included were public versus private and rural versus urban school status, and both these variables were significantly related to daily smoking in all analyses. Based on the preliminary analyses, the hierarchical models only examined daily smoking, and only policy for staff outdoors for 13-year-old girls, and policy only for staff indoors for 16-year-old boys. Staff being permitted to smoke outdoors was significantly related to 13-year-old girls daily smoking prevalence (p<0.05). Staff being permitted to smoke outdoors was not significantly related to daily smoking among the 16-year-old boys. The authors emphasise the sex differences, but concluded that smoke-free schools might aid in the prevention of adolescent smoking.

Summary

To date there are only a few studies that have addressed the possible effect of a completely smoke-free school campus for everyone, including teachers and other adults, on youth smoking behaviour. All of the studies were cross-sectional. Because school level characteristics are related to student smoking prevalence, hierarchical analyses that properly account for such potential confounding factors are most appropriate for evaluating the effect of a smoke-free school policy. While the results from the few such studies employing this approach appear somewhat promising, more research is required. Nevertheless, regardless of the effect of a smoke-free school on smoking behaviour, such restrictions can be justified on the grounds that they potentially reduce exposure to SHS in the school setting.

Chapter summary

Smoking restrictions as one component of a comprehensive tobacco control programme

In localities where new laws were part of multiple tobacco control efforts, there was clear and consistent evidence for a change from prior ongoing trends. However, if multiple tobacco control measures are instituted simultaneously, attribution of the change to a new law restricting smoking is not possible.

Pre-post new law studies

Reviewed studies that assessed smoking behaviour before and after the implementation of new laws restricting smoking in public and workplaces were analytically weak and produced mixed results; some provided no statistical evaluation even though differences or trends appeared to be present.

Correlative studies

Nearly all the studies correlating the extent and strength of laws restricting smoking with various aspects of smoking behaviour found the expected associations. Localities with relatively stronger restrictions in more places, or that covered a greater proportion of the population generally showed lower adult and youth prevalence rates and reduced cigarette consumption. Whether localities with strong anti-smoking norms were more likely to pass such regulations or the regulations led to reduced smoking, is unknown.

Workplace studies

At a more individual level, studies of workers subject to restrictions in the workplace indicate that new restrictions reduce smokers' cigarette consumption by 2-4 CPD. Whether or not the reduction in daily cigarette consumption is sufficient to make the smokers less addicted, and therefore more likely to quit in the future, is unknown, but some evidence exists that the cuts in consumption in the shorter-term may lead to increased cessation in the longer-term.

Population studies

Population studies, even the cross-sectional ones, that adjusted for worker characteristics, including demographics and occupation, are likely minimally biased. Nearly all these studies found that smoke-free workplaces were more associated with decreased smoking among workers than partial restrictions.

Smoke-free school policies

To date, there are limited data concerning the effect of a completely smoke-free campus for everyone, students and adults, on adolescent smoking behaviour. Not witnessing teachers smoking on campus may reinforce school level anti-smoking norms and lead to reduced adolescent smoking initiation, but further research is required to explore this issue.

Conclusions

1. The different lines of evidence reviewed indicate that workplace smoking restrictions reduce cigarette consumption among continuing smokers.

2. The evidence from earlier studies concerning reduced prevalence and/or increased cessation is less clear. However, more recent evidence suggests that smoke-free workplaces reduce prevalence and increase quitting.

3. Correlative studies indicate an association between the strength and scope of laws restricting smoking in public and workplaces and reduced youth tobacco use.

4. When smoking restrictions are part of a comprehensive tobacco control programme, significant declines in smoking behaviour are observed. However, not all of the decline can be attributed to the smoking policies.

5. Few appropriate studies have assessed whether a smoke-free school campus for everyone, including adults and visitors, reduces smoking among students.

Recommendations

1. Smoking restrictions for public or workplaces should prohibit smoking completely if they are to have an optimal impact on reducing smoking behaviour, as well as reducing exposure to SHS.

2. To have optimal effect, smoke-free policies should be part of comprehensive tobacco control programmes aimed at reducing the adverse health effects from tobacco use.

3. Since much of what is known regarding the effect of smoking restrictions on smoking behaviour is from developed countries, further research on this topic is needed that involves multiple nations from different stages of the tobacco epidemic.

Chapter 8
Home smoking restrictions: effects on exposure to SHS and smoking behaviour

Introduction

The concept of smokers refraining from smoking in their own homes is a new one in many parts of the world. Two lines of evidence suggest that this phenomenon will become more commonplace worldwide in the years to come. As documented below, localities well along in their battle of the tobacco epidemic with laws prohibiting smoking in public and workplaces have observed increases in the percentage of smokers reporting smoke-free homes (Borland *et al.*, 1999; Al-Delaimy *et al.*, 2007; Lund & Lindbak, 2007). Other studies have found a positive association between smokers working in smoke-free workplaces and reporting that they live in smoke-free homes (Farkas *et al.*, 1999; Gilpin *et al.*, 2000; Gower *et al.*, 2000; Merom & Rissel, 2001; Shopland *et al.*, 2006; Thomson *et al.*, 2006). Workplace smoking restrictions may make people more aware of the dangers to nonsmokers of secondhand smoke (SHS), and help establish norms regarding the inappropriateness of smoking around nonsmokers. After learning to cope with workplace smoking restrictions, a smoker may be more agreeable to having them in the home as well.

Prohibitions against smoking in the home setting are generally not mandated by law, and thus, could be considered "voluntary." A situation in which a home may be mandated to be smoke-free is in child custody cases; the court orders a parent to maintain a smoke-free home so that the child, often with asthma or other health problems, is not exposed to SHS (Sweda, 2004). Further, as population knowledge about the health dangers of SHS becomes more widespread, nonsmokers living with smokers may demand that the smoker not smoke inside the home. A smoker may feel coerced into adhering to this demand and not feel that it is voluntary. However, concern on the part of smokers for the health of nonsmoking family members, including children, may lead them to voluntarily agree to a smoke-free home. Also, if the smoker feels that a smoke-free home can directly benefit them (e.g. facilitate cessation) they may voluntarily implement a smoke-free home policy.

The purpose of this chapter is to examine the potential for this relatively new situation of smokers living in smoke-free homes to: (1) reduce child exposure to SHS, and (2) influence the smoking behaviour both of adults and youths.

Methodological issues

The reader is referred to Chapter 7 for a discussion of methodological issues including the literature review procedures, typical study designs, and conventions for reporting results. Also, Appendix 2 provides common definitions of smoking behaviour.

The studies described in this chapter differed considerably in how a smoke-free home was analysed. In some cases there were one or more categories included for partial restrictions, but in other cases smoke-free homes were contrasted to all others, regardless if the home was less than completely smoke-free. Including those with partial restrictions with those reporting no restrictions would reduce the chance of finding an association of a smoke-free home with the outcome of interest.

Scope of chapter

This chapter begins by reporting the prevalence of home smoking restrictions among smokers in various localities worldwide and summarising the available data characterising which smokers live in homes with smoking restrictions. Next, it presents evidence that smoke-free homes can reduce childhood exposure to SHS, even in households with adult smokers. This section also summarises previous reviews of interventions designed to reduce children's exposure to SHS in the home. The last main section reviews all the studies located to date regarding the effect of home smoking restrictions on adult and youth smoking behaviour.

The phenomenon of home smoking restrictions

Prevalence of smoking restrictions among smokers

There are data on the prevalence of smoke-free homes from respondents to population surveys, and these rates are highly related to smoking prevalence. However, some homes without smokers do not report that their home is smoke-free, as they never considered the necessity for a formal policy.

A more important measure reflecting progress in tobacco control in general and protection of nonsmokers from SHS in particular, is report of a smoke-free home among smokers (Table 8.1). Among studies that provide data on smoke-free homes among smokers, most still show a minority reporting a smoke-free policy. However, in some localities in recent years, a majority do report having smoke-free homes (e.g. 52.8% in a New Zealand study in 2004 (Gillespie et al. 2005), 58% of daily smokers and 80% of occasional smokers in Norway in 2006 (Lund & Lindbak, 2007), 58% in California in 2005 (Al-Delaimy et al., 2008), 67% in Finland in 2005 and 55% in Sweden (European Commission, 2007)).

A survey conducted in the fall of 2005 covering the 25 European Union Countries and three additional European countries (Bulgaria, Croatia, and Romania) asked smokers whether they ever smoked when alone in their home (European Commission, 2007). This question is a fairly good proxy for identifying those who adhere to a completely smoke-free home policy. Overall, 18% of respondents claimed they never smoked at home when alone. This ranged from 67% of smokers in Finland to just 7% in Hungary and Croatia. Six countries had reported levels of 30% or higher (Finland, Sweden, Slovak Republic, Czech Republic, and Malta), and eight reported levels of 15% or less (Hungry, Croatia, Estonia, Greece, Belgium, Denmark, Estonia and Austria). These results underscore the disparities among countries.

Another key point is that for all countries with trend data, the proportion of smoke-free homes has increased over time both for the total population and for smokers. These trends may have been partly driven by reductions in smoking prevalence (U.S. Department of Health and Human Services, 2006), but there is evidence that other factors are involved. One review considered that comprehensive tobacco control programmes are likely to be important to changing social norms about where it is appropriate for smokers to smoke (Thomson et al., 2006). Also, mass media educational programmes, that are part of such tobacco control programs and that address the SHS hazard or specifically promote smoke-free homes, may have played an important role. In California, there was a particularly sharp increase in smoke-free homes (everyone not just smokers) in just one year (1992 to 1993) from 38% to 51% (Gilpin et al., 1999). During that time, the California Tobacco Control Programme's media campaign placed particular emphasis on protection of children from SHS in the home. Television spots depicted children coughing and breathing SHS from adults in the household.

There has been some speculation that smoking restrictions in public venues might lead to increases of smoking in private venues, such as homes. However, no evidence for such an effect was found in Ireland (Fong et al., 2006) or New Zealand (Edwards et al., 2008).

Who has a smoke-free home?

The question addressed in this section is: What are the characteristics of the population in general, and of smokers in particular, that report that smoking is not allowed in their homes?

Few studies addressed this question in a multivariate manner for the entire population. Univariate examinations of factors related to having a smoke-free home in Canada and the USA (Ashley et al. 1998; U.S. Department of Health and Human Services, 2006) provide some insight.

Table 8.1 Population prevalence of home smoking restrictions among *smokers*

Reference	Locality	Population	Year	Type of restriction	Prevalence %
Ashley *et al.*, 1998	Canada	443 adult smokers	1996	Partial Smoke-free	21.8 14.4
Norman *et al.*, 1999	California (USA)	Survey of 1245 adult smokers	1996/97	Smoke-free	43.3
Borland *et al.*, 1999	Victoria, Australia	800-900 adult smokers per survey year	Surveys 1995 1996 1997	Smoke-free 1995 1996 1997	 20.0 23.5 28.0
McMillen *et al.*, 2003	USA	362 & 669 smokers	Surveys 2000 2001	Smoke-free 2001 2002	 28.5 30.2
Pizacani *et al.*, 2003	Oregon (USA)	567 adult smokers	1997	Smoke-free	30.4
Gillespie *et al.*, 2005	New Zealand	1507 adult current smokers	2004	Smokers who do not smoke indoors at home	52.8
Borland *et al.*, 2006a	Canada, USA, UK, Australia	9046 adults in 4 countries	2002	Canada, partial / Smoke-free USA, partial / Smoke-free UK, partial / Smoke-free Australia, partial / Smoke-free	34.1 / 31.5 32.0 / 27.9 49.5 / 19.0 43.1 / 32.6
Fong *et al.*, 2006	Ireland and UK	Adults surveyed before (n=1679) and after (n=1185) law banning smoking in public places	2003/04 and 2004/05	Smoke-free 2003/04 2004/05	Ireland UK 15 18 20 24
Centers for Disease Control and Prevention, 2007a	USA	Current Population Surveys	Surveys 1992/93 2003	Smoke-free 1992/93 2001	 9.6 31.8
Al-Delaimy *et al.*, 2007	California (USA)	Survey of adult smokers 4558 in 1992 8581 in 1996 5470 in 1999 5278 in 2002 3821 in 2005	Surveys 1992 1996 1999 2002 2005	Smoke-free 1992 1996 1999 2002 2005	 19.4 35.9 46.8 51.9 57.8
Lund & Lindbak, 2007	Norway	Annual surveys	1995-2006	Smoke-free 1995 1996 1997 1998 1999 2000 2001 2002 2003 2004 2005	Occasional, Daily 26 10 26 12 45 20 52 21 46 19 49 24 53 26 66 25 64 42 75 43 80 58
European Commission, 2007	25 European Union countries and three other European countries	Survey conducted by Directorate-General Health and Consumer Protection of the European Commission	2005	Answer "no" to: Do you smoke inside your home when you are alone?	Mean: 18% Range: 7% to 67% 6 countries ≥ 30% 8 countries ≤ 15%

In Canada, in 1996, 34.6% (95% CI=32.3-36.9) of households were smoke-free (Ashley *et al.*, 1998). This percentage ranged from 42.9% (95% CI=39.6-46.2) in households with never smokers to 38.4% (95% CI=33.9-42.9) in households with former smokers to only 14.4% (95% CI=11.1-17.7) in households with current smokers. The number of daily smokers in the household was also related to the household being smoke-free: 44.3% (95% CI=41.5-47.1) smoke-free for no smokers, 17.5% (95% CI=13.7-21.3) for one smoker, and 7.4% (95% CI=3.7-11.1) for more than one smoker. Households with children 0-5 years were smoke-free 47.3% (95% CI=39.4-55.2) of the time, with children 0-17 years 42.5% (95% CI=32.9-52.1) were smoke-free, and with children 6-17 years 41.9% (95% CI=36.6-47.2) were. If no children were present, only 28.4% (95% CI=25.4-31.4) of households were smoke-free.

Data from the Current Population Survey, which was conducted in the USA, indicate that in 2001-2002, 66.03% of households were smoke-free (U.S. Department of Health and Human Services, 2006). Such homes were more prevalent among those of high (67.4%) versus low (57.8%) socioeconomic status. There were regional differences as well: northeast (64.9%), midwest (59.5%), south (65.2%) and west (75.2%). The states with the highest levels included Utah (83.1%), California (77.5%), and Arizona (75.9%), and those with the lowest percentages were Kentucky (50.9%), West Virginia (50.2%), and Tennessee (56.1%). Smoke-free homes were more prevalent among households without smokers (78.9%)

than with smokers (25.6%). In households with a child younger than 13 years of age, overall 72.8% were smoke-free. However, if there was a smoker in the home, only 36.5% of such households were smoke-free compared to 85.2% if there were no smokers and a child younger than 13 years in the household.

Tables 8.2 and 8.3 present the correlates of persons reporting smoke-free homes in four countries (the USA, Canada, the UK, and Australia). Only a few studies examined the multivariate association and only in subgroups of the general population (Table 8.2), but many more considered the associations of reporting smoke-free homes among smokers (Table 8.3). There is evidence that in households with both adult nonsmokers and smokers, that there is some discrepancy in reporting home smoking rules (Mumford *et al.*, 2004), with smokers in mixed households less likely than nonsmokers in the same household to say the household is smoke-free. However, if smokers behave according to their own perceptions, their reports may be more relevant. In both Tables 8.2 and 8.3, the studies summarised examined a variety of factors, but none examined them all. Omitted factors, either because the data were not gathered or not used, can lead to significant multivariate correlates that might have lacked significance had the missing factors been included.

The studies summarised in Table 8.2 pertain to subgroups of the general US population (women, households with children, African Americans, and Hispanics). These studies all presented the results of

multivariate analyses of a variety of factors that might be expected to be associated with having a smoke-free home. One study examined change over time in the proportion of families with children aged 18 years or younger, in which no one smoked on any days of the week in the home (Soliman *et al.*, 2004). This measure implies a smoke-free home, as it was in any week not just the most recent one. The authors compared data from the 1992 and 2000 National Health Interview Surveys, and found a decline in the "prevalence of exposure" in these families from 35% to 25%; this decline was demonstrated statistically to be greater than would be expected from the change in adult smoking prevalence over this period. The pattern of exposure among demographic and other groups was similar both years (combined year results are shown in Table 8.2), and the decline was observed among all the groups, but with higher educated groups showing somewhat greater declines.

Theses studies confirm that being a smoker is associated with a lower likelihood of reporting a smoke-free home (King *et al.*, 2005; Martinez-Donate *et al.*, 2007; Gonzales *et al.*, 2006; Shopland *et al.*, 2006). Three of the studies did not limit their population to families with children (King *et al.*, 2005; Shopland *et al.*, 2006; Martinez-Donate *et al.*, 2007), and two of them found that a young child in the home was correlated with report of a smoke-free home (Shopland *et al.*, 2006; Martinez-Donate *et al.*, 2007).

Table 8.2 Population studies reporting factors associated with having a smoke-free home from multivariate analyses

Reference/ location	Population / year of study	Factors associated with a smoke-free home								
		Odds Ratios, 95% CI								
		Smoking status	Young children present	Adult nonsmoker present	Believes SHS harmful	Age	Education	Race/ ethnicity	Employed in smoke-free workplace	Friends smoke
Soliman et al., 2004 USA	15 601 families with children ≤ 18 years Model predicted smoking inside house 1992; 2000	NA	NA	NA	0.27 0.23-0.32	NA	<HS: 1.18 1.03-1.35; some college: 0.64 0.57-0.71; college grad: 0.36 0.30-0.43; post grad: 0.28 0.21-0.37; Reference: High school graduate	Hispanic: 0.36 0.30-0.42; Black: 0.74 0.65-0.84; Native American: 1.12 0.74-1.69; Asian: 0.57 0.41-0.80; Reference: Non-hispanic whites	NA	NA
King et al., 2005 USA	1000 African Americans 2000-01	Former: 0.59 0.36-0.96; Current: 0.11 0.07-0.18; Reference: Never	NS	Marital status: Married: 2.89 1.76-4.73; Single: 1.79 1.03-3.1; Reference: Never married	Public should be protected: 2.69 1.36-5.34	NS	NA	NA	NA	Few: 0.45 0.28-0.73; Half: 0.28 0.16-0.47; Reference: None
Shopland et al., 2006 USA	128 024 employed females who do not live alone 2001-02	Never: 3.80 3.40-4.25; Former: 3.04 2.69-3.43; Occasional: 2.79 2.39-3.25; Reference: Daily	<5 years: 1.37 1.24-1.52; Ref: none or <5	All never: 7.58 6.44-8.92; All former: 5.12 4.37-5.99; Mixed (1+ smokers): 1.38 1.20-1.59; Reference: All smokers	NA	25-44 years 0.87 0.78-0.98; 45-64: 0.79 0.71-0.88; 65+: 0.89 0.72-1.10; Reference: 18-24 years	HS:1.40 1.30-1.51; College:1.68 1.56-1.82; Reference <HS	Hispanic: 1.81 1.56-2.09; Black: 0.78 0.71-0.86; Asian: 1.42 1.15-1.76; Reference: White	1.41 1.33-1.50; Service: 0.92 0.85-1.00; Blue collar: 0.78 0.70-0.86; Reference: White collar	NA

Table 8.2 Population studies reporting factors associated with having a smoke-free home from multivariate analyses

Reference/ location	Population/ year of study	Smoking status	Young children present	Adult nonsmoker present	Believes SHS harmful	Age	Education	Race/ ethnicity	Employed in smoke-free workplace	Friends smoke
					Factors associated with a smoke-free home					
Gonzales et al., 2006 Albuquerque, New Mexico, USA	269 Hispanic mothers of children 2-12 years 2003-04	Non-smoker: 5.47 2.50-11.95 Reference: Smoker	NA	11.17 4.56-27.38	NA	NS	NS	Born in the USA 0.17 0.06-0.50 Reference: In Mexico	NA	NA
Yousey, 2006 Midwestern USA	226 parents of children in Head Start programmes	NA	NA	Marital status and number of residents: NS	Attitude scale 0.83 0.76-0.91 Higher value implies lower agreement	NS	NS	English: 19.9 3.0-131.6 Reference: Spanish question-naire	NA	NA
Martinez-Donate et al., 2007 San Diego, California, USA	1103 adults of Mexican decent 2003-04	Former: 2.47 1.27-4.81 Never: 2.55 1.14-5.75 Reference: Smoker	2.03 1.18-3.51	Smoker: 0.45 0.26-0.78 Reference: Nonsmoker	Aversion to SHS: 2.82 1.41-5.63	Per year 0.98 0.96-0.99	Per year 0.81 0.70-0.95	Accultu-ration 1.50 1.10-2.05	NS	NA

NA = Not analysed or not applicable
NR = Not reported, but included in multivariate model
NS = Not significant
HS = High school education

Table 8.3 Population studies reporting factors associated with smokers living in a smoke-free home from multivariate analyses

Reference, sample size, study year	Factors associated with a smoke-free home									
	Child present	Adult Non-smoker present	Believes SHS harmful	Household income	Age	Sex	Education	Race/ ethnicity	Intention to quit, cigarette consumed	Friends smoke
					Odds ratios, 95% CI					
Gilpin et al., 1999 California, USA N=8904 1996	Child and adult: 5.7 4.6-7.0 Child, no adult: 2.7 2.1-3.4 Versus no child no adult	Adult nonsmoker only: 4.0 3.3-4.8	5.1 2.3-10.9 NA	NA NA	NR 25-44 years 0.8 0.6-0.9 45-64: 0.4 0.3-0.5 65+: 0.3 0.2-0.4 Versus 18-24 years	NR F: 0.7 0.6-0.8	NR NS	NR Hispanic: 2.5 2.0-3.1 Black: 0.6 0.5-0.9 Asian: 1.4 1.1-1.8 Versus White	NA NA	NA NA
Norman et al., 1999 California, USA N=1245 1996	6.1 2.8-13.7	NA	NA	1.19; 1-1.4	18-24 years 4.5 1.6-12.6 25-34: 2.1 1.1-4.0 35-54: 0.8 0.4-1.5 Versus 55+ years	F: 0.6 0.4-0.9	NA	Hispanic: 1.5 0.8-2.8 Black: 0.3 0.1-0.8 Other: 0.8 0.4-1.9 Versus White	NA	No friends smoke: 4.1 1.2-13.5 Few smoke: 4.1 2.0-8.3 <Half smoke: 1.7 0.8-3.9 Half smoke: 1.3 0.6-2.8 Versus Most smoke

Table 8.3 Population studies reporting factors associated with smokers living in a smoke-free home from multivariate analyses

Reference, sample size, study year	Factors associated with a smoke-free home									
	Child present	Adult Non-smoker present	Believes SHS harmful	Household income	Age	Sex	Education	Race/ethnicity	Intention to quit, cigarette consumed	Friends smoke
					Odds ratios, 95% CI					
Merom & Rissel, 2001 Australia N=4270 1998	<6 yrs: 3.8 3.1-4.7 ≥6 yrs: 1.9 1.5-2.3 Other adult: 0.9 0.7-1.1 Versus lives alone		NA	NA	35-54: 0.7 0.6-0.9 55+: 0.8 0.6-0.9 Versus 16-34 years	F: 0.8 0.7-1.0	HS: 1.3 1.1-1.5 College: 1.4 1.1-1.7 Versus <HS	Non-English background: 1.5 1.2-1.9	NA	NA
Kegler & Malcoe, 2002 Oklahoma, USA N=200 2000	NA	NS	4.56 1.3-16.2	NS	NS	NS	NA	NS	Quit attempt in last year: 2.5 1.2-5.4 <10/day: 3.3 1.5-7.7	NS
Okah et al., 2002 Inner city (Kansas City, Kansas, and Missouri) USA N=598 2000	2.6 1.7-4.1	2.1 1.8-3.6	NA	NA	0.98 0.96-1.00	NS	NS	NS	NS	NS
Pizacani et al., 2003 Oregon, USA N=147 1997	3.0; 2.1-4.4	4.3 2.5-7.3	6.6 3.6-12.3	>$35K 2.5 1.7-3.5	NA	NA	NA	NA	NA	NA

Factors associated with a smoke-free home

Reference, sample size, study year	Child present	Adult Non-smoker present	Believes SHS harmful	Household income	Age	Sex	Education	Race/ethnicity	Intention to quit, cigarette consumed	Friends smoke
					Odds ratios, 95% CI					
Okah et al., 2003 Inner city (Kansas City, Kansas, and Missouri, USA) N=383 2001	1.7 1.0-3.0	2.3 1.2-4.6	NA	NA	NS	NS	NA	NA	Preparation: 3.3 1.7-6.2 Versus Contemplation Progression: 4.2 2.2-7.9 Versus no progression	NA
Borland et al., 2006a USA, UK, Canada, Australia N=4053 2002	Infant: 3.7 2.1-6.4 Pre-school: 1.4 1.0-2.1 Preteen: 1.1 0.8-1.6 Teen: 1.2 0.9-1.8 Versus none	Non-smoker: 5.2 2.3-11.6 Other smoker: 2.2 0.8-6.1 Versus lives alone	NS	NS	18-24: 3.6 1.3-10.4 25-39: 1.7 0.8-3.5 40-54: 1.2 0.6-2.5 Versus 55+ years	NS	NS	Minority status: NS	NS Heaviness of smoking: 0.8 0.7-0.8	Intend to quit: In one mo: 1.6 1.0-2.5 In six mo: 1.4 1.0-2.0 >6 mo: 1.5 1.1-2.0 Versus No intent
Berg et al., 2006 Rural Kansas, USA N=472	2.2 1.1-4.3	1.6 1.1-2.5	NA	NA	NS	M: 1.4 1.0-2.2	NA	NA	Motivation scale: 1.03 1.01-1.05	3-5 of five best friends smoke: 0.6 0.4-0.9 Nicotine dependence scale: 0.8 0.7-0.9

217

Table 8.3 Population studies reporting factors associated with smokers living in a smoke-free home from multivariate analyses

Reference, sample size, study year	Child present	Adult Non-smoker present	Believes SHS harmful	Household income	Age	Sex	Education	Race/ ethnicity	Intention to quit, cigarette consumed	Friends smoke
				Factors associated with a smoke-free home						
					Odds ratios, 95% CI					
Shields, 2007 Canada N=4394 2005	2.7 2.2-3.3	NA	NA	NA	15-24: 3.1 2.0-4.9 25-34: 2.0 1.9-2.1 Versus 35-44 years	M: 1.3 1.1-1.6	HS: 1.9 0.6-5.8 College: 2.4 1.3-4.3 Versus <HS	NA	NA	NA

NA = Not analysed or not applicable
NR = Not reported, but included in multivariate model
NS = Not significant
HS= High school education
F=Female
M=Male

Attitudes and beliefs about the danger posed by SHS were examined in four of the studies, and all found an association with report of a smoke-free home (Soliman *et al.*, 2004; King *et al.*, 2005; Yousey, 2006; Martinez-Donate *et al.*, 2007). While all but one of the studies examined age, just two found an association. Employed women 25-64 years were less likely to report restrictions than younger women 18-24 years (Shopland *et al.* 2006), and among San Diego residents of Mexican decent, younger age was associated with less likelihood of a smoke-free home (Martinez-Donate *et al.*, 2007). Only one of the three studies that included both sexes examined the association of respondent sex (not shown in Table 8.2) with report of a smoke-free home, and found no association (Martinez-Donate *et al.*, 2007). In three of the five studies that examined educational attainment, having a high school education or greater was associated with report of a smoke-free home than not graduating from high school (Soliman *et al.*, 2004; Shopland *et al.*, 2006; Martinez-Donate *et al.*, 2007). The study by Martinez-Donate *et al.*, 2007 also found that persons of higher acculturation were more likely to have smoke-free homes. This is in contrast to all four studies where persons of Hispanic ethnicity/lower acculturation could be compared to non-Hispanic whites. In these studies, Hispanic ethnicity or less acculturation (immigrant or need to take the survey in Spanish) was associated with greater levels of smoke-free homes (Soliman *et al.*, 2004; Gonzales *et al.*, 2006; Shopland *et al.*, 2006; Yousey, 2006).

Asian households were also more likely to be smoke-free than non-Hispanic white households (Soliman *et al.*, 2004; Shopland *et al.*, 2006). It was found that report of employment in a smoke-free workplace and type of occupation were correlated with having a smoke-free home (Shopland *et al.*, 2006). In the study of US African Americans, having friends who smoke was associated with a report of a smoke-free home.

Another group of studies involving only smokers considered the presence of children or nonsmoking adults in the home (Table 8.3). In general, these factors were highly correlated with the smoker reporting a smoke-free home. In studies that examined attitudes or beliefs about the harmfulness of SHS (see also Chapter 5), with the exception of one study (Borland *et al.*, 2006a), there was a relationship with these factors and having a smoke-free home.

Since household income and educational attainment are related, studies tended to include one or the other of these factors, but not both. While respondents tend to freely report their educational status, many will not divulge their income, so most studies analysed education. Only one study in Table 8.3 included both (Borland *et al.*, 2006a); and neither was significantly related to having a smoke-free home. In the majority of studies, higher income or higher educational attainment was associated with the smoker having a smoke-free home. Many of the studies examined age and sex. In the studies that showed a significant effect for the age of the respondent, younger smokers were more likely to report a smoke-free home, and in

those that showed a significant effect for sex, female smokers reported having a smoke-free home less often than male smokers. Younger smokers may be more open to adoption of a smoke-free home, as they have not yet solidified their smoking behaviour, and tend to smoke fewer cigarettes per day (CPD) than older smokers (Al-Delaimy *et al.*, 2007). Heavier smokers might find it more inconvenient than lighter smokers to tolerate not smoking inside the home. If women are at home more than men, a smoke-free rule might be more difficult for them to tolerate as well.

In California, smokers of Hispanic ethnicity were more likely to report a smoke-free home, and African Americans were less likely to report one than non-Hispanic whites (Gilpin *et al.*, 1999; Norman *et al.*, 1999). Few Hispanic women (mostly of Mexican descent in California) smoke, and occasional smoking among Hispanic men is prevalent (Palinkas *et al.*, 1993). In Australia, a non-English background was significantly associated with greater report of a smoke-free home (Merom & Rissel, 2001). However, a four-country study that examined "minority status" failed to find an independent correlation (Borland *et al.*, 2006a). One study that included working in a smoke-free workplace (factor not included in Table 8.3) (Merom & Rissel, 2001) found that it was associated with a higher likelihood of reporting a smoke-free home compared to not being employed. Employment in a non smoke-free workplace showed a marginally higher likelihood of reporting a smoke-free home than the unemployed. Half the studies that examined having friends who smoke (Norman *et al.*, 1999; Kegler & Malcoe, 2002; Okah *et al.*, 2003; Berg *et al.*, 2006) found that smokers with friends who smoke were less likely to have a smoke-free home (Norman *et al.*, 1999; Berg *et al.*, 2006).

Two studies specifically looked longitudinally at factors predictive of adoption of a smoke-free home (Okah *et al.*, 2003; Borland *et al.*, 2006a). One study was clinic-based and participants were part of a smoking cessation program (Okah *et al.*, 2003). Being in the preparation stage for quitting (defined in this study as intending to quit in the next month and having a quit attempt of a day or longer in the past year) at baseline or advancing their stage of quitting by follow-up were both associated with adopting a smoke-free home. The other study was a population-based longitudinal study, and it found baseline intention to quit was associated with adoption of a smoke-free home (Borland *et al.*, 2006a). This study also included an index for "heaviness of smoking," which was inversely related to adoption of a smoke-free home. Two cross-sectional studies included variables related to heaviness of smoking: daily cigarette consumption (Kegler & Malcoe, 2002) or addiction level (Berg *et al.*, 2006). Both were similarly inversely related to adoption of a smoke-free home.

The two longitudinal studies of adoption of smoke-free home policy suggest that smokers thinking about quitting are more likely to institute a smoke-free policy; they may adopt a smoke-free home policy when they make a quit attempt. Personal desire

to quit, concern for the health of others in the household, and cultural factors may all play a role in smokers' adoption of a smoke-free home.

Protection of children from exposure to secondhand smoke in the home

Protection of children and adult nonsmokers from secondhand smoke (SHS) in the household is an important public health goal (WHO, 1999; U.S. Department of Health and Human Services, 2000). By 2010, the US goals are to reduce to 10% the fraction of children age 6 years or younger who are exposed to SHS in the home, and to reduce to 45% the fraction of nonsmokers age 4 years and older who exhibit a serum cotinine level >0.10 ng/ml (Healthy People 2010 initiative, http://www. healthypeople.gov/).The goal outlined by the WHO emphasised educational strategies to reduce SHS exposure in the home, recognising that smoke-free workplace legislation will help smokers accept that they should not smoke in their homes as well (WHO, 1999). Since children, especially pre-school aged, spend most of their time in the home or in the family automobile, having these settings smoke-free is the most effective step parents can take to reduce their children's exposure to SHS (see also Chapters 5 and 6).

Methods available to assess exposure to SHS are mentioned in Appendix 1. It can be costly and logistically complicated to obtain biological samples for determination of cotinine levels, or other biologic markers, on a large-scale population basis. Thus, many surveys ask

respondents to estimate hours of SHS exposure that they and/or their children have experienced in the home or in other settings, and these reports, along with other data describing smoking habits, have been compared to various biologic measures and found to correlate reasonably with them as in the example study described below.

This study compared detailed parental reports of smoking to their child's urinary cotinine levels (Wong *et al.*, 2002). It included 146 asthmatic children (7 years and older) and parent/guardian pairs from low-resource homes (Los Angeles, California) in which at least one adult smoked. Log transformed urine cotinine level was used as the dependent variable in a multivariate regression analysis with independent variables describing factors related to child exposure. These included number of smokers in the household, maternal and paternal smoking status, total number of cigarettes smoked per day in the home, total number of hours smoked per week by all household smokers in three locations (inside, directly outside the home, and in the car), and total number of hours the child was present when smoking occurred in each of these locations. In addition, a three-level variable for home smoking restrictions was included: no smoking ever allowed inside, partial restrictions (some rooms, some circumstances), and no restrictions on smoking indoors. Results indicated that the smoking restriction variable was the most important determinant of urinary cotinine level, followed by maternal smoking, total number of cigarettes smoked indoors at home, and paternal smoking. The first three factors accounted for 45% of the variance in urinary cotinine levels. The authors conclude that questionnaires can be kept relatively simple and ask only about these factors. While prediction of the biologic marker was not perfect, the questionnaire data provides a useful indication of a child's exposure to SHS in the home.

This section first examines levels of exposure typically experienced by children in the home. It then presents the evidence to support the assertion that a smoke-free home can protect children from SHS. Next, it summarises reviews of interventions designed to protect children from exposure to SHS in the home.

Prevalence of child exposure to SHS in the home

The largest international study that provides information regarding exposure to SHS in the home is the Global Youth Tobacco Survey (GYTS) (GTSS Collaborative Group, 2006). Students aged 13-15 years from 132 countries participated in the GYTS, from 1999 through 2005, and were asked if they had been exposed to SHS on one or more days in the past seven days. The data presented in Table 8.4 may not be representative of entire countries or regions, since the surveys were conducted in selected localities within the respective countries. The collective results of this survey suggest that worldwide nearly half of young people aged 13-15 years who are never smokers were exposed to SHS at home (43.9%) in the last seven days (Table 8.4).

Table 8.4 Any exposure to SHS at home in the last seven days according to results from Global Youth Tobacco Survey between 1999-2005 (GTSS Collaborative Group, 2006)

WHO region (by descending level of home SHS exposure)	Number of sites sampled	Percentage reporting exposure to SHS at home	95% CI	Had one or more parents who smoke (%)	Range for SHS exposure at home for jurisdictions within each region (and selected results)	Proportion of jurisdictions with ≥ 50% exposed (n)
Europe	29 in 26 countries	78.0	±2.6	59.6	Sarov, Russia (36.5%) to Republic of Serbia (97.7%)	89.7% (26/29)
Western Pacific	30 in 16 countries	50.5	±3.2	59.7	Puyang, China (32.6%) to Denang, Viet Nam (65.8%)	50.0% (15/30)
Americas	98 in 37 countries	41.6	±2.6	41.0	Virgin Islands (British) (10.4%) to Buenos Aires, Argentina (71.0%)	13.3% (13/98)
Eastern Mediterranean	25 in 21 countries	37.6	±3.5	35.6	Oman (21.0%) to Gaza Strip (87.0%)	28.0% (7/25)
South East Asia	11 in 7 countries	37.0	±1.6	43.5	Bhutan (29.2%) to Biratnagar, Nepal (84.7%)	54.5% (6/11)
African	37 in 25 countries	30.4	±3.8	22.7	Addis Ababa, Ethiopia (14.9%) to Bamako, Mali (59.9%)	2.7% (1/37)
Total	230 in 132 countries	43.9	±2.5	46.5	Virgin Islands (British) (10.4%) to Republic of Serbia (97.7%)	29.6% (68/230)

221

The WHO region with the highest level of SHS exposure at home was Europe (mean of 78.0%) and the lowest level was in Africa (mean of 30.4%).

Overall, the GYTS results show that there was only a small difference between those reporting SHS at home (43.9%) and those reporting that they have one or more parents who smoke (46.5%), suggesting that exposure to SHS at home is correlated with population smoking prevalence. It might be expected that countries with relatively higher levels of smoke-free homes among smokers would show a gap in these figures, with lower exposure rates than parental smoking prevalence. Worldwide, relatively few sites showed home SHS exposure rates much lower than parental smoking rates. In fact, in many cases the exposure percentage was somewhat higher than the rate of parental smoking, perhaps because of household members, other than parents, who were smokers.

Other studies of child or youth exposure to SHS in the home are described in the Table 8.5. The measure of exposure to SHS varies considerably so that the studies are not directly comparable. Report of a smoke-free home may not mean that exposure does not take place inside the home, particularly if the question asking about home smoking rules did not include an alternative for partial restrictions allowing smoking under particular circumstances (e.g. by visitors, in bad weather, only in some rooms, when children not present, etc.). As mentioned previously in the chapter, the prevalence of smoke-free homes is increasing over time, particularly in localities with a tobacco control programme with a media component emphasizing the importance of protecting children from SHS.

Do rules about smoking in the home reduce children's exposure to SHS?

All of the studies summarised in Table 8.6 concern exposure of children to SHS in households with and without some rules or measures being taken to protect them. Children with asthma whose parents smoke are a group of particular concern; Table 8.6 separates the studies dealing with asthmatic children. The studies reviewed include diverse measures of exposure, ranging from estimated hours of exposure per day or week to biochemical measures of cotinine (urine, serum, hair) or nicotine (hair). Further, the variable capturing rules about smoking inside the home sometimes included precautions, such as only smoking by an open window and not in the presence of a child, along with more strict rules up to a completely smoke-free policy. Also, while some studies included covariates related to sociodemographic factors and the smoking behaviour of the household adults, others did not.

Nevertheless, only one study reviewed failed to find a direct relation between increased SHS exposure to children and smoking allowed inside the home (Al-Delaimy et al., 2001b). Children 3 months to 10 years of age (n=112) were the subject of this study that compared hair nicotine levels in children in households with and without smokers, as well as in households with smokers but a smoke-free policy. In children reportedly exposed to smokers, hair nicotine levels were higher than in those not exposed to smokers (median 0.80 ng/mg of hair versus <0.10 ng/mg, respectively, p<0.0001). An even greater difference was observed for smoking mothers versus nonsmoking mothers (median 1.38 ng/mg versus <0.10 ng/mg, p<0.0001). The difference was less pronounced if the father smoked or not (0.61 ng/mg versus 0.10 ng/mg, p=0.0085). Typically, young children would be expected to spend more time in the home with the mother present than the father. In families with smokers who smoked only outside, the distribution of hair nicotine levels was reported to be similar (but data not presented) to that in families in which smokers smoked inside. The length of time the child spent inside the home was also related to hair nicotine levels. No multivariate analysis was performed, so it is unknown what effect time spent away from home might have on the relationship between smokers smoking only outside on hair nicotine levels.

An example of a positive study with a multivariate analysis was presented in the introduction to this main section (Wong et al., 2002). The purpose of this study was to determine whether questionnaires designed to capture information about exposure of children to SHS in the home needed to be brief or detailed. However, a number of the other studies (Table 8.6) used similar measures, and like the Wong et al. (2002) study, besides home smoking rules, some measure of intensity of smoking in the home was significantly associated with the particular biomarker being analysed

Table 8.5 Exposure of children to SHS in the home

Reference/location	Population	Year data collected	Measure of SHS exposure	Results	Comments
Jarvis et al., 2000 UK	Nationally representative cross-sectional surveys of secondary school children (11-15 years)	1988, 1998	Saliva cotinine concentrations	Saliva cotinine decreased from OR=0.96; 95% CI=0.83-1.11 ng/ml in 1988 to OR=0.52; 95% CI=0.43-0.62 ng/ml in 1998.	The authors attributed the decline to an increase in nonsmoking households and cessation among parents. Among those living with a smoking parent, there was little change.
Wakefield, et al., 2000a USA	Survey of 17 287 high school students aged 14-17 years	1996	Report of having a smoke-free home or partial restrictions regarding smoking inside the home	Close to half (48.2%) of students reported having a smoke-free home, and another quarter (27.2%) reported partial restrictions.	
Helgason & Lund, 2001 5 Nordic countries (Sweden, Norway, Denmark, Iceland, and Finland)	A mailed cross-sectional community-based survey of parents of children aged 3 years; 3547 households participated	1995-1996	At least weekly exposure inside the home	The reported levels of no SHS exposure in these homes was 63% in Denmark, 63% in Iceland, 76% in Norway, 89% in Sweden, and 95% in Finland.	Exposure to SHS was related to parent educational status and attitudes and awareness of the health effects of SHS on children.
Stephen et al., 2003 Nogales, Arizona, USA	Survey of students (10-12 years) and parents (n=631 pairs)	1996	Report of smoking inside the home	A majority of Mexican students (59.3%) had smokers living in their homes. Someone smoking inside was somewhat less common (50.0%). These numbers were lower for the Arizona students, 43.0% and 42.0%, respectively.	A larger proportion of homes with smokers appeared to be smoke-free in Nogales, Sonora than in Nogales, Arizona.
Soliman et al., 2004 USA	National Health Interview Surveys. Homes with children aged ≤ 18 years; 4418 families in 1992 and 11 183 in 2000	1992, 2000	Adult report of smoking inside the home	SHS exposure in homes with children declined from 35.6% to 25.1% from 1992 to 2000. This was greater than the decline in smoking prevalence (26.5% to 23.3%).	Home SHS exposures were more prevalent among non-Hispanic whites than among African Americans, Asian Americans, and Hispanics. Exposures declined across all groups, but with greater gains in higher education and income groups.
Leung et al., 2004 Hong Kong	Population-based birth cohort of 8327 newborn infants followed for 18 months	1997	Having a smoker in the household. Household smokers reported to smoke within 3 meters or beyond 3 meters of the infant.	41.2% of infants were exposed to a smoker in the household. 25.6% of these smokers smoked within 3 meters of the infant.	

Table 8.5 Exposure of children to SHS in the home

Reference/location	Population	Year data collected	Measure of SHS exposure	Results	Comments
Lund & Helgason, 2005 Norway	National random samples of households with children aged 3 years old. In 1995, 609 households participated. In 2001, 613 households participated.	1995, 2001	If smokers resided in the home, the respondent was asked how often they or their partners smoked indoors when their children were present. Respondents could answer every day, several times a week, about once a week, less than once a week, and never. Whether the home had some sort of rule restricting smoking.	In these households reported exposure of children (any, even less than once a week) to SHS was 18% in 2001. This was down from 32% in 1995. In 1995, 67% of families had imposed some sort of rule to limit smoking by family members or others indoors. This increased to 85% in 2001.	The prevalence of parental smoking was not significantly different between the two survey years.
Health Canada, 2006 Canada	Canadian Tobacco Use Monitoring Survey Households with children under the age of 12 years from over 21 976 respondents age 15 years and older	2006	Smoking inside the home every day or almost every day	The survey found that 15% of households reported at least one person who smoked inside the home every day or almost every day. Also, 9.2% of children under 12 were regularly exposed to SHS at home. This varied from 3.0% in British Colombia to 18.4% in Quebec.	
Healton et al., 2007 USA	American Legacy Foundation national survey of young people 12-17 years	2003	Report of daily exposure	Altogether, 13% of young people aged 12-17 were exposed to SHS daily in homes.	
Bird et al., 2007 Mexico	506 students (11-13 years old) from randomly selected schools, Ciudad Juarez	2000	Report of any exposure in past seven days	Overall, 41.3% were exposed to smoking in the home in the past seven days, and over 38% had one or more parents who smoked.	Exposure was highest in students from public low-socioeconomic status (SES) schools (57.4%) versus private high-SES schools (26.3%). Only students attending school in a high-SES setting reported SHS exposure at home (27.5%) that was lower than tobacco use by their parents (32.6%) (i.e. suggestive of some impact from smoke-free home rules).
Al-Delaimy et al., 2007 California	Households from the California Tobacco Surveys with children under 6 years	1993, 1996, 1999, 2002, 2005	No adult smoker in home, or if adult smokers live in home, home is reported to be smoke-free (no one smoked indoors at any time or under any circumstances).	In homes where all adults smoke, the percentage of children unexposed to SHS increased from 18% in 1993 to 57.8% in 2005. If mixed households (adult smokers and nonsmokers) the percentage of children protected increased from 43.2% in 1993 to 79.6% in 2005.	Having a nonsmoking adult in the household may provide advocacy for making the home smoke-free.

(Bakoula *et al.*, 1997; Wakefield *et al.*, 2000a; Blackburn *et al.*, 2003; Spencer *et al.*, 2005). In another study of reported hours of SHS exposure, the number of smokers in the household was significant in the multivariate analysis (Biener *et al.*, 1997).

A study that examined multiple measures of infant (≤ one year) exposure to SHS in 49 families is worth noting because of the consistency of findings across measures (Matt *et al.*, 2004). Three types of families were compared: all adults in the family were nonsmokers (n=17); at least one adult smoker in the family, but the smoker only smoked outside or in the absence of the infant (n=17); and at least one adult smoker and no steps were taken to protect the infant (n=15). Families were recruited in San Diego County by advertisements in clinic sites and the local news media. The families were eligible only if the infant was not being breast fed. Exposure to toxins from SHS was measured at multiple times in a variety of ways, including nicotine in household dust, indoor air, infant hair, and on household surfaces, and cotinine levels in infant urine and hair. Infant urine cotinine was 0.32 (95% CI=0.19-0.47) ng/ml in the nonsmoking households, 2.88 (95% CI=1.22-5.79) ng/ml in the protective households, and 13.02 (95% CI=8.01-20.81) ng/ml in the smoking households. Hair cotinine was 0.08 (95% CI=0.05-0.11) ng/mg in the nonsmoker households, 0.52 (95% CI=0.20-0.92) ng/mg in the protective, and 1.05 (95% CI=0.55-1.72) ng/mg in the smoking households. Hair nicotine was 0.53 (95% CI=0.25-0.86) ng/mg in the

nonsmoking households, 2.65 (95% CI=1.10-5.34) ng/mg in the protective, and 5.95 (95% CI=3.25-10.37) ng/mg in the smoking households. There was no measurable surface contamination in homes without smokers. In homes with smokers but protective of infants, mean surface contamination in the living room was 10.08 (95% CI=0.01-21.10) $\mu g/m^2$, and it was 8.19 (95% CI=2.69-14.98) $\mu g/m^2$ in the infant's bedroom. In non-protective homes, these levels were 51.33 (95% CI=19.17-32.16) $\mu g/m^2$ and 41.85 (95% CI=24.71-59.09) $\mu g/m^2$, respectively. The other measures of contamination were nil in the nonsmoking families, and generally much higher (up to a factor of 7) in the families not trying to protect their infants compared to the families that did. It appears that infants in families with smokers who try to protect their child are still exposed to between 5 and 10 times more SHS toxins as in families without smokers. These concerned families do, however, manage to at least halve their infant's exposure when compared to those who take no steps to protect their infants. When smokers smoke in the home when the infant is not present, contaminants accumulate; they may even accumulate from contact with the smoker's skin and clothing, even when the smoker does not smoke inside the home.

A large international study conducted in 2006 examined 1284 households from 31 countries fairly evenly distributed in three regions: Latin America, Asia, and Europe and the Middle East (Wipfli *et al.*, 2008). Households had at least one child younger than 11 years; hair samples were collected for determination

of hair nicotine concentrations if smoking was not permitted inside the household (smoke-free). A multilevel linear model of households with male smokers allowed for a country-specific intercept, and with child hair nicotine concentrations as the dependent variable it examined the following independent variables: whether the household was smoke-free, the number of smokers in the household, whether the mother smoked, cigarettes smoked per day by all smokers and by female smokers only, whether at least one smoker smoked near the child, and the child's age. The model estimated that hair nicotine concentrations were 2.6 (95% CI=2.0-3.3) times higher in children residing in non smoke-free households compared to those that were smoke-free. A similar analysis of air nicotine concentrations, that included the number of smokers in the household, the number of cigarette smoked per day by all smokers, whether the household was smoke-free, and mean outdoor temperature, showed homes without a smoke-free policy to have 12.9 (95% CI=9.4-17.6) times the air nicotine concentration as those with such a policy.

The results of these studies (Table 8.6) suggest that while partial restrictions on smoking indoors in the home might reduce exposure of children to SHS toxins compared to no restrictions at all, a smoke-free home provided the best protection to children in homes with an adult smoker present. When analysing the factors related to SHS exposure, besides the presence of smoking restrictions, measures of the intensity of smoking in the household appeared to be significantly related.

Table 8.6 Clinic-based (unless otherwise indicated) studies reporting exposure of children to SHS in homes with and without smoking restrictions

Children in general

Reference/ location	Population/ year data collected	Analysis	Exposure measure(s)	Home smoking restriction variable	Results	Comments
Bakoula et al., 1997 Athens, Greece	2108 Children ≤ 14 years who attended hospital outpatient clinics 1991-92	Multiple linear regression of log cotinine to creatinine ratio. Model included child's age and gender, day of the week sample taken, home floor area, non-central versus central heating, and maternal and paternal daily cigarette consumption	Urinary cotinine to creatinine ratio (CCR)	Precautions by parents taken to reduce exposure: never smoking in presence of child, or only in certain areas, or with the windows open	Less by 38% (24-54%) if precautions taken by parents. Also significant: cigarettes smoked when the child was at home, child's age, sample taken any day but Monday, floor area of the home, heat central versus noncentral, maternal education, paternal education.	Having a smoke-free home could not be evaluated separately.
Biener et al., 1997 Massachusetts	Population survey of 1606 adolescents 12-17 years Analysis in subset of 679 families with at least one adult smoker 1993-94	Multiple linear regression of log hours exposed to SHS. Model included teen age, adult educational attainment, and number of adult smokers in the household.	Reported hours of exposure to SHS in the home in the past week	Full, partial, or no smoking restrictions: Restrictions: None 53% Partial 22% Full 25%	Model-adjusted mean number of hours of SHS exposure was: 33.2 12.7 2.4 (p<0.001). Also significant: Number of smokers in household, and in households without smokers, whether visitors smoked	Even with a supposedly smoke-free home, exposure was not zero, indicating incomplete resident/visitor compliance to the smoke-free policy.
Al-Delaimy et al., 2001b Wellington, New Zealand	117 children aged 3 months to 10 years in households with an adult smoker 1996	Wilcoxon ranksum test of log transformed hair nicotine concentration	Hair nicotine concentration	Ban on smoking indoors in households with smokers	Authors reported that distribution of hair nicotine concentrations similar in those with and without a smoke-free policy indoors, but no data given. Other factors examined: Unvariately significant were whether the mother smoked, the father smoked, and the time per week that the child spent away from the home	No multivariate analysis.

Reference/ location	Population/ year data collected	Analysis	Exposure measure(s)	Home smoking restriction variable	Results	Comments
Children in general						
Blackburn *et al.*, 2003 Coventry and Birmingham, England UK	164 households with smokers and bottle fed infants 4 to 24 weeks of age Not reported	Linear regression of log CCR including parent's daily cigarette consumption, partner's daily consumption, housing tenure, overcrowding, and a smoke-free home contrasted to all others	Urinary CCR	No protective measurers used (12%) Some measures used but not a prohibition on smoking inside (69%) Ban on smoking inside (18%) The mean log cotinine to creatinine ratio was 1.26 (range 0.68-1.82) for infants in smoke-free households vs. 2.58 (2.38-2.78) others. No differences in groups using no measures (2.43 [1.83-3.03]) or weak measures (2.61 [2.41-2.81]).	When a smoke-free home was contrasted to all others it was independently significant (p<0.001). Also significantly related were parent's daily cigarette consumption (p<0.001), and housing tenure (p=0.003).	
Johansson *et al.*, 2004 Southeastern Sweden	366 children 2.5-3 years with smoking parents from a population cohort study were compared to a control group of 433 age-matched children with nonsmoking households 1997-99	Logistic regression of < 6 versus ≥ 6 cotinine value in households with smokers	Urine samples were obtained after family approval to participate, but before a detailed survey assessed smokers' behaviour regarding protection of their children from exposure to SHS.	Multi-level variable: Smoke only outdoors with door closed (56%) Smoke outdoors with door open (12%) Smoke by kitchen fan or outside with door closed (14%) Smoke by kitchen fan, outdoors with door closed or by the open door (7%) Take no protective measures (8%)	The odds of a high urinary cotinine level compared to controls were: OR=1.99; 95% CI=1.1-3.6 OR=2.39; 95% CI=0.9-6.1 OR=3.23; 95% CI=1.3-7.9 OR=10.32; 95% CI=4.3-24.8 OR=15.09; 95% CI=6.6-35.3	Logistic regression analysis did not adjust for other factors possibly related to exposure.
Matt *et al.*, 2004 San Diego, California, USA	49 families with infants ≤ 1 year recruited from advertisements Not reported	Tobit regression for data with minimal detectable concentrations	Urinary and hair cotinine and nicotine in hair, as well as nicotine in dust, on surfaces ,and in the air measured at multiple different times	Nonsmoking households contrasted with smoking households where smokers did not smoke inside, or did smoke inside	All exposure measures significantly different in households with smokers with versus without smoking restrictions (see text for details).	No multivariate analysis performed.

Table 8.6 Clinic-based (unless otherwise indicated) studies reporting exposure of children to SHS in homes with and without smoking restrictions

Reference/ location	Population/ year data collected	Analysis	Exposure measure(s)	Home smoking restriction variable	Results	Comments
Children in general						
Groner et al., 2005 Columbus, Ohio, USA	291 children 0-3 years attending pediatric primary care facility 1999-2000	Chi-square tests conducted across groups defined by hair cotinine concentration level	Hair cotinine level : <0.3 ng/mg 0.3-0.7 ng/mg >0.7 ng/mg	A smoke-free home policy present or not	Percentage with policy present 78.6% 54.4% 23.5% p<0.001	The cigarette consumption of the smoking mother was not related to concentration group.
Rise & Lund, 2005 Norway	Mailed questionnaire to random sample of households. Present analysis included children age 3 years with a parent who smokes 1995; 2001	Multiple linear regression of exposure index included household education, attitudes toward SHS, and awareness of SHS risk. Separate analyses for each year.	Index of exposure constructed from parental report of frequency of child exposure to a smoker in a car, TV-room, dining room, elsewhere in the home. The higher the score, the less the child was exposed.	Household had rules about smoking or not	Percentage of households with rules increased from 71% in 1995 to 91% in 2001. In 1995, rules about smoking were more strongly associated with exposure than the other factors in the model, p<0.0001. Rules not significant in 2001.	Rules may have involved less than a smoke-free home
Spencer et al., 2005 Coventry, England, UK	Baseline data for 309 infants 18-30 months in households with smokers from the Coventry Cohort study Not reported	Multiple linear regression of log CCR. Model included mothers' and fathers' average daily cigarette consumption, length of time in home and overcrowding and a smoke-free home contrasted to all others	Urinary CCR	Smoke-free home (13.9%) versus all others	A smoke-free home was found to be significant at the p<0.001 level. Also significant were mothers' average total daily cigarette consumption (p=0.008) and fathers' average total daily consumption (p<0.001). The length of time the family lived in the home and over-crowding, were not significant.	No adjustment was made for demographic variables.
Yousey, 2006 Midwestern, USA	Convenience sample of 202 English speaking and Spanish speaking adult smokers living with a child younger than 6 years of age Not reported	Multivariate logistic regression included number of smokers in home, and potential correlates of a smoking ban (last time someone smoked in home, number of cigarettes smoked in home in last week, other.	Urine cotinine ≤ 30ngdL versus >30 ng/dL.	Smoke-free home versus all others	Even with other variables potentially related to having a completely smoke-free home in the analysis, children living in a smoke-free home had less exposure compared to those in a non-smoke-free home. OR=0.224; 95% CI=0.056-0.902	

Reference/ location	Population/ year data collected	Analysis	Exposure measure(s)	Home smoking restriction variable	Results	Comments
Children in general						
Hughes et al., 2008 Seoul, Korea	207 adult respondents to a population survey living with at least one child under 18 years of age 2002	Multivariate logistic regression adjusted for age, adult smoking, grand-parents smoking, other groups discourage smoking	Adult estimate of number of cigarettes child exposed to in the home in a typical week.	Smoke-free home versus all others	Exposure increased in non-smoke-free households compared to all others. OR=9.13; 95% CI=2.06-40.4	
Wipfli et al., 2008 3 regions: Latin America, Asia, and Europe and the Middle East	1284 households (not randomly selected) from 31 countries with at least one child younger than 11 years 2006	Separate multi-level linear model of each SHS exposure measure for households with male smokers. (See text for variables included).	Hair nicotine levels Air nicotine concentrations	Smoke-free versus all others	Compared to a smoke-free home: Hair nicotine OR=2.6; 95% CI=2.0-3.3 Air nicotine OR=12.9; 95% CI=9.4-17.6 times higher	
Children with asthma						
Winkelstein et al., 1997 Baltimore, Maryland, USA	108 inner city asthmatic children aged 1-19 years attending allergy clinics 1993-94	Analysis of variance of log CCR	Urinary CCR	Households with smokers with a smoke-free home versus Households with smokers with smoking permitted indoors	8.5 ng/mg (median, 5.5 ng/mg) 73 ng/mg (median, 25 ng/mg)	p=0.0005 for log transformed CCR
Wakefield et al., 2000b Adelaide, Australia	249 asthmatic children aged 1 to 11 years with at least one smoking parent attending hospital outpatient clinics 1998-99	Multivariate regression of log CCR. Model also included child's age, mother's smoking status, and total parental daily cigarette consumption.	Urinary CCR	Smoke-free (40.2%) mean CCR: 7.6 nmol/mmol Some exceptions allowed to the policy: (16.5%): 14.9 nmol/mmol Allowed in rooms where child rarely present: (16.8%): 14.1 nmol/mmol No restrictions (26.5%): 26.0 nmol/mmol	In the multivariate regression analysis of the log transformed ratios there was an effect of home restrictions, p<0.001. The type of partial restrictions (visitors, when child absent, cold weather, etc.) did not appear to make a difference. Other significant variables were child's age and total daily household cigarette consumption.

Table 8.6 Clinic-based (unless otherwise indicated) studies reporting exposure of children to SHS in homes with and without smoking restrictions

Reference/ location	Population/ year data collected	Analysis	Exposure measure(s)	Home smoking restriction variable	Results	Comments
Children with asthma						
Wong et al., 2002 Los Angeles, California, USA	146 asthmatic children (7 years and older) and parent/ guardian pairs from low income homes in which at least one adult smoked. Not reported	Multivariate regression analysis of log urinary cotinine. Independent variables: number of smokers in household, maternal and paternal smoking status, total number of cigarettes per day in the home, number of hours smoked / week by all household smokers in three locations (inside, directly outside the home, in the car), and total number of hours the child was present when smoking in each of these places.	Urinary cotinine	No smoking ever allowed inside versus partial restrictions (some rooms, some circumstances), versus no restrictions on smoking indoors.	In the multivariate analysis, the smoking restriction variable was the most important significant determinant of urinary cotinine level (p<0.001), followed by maternal smoking (p<0.001) and total number of cigarettes smoked indoors at home (p<0.001), and paternal smoking (p=0.015). Importance ranked by proportion of variance explained by each factor in univariate analysis.	The authors conclude that only a limited amount of information about smoking in the home is needed to characterise children's SHS exposure.
Berman et al., 2003 Los Angeles, California USA	242 asthmatic children 2-14 years who live in households with smokers identified from schools, clinics and agencies serving low income families 1996-98	Kruskal-Wallis analysis of variance	Parental report of hours exposed, air nicotine concentration, urinary cotinine concentration	Smoke-free (47%): 0.0 hours/week; air 0.01 g/m³, urine 0.37 ng/ml Partial restrictions (42%): 0.0 hours/week; air 0.06 g/m³, urine 1.32 ng/ml No restrictions (10%): 5.0 hours/week; air 0.66 g/m³, urine 2.92 ng/ml	Hours/week (p<0.001). Air nicotine concentrations p<0.001. Hair nicotine concentrations p<0.001.	No multivariate analysis performed. In these California homes, even a partial restriction was linked to a drastically lower exposure.
Wamboldt et al., 2008 USA	91 asthmatic children 6-12 years matched by age, gender, and race/ethnicity to 91 healthy children, all with at least one current smoker in household	Bivariate ANOVA and chi-square analyses	Nicotine dosimeters worn by child and placed in bedroom and family room. Salivary cotinine, self-report by adult of number of cigarettes smoked in presence of child.	Smoke-free home versus all others	Just over 40% of children lived in smoke-free households. All exposure measures were significantly related to reduced exposures in a smoke-free home (p<0.0001). No multivariate analysis of exposure conducted.	Main analysis (logistic regression) was to identify predictors of smoke-free homes.

A smoking mother (likely to expose a child more than a smoking father), the total number of smokers in the home, or the total daily cigarette consumption by smokers in the household are all measures that capture the intensity of smoking in the home.

Can interventions aimed at families with smokers reduce children's SHS exposure?

A number of interventions have been designed to increase the protection of children from SHS. Nearly all have focused on getting smoking parents to quit. Although cessation would be best for all concerned, it is difficult to achieve. A later section of this chapter suggests that implementation of a smoke-free home might facilitate cessation in the longer-term, and as the evidence presented above (Table 8.6) indicates, in the shorter-term a smoke-free home will help to minimise children's exposure to SHS.

Family-level interventions

Reviews of trials of interventions at the family level to protect children from SHS include Hovell *et al.*, 2000; Hopkins *et al.*, 2001; Wewers & Uno, 2002; Gehrman & Hovell, 2003; Roseby *et al.*, 2003; Klerman, 2004; and the U.S. Department of Health and Human Services, 2006. The trials were generally of modest scale (<300 families), involved (at a minimum) provision to the intervention group of written educational material about smoking cessation (during pregnancy and for parents of young children), and in some instances, information on the health dangers

of smoking in the presence of an infant or child. On the whole, minimal interventions of this kind have not been found to be effective. More intensive interventions have involved brief counseling sessions by a health care provider with or without written materials, and the reviews find little evidence of an impact on childhood exposure to SHS.

Other studies involved multiple clinic-based or in-home counseling sessions, sometimes with follow-up calls or written reminders delivered over months. A few of these more intensive interventions found greater reductions in SHS exposure had occurred among children in the intervention groups compared to controls (Greenberg *et al.*, 1994; Groner *et al.*, 2000; Hovell *et al.*, 2000, 2002; Emmons *et al.*, 2001). However, the evidence from biomarkers in the studies that included them was weak. The review articles concluded that fairly intensive interventions are necessary to bring about the desired result in individual households. An editorial commenting on such programs questioned whether they were worth the modest results observed given the effort (Berman, 2003).

It is possible that clinic- or home-based methods aimed at families are too personally intrusive. A somewhat less personal approach used educational materials and one telephone counseling call in the US state of Oregon (Lichtenstein *et al.*, 2000; Glasglow *et al.*, 2004). Coupons to obtain a radon test kit were sent out in utility bills to 14 000 households. Kits and a brief survey were sent to those returning the coupons (n=1220). From the survey responses,

714 households with smokers were randomised to receive: (1) a copy of the Environmental Protection Agency pamphlet on protection from radon (control group), (2) a copy of a special pamphlet that emphasised that even in low radon households smoking put household members at increased risk of disease, or (3) the special pamphlet and a single telephone counseling call reinforcing the pamphlet by emphasising that smoking cessation or a smoke-free home policy would optimally protect household members. There was a nonsignificant trend for more smoking cessation in the counseling call group compared to the other groups, and this group had significantly more newly implemented home smoke-free policies in place at 12 months follow-up: group 3 -17.2% versus group 1 -14.2% and group 2 -9.9%, p<0.05. At baseline, over one-quarter of these households were already smoke-free; Oregon has an ongoing comprehensive tobacco control program.

Population-level interventions

Some of the review articles concerning the clinic- and home-based interventions have suggested that standard population-based tobacco control efforts, including legislation to increase cigarette taxation, include warning labels on cigarette packages, implement advertising restrictions, initiate anti-tobacco media campaigns, and to prohibit smoking in public and workplaces, might reduce the exposure of nonsmokers to SHS simply by reducing population smoking prevalence (Hovell *et al.*,

2000; Wewers & Uno, 2002; Klerman, 2004). Chapter 6 looks specifically at reduction in SHS exposure following new laws restricting smoking. Chapter 7 addresses the implication of smoking restrictions in public places on smoking behaviour, and concludes that comprehensive laws prohibiting smoking in all workplaces reduces smoking; therefore, exposure of nonsmokers to SHS would be reduced.

A review of studies evaluating such policy level options concluded that they might prove to be the most effective option for increasing the prevalence of smoke-free homes (Thomson et al., 2006). This review reported on studies relating greater exposure to tobacco control efforts to a higher prevalence of smoke-free homes. To date, there is no evidence that restricting smoking in public places makes smokers more likely to smoke in their homes (Hyland et al., 2008b), and such policies appear to reduce children's exposure to environmental tobacco smoke overall (Akhtar et al., 2007).

Barriers and triggers for smoke-free homes

Several qualitative studies have examined what messages might best encourage smokers to adopt smoke-free policies at home or how such policies had been adopted (Gupta & Dwyer, 2001; Kegler et al., 2007; Robinson & Kirkcaldy, 2007; Escoffery et al., 2008). Results from one study suggested that themes emphasising child health, but at the same time respecting smokers, might be effective (Gupta & Dwyer, 2001). Language should not be patronising

and should encourage smokers not to smoke rather than criticising them for smoking. Messages should not make smokers feel guilty or imply a criticism of bad parenting. Participants preferred the slogan "welcome to a smoke-free home" to the slogan "our home is smoke-free because we care." One study found that it was almost always a female caregiver that broached the subject of adopting a smoke-free home, usually a nonsmoker, and at least half the time this person was also the one in the family seen as having the power to do it (Kegler et al., 2007). Triggers for adopting a smoke-free home included a new baby, a move to a new home, someone moving in or out, physician recommendation, or a health problem of a household member. Reasons for adopting a smoke-free home centered on protecting children, but also included aversion to smoke by adults and children, as well as the smell of cigarettes permeating the household. Whether smoke-free home policies would be lifted after children grow up and leave home is a matter for further research. Participants generally believed that allowing or not allowing smoking in the home was a private matter.

In 2004, focus groups in the UK, with 54 disadvantaged smoking mothers of children 0-4 years of age, revealed not all mothers understood the dangers of SHS to their children (Robinson & Kirkcaldy, 2007), and that knowledge did not necessarily mean the mother took steps to protect her children. Nearly all mothers agreed that they never would smoke in their child's bedroom. While some indicated that no smoking

was allowed inside their homes, they went on to describe significant exceptions, such as smoking only in the bathroom or kitchen with the door closed and window open, or smoking inside at night if they felt unsafe going outside. Many mothers smoked in the doorway or outside, but noted that their small children tended to follow them and so were exposed anyway. Some tried to smoke only when the child was not present in a particular room, but wondered whether the smoke lingered or dispersed into adjacent rooms. Small homes limited the distance mothers could maintain between themselves and their children when they smoked. Often attempts to limit their children's exposure were transitory, because the mother did not believe her efforts were making a difference. How to overcome these barriers for disadvantaged families remains a subject for further research.

Another study conducted interviews with adults in 102 households with smokers and with young adolescent children in rural areas of the US state of Georgia (Escoffery et al., 2008). Thirty-five (34%) of these households had a smoke-free home, 55 (54%) had partial restrictions, and 12 (12%) no restrictions. Enforcement of a smoke-free policy was problematic for about a third of the households; visitors and bad weather accounted for most of the infractions. Those without a smoke-free policy might consider implementing one if someone, particularly a child, became ill. Smokers in households with a smoke-free policy or partial restrictions discussed their family's desire that they quit. Ideas for implementing a completely smoke-free home included putting up signs indicating the home was smoke-free, getting rid of ashtrays, and creating a place outside for smoking. The author supported these ideas of ways to create and maintain smoke-free households.

While some attention has been devoted to the idea of legislation making it illegal to smoke in homes and cars with children (Ezra, 1994; Ashley & Ferrence, 1998), it is unlikely that such laws affecting homes will become widespread. In the USA, such a law would be unconstitutional, but this may not be the case in other countries. Perhaps enforcement of such a law would involve too great an invasion of privacy, superseding a public obligation to protect the health of children. However, enforcement of a law prohibiting smoking in cars in which children are passengers may be no more difficult than enforcement of laws regarding seatbelt use. There appears to be substantial popular support for a law prohibiting smoking in cars when children are present in many localities, including in a number of US states (see Chapter 6).

A recent study examined how families establish and enforce smoking rules in family cars (Kegler et al., 2008). Like the Escoffery et al. (2008) study described above, this study summarised findings from interviews of 136 Black and White families in rural Georgia. Just under half (46.3%) of the families had a smoker. Fewer than half the families had ever discussed car smoking rules, but 36.8% reported a smoke-free car rule, 40.4% partial restrictions, and 22.8% reported no rules against smoking in the car. Reasons stated

for having a smoke-free car included protecting nonsmoking passengers from SHS, that the closed in nature of a car makes smoke stifling, the smell of smoke, and not wanting damage to the car from burns or smoke. Besides prohibiting smoking, respondents suggested only smoking with the windows open or when nonsmokers (including children) were not present. Families with rules generally had some difficulty enforcing them. Smokers were agreeable at least half the time they were asked not to smoke, but a few were resentful. Participants without a smoke-free policy indicated that they might consider adopting one if the smoker(s) in the family quit or the family got a new car.

Summary

In localities with relatively high adult smoking prevalence, protecting children and youth from exposure to SHS remains problematic. Often the reported prevalence of exposure to SHS and parental smoking prevalence are similar. In some localities, there have been marked increases in the fraction of children protected from SHS smoke in the home; these trends are more rapid than what would be expected to result from a decline in population smoking prevalence. These locales tend to be places where there are laws prohibiting smoking in public and workplaces. Increased awareness of the dangers of SHS, resulting from passage and implementation of these laws, might influence people to adopt such rules for their homes as well.

Observational studies show that children are less exposed to SHS in households in which smoking

is restricted than in those allowing smoking inside. A smoke-free home policy appears to provide greater protection than partial restrictions. Even then, protection may not be complete because of breaches in compliance and exposure of children to SHS in settings outside the home. In multivariate analyses relating exposure of children to SHS to smoking habits of adults, besides the presence of smoking restrictions, some measure of the intensity of smoking in the home is an important correlate.

Home smoking policies appear to be more prevalent in homes with children or other nonsmokers, among those of higher socioeconomic status or education, among those who believe that SHS is dangerous, among younger smokers and in some ethnic groups (for instance, in the USA, smoking in the home is less common among Hispanics and Asians). Women smokers, perhaps mostly stay-at-home mothers, appear less likely to have a smoke-free home because they spend so much of their time there. Smokers interested in quitting or who have made a quit attempt also may be more likely to have smoke-free homes.

Increasing the number of smoke-free homes in general is an important public health goal, but only a very small minority of trials designed to protect children from SHS have shown positive results. These trials have tended to focus more on parental smoking cessation than promoting smoke-free homes. Bringing about behaviour change on an individual level has proved difficult.

Laws prohibiting smoking in public settings and workplaces may prove to be the most effective way to stimulate adoption of such polices in the home. Such laws both establish and reinforce a population norm that smoking around nonsmokers is unacceptable. Smokers tend to increase their support for such smoke-free laws after they are implemented (see Chapter 5), and as a result, may extend such policies voluntarily to their homes. Other common tobacco control measures might also reinforce population norms against smoking.

Smoke-free home effect on smoking behaviour

There have been no previous reviews of studies addressing the potential effect of home smoking restrictions on adult or youth smoking behaviour. For this reason, all, rather than only selected studies located in the literature on this topic, are described below. First, there is a discussion of how smoking restrictions in the home might alter smokers' smoking behaviour, leading them to smoke less and perhaps eventually quit. This section also addresses the effect home smoking restrictions have on smoking uptake among adolescents.

Whereas smoke-free workplaces are generally imposed by law or by an employer, smoking restrictions in the home generally need to be by agreement among household adults. Often a nonsmoking adult in the household will negotiate a smoking policy to protect themselves and/or children in the household from exposure to SHS. However, even in a household where all adults smoke, residents may agree that not smoking inside is important for the health of their children. In households without

children where all adults smoke, residents may want to maintain a home free of stale cigarette smoke and that is inviting to their nonsmoking relatives and friends.

The studies described below involve data from population surveys and are subject to the limitations inherent in the resultant data. Smoking behaviour and information on smoking restrictions are by self-report. In general, biochemical validation, or validation by report from a significant other, have indicated self-report to be reliable (Hatziandreu et al., 1989; Gilpin et al., 1994).

Effect on adults

Why home smoking restrictions might affect adult smoking behaviour

Having a smoke-free home may be a sign of a smoker's motivation to quit or it may lead to an increase in a smoker's level of motivation to quit. Some smokers may initially agree to the imposition of a smoke-free home policy because of pressure from nonsmokers in the household to protect the health of family members and to eliminate annoyance and odor from tobacco smoke in the home. However, for such smokers, the barriers to smoking intrinsic in having a smoke-free home may also lead to changes in smoking behaviour that increase the chances for future successful cessation.

For many moderate to heavy smokers, the most important cigarette is the first one in the morning (after a night without nicotine). A sizable majority of these smokers have their first cigarette within the first half-hour of awakening, which is one of the

main indicators of nicotine addiction (Fagerstrom & Schneider, 1989). Smokers with smoke-free homes must cope with the inconvenience of going outside soon after awakening or postponing their first cigarette. A smoke-free home also creates a barrier to other cigarettes, such as the one after a meal. Thus, the smoke-free home policy may disrupt some psychologically addictive behaviour patterns commonly cited as the most difficult situations in which to avoid smoking (Best & Hakstian, 1978; U.S. Department of Health and Human Services, 1988; Payne et al., 1996; Shiffman et al., 1996; Drobes & Tiffany, 1997). Eventually, because of these barrier-induced behavioural changes, smokers may smoke less, thereby lessening their addiction, and have increased self-efficacy with respect to managing their smoking behaviour. Together with the inconvenience of having to go outside to smoke, these factors may increase the smoker's motivation to quit. In fact, having a smoke-free home has been associated with higher smoking abstinence, self-efficacy, and motivation to quit (Berg, et al., 2006; Shields, 2007).

Once quit, a smoke-free home may be effective in preventing relapse. Especially when there is another smoker in the household, a smoke-free home can reduce smoking temptations; quitters will not have to witness people smoking in their immediate environment, which can induce cravings in recent ex-smokers (Mermelstein et al., 1983; Coppotelli & Orleans, 1985; Horwitz et al., 1985; Brownell et al., 1986; Marlatt et al., 1988; Garvey et al., 1992).

To the extent that smoke-free homes can lead to reduced nicotine addiction and encourage and prolong quit attempts, they will likely foster eventual successful cessation (Farkas et al., 1996; Pierce et al., 1998d). However, reduced cigarette consumption does not always translate to reduced addiction. Some smokers may maintain their accustomed nicotine levels by increasing the number of puffs they take from each cigarette they smoke or inhaling more deeply (McMorrow & Foxx, 1983; Scherer, 1999). To the extent that smokers derive more from each cigarette they smoke, the potential to diminish addiction is less. A recent study compared reducers to habitual light smokers (Hatsukami et al., 2006). Both groups smoked on average the same number of CPD (5-6). However, the levels of toxins in the reducers' blood was about 20% higher than measured in the blood of the habitual light smokers. Further, the variability of toxin level in the reducers was much greater than for the habitual light smokers, indicating that while some managed to reduce their addiction level by reducing their consumption, others likely had maintained it.

Results for studies examining the effect of home smoking restrictions on adult smoking behaviour

The published findings summarised in Table 8.7 and presented in detail in Appendix 6 all show some relationship between home smoking policies and characteristic(s) of adult smoking behaviour. Whether studies investigating this topic that failed to find such an effect were not submitted or not accepted for publication is unknown.

Seven of these studies were longitudinal and all showed reduced relapse, increased quitting, or progress toward cessation by follow-up for smokers living in a smoke-free home compared to those without such a policy or no policy. In the five studies that examined consumption among continuing smokers, all but one noted a decline for those in smoke-free homes that was greater than that observed among those not living in a smoke-free home. The exception (Hyland et al., 2009) found a significant effect if baseline consumption was not included in the model. Several of the other studies included this variable, but still found an effect (Shields, 2005, 2007; Messer et al., 2008a).

The other studies were all cross-sectional, so that while it is possible to demonstrate a relationship, the direction is not clear. Do people who modify their smoking behaviour institute home smoking rules to help them maintain their changes, or do such restrictions lead to modifications in smoking behaviour, including quitting? Again, among the cross-sectional studies that examined the relationship between home smoking restrictions and cessation and/or cigarette consumption, such a relation was found in all but one (Norman et al., 2000). It should be noted that many of the researchers examined the same surveys, although perhaps in different years: three looked at the California Tobacco Surveys, seven the Current Population Surveys, and two Canadian national surveys. It would be expected, therefore, that the results would be concordant because the same survey instruments were used in the same locales. However, as the prevalence of smoke-free homes increases, it is possible that the strength of the association may change (Shopland et al., 2006; Pierce et al., 2009). A number of these studies examined workplace smoking policies, as well as home smoking restrictions (Pierce et al., 1998c, Farkas et al., 1999; Gilpin et al., 2000; Gilpin & Pierce, 2002b; Shavers et al., 2006; Shopland et al., 2006; Burns et al., 2007; Shields, 2005, 2007; Lee & Kahende, 2007; Messer et al., 2008b). These studies are also included in Chapter 7, but only the results regarding workplace policies are discussed. The present chapter presents both the results for home and workplace smoking restrictions.

Longitudinal. The earliest long-itudinal study investigating the effect of home smoking restrictions was from California. Although home and work area smoking restrictions and having cessation assistance were only assessed at follow-up, this study (n=1736) related these factors to changes in smoking behaviour over an average 18-month period between 1990 and 1992 (Pierce et al., 1998c). The outcome variable was advancement along a quitting continuum (high addiction and no quitting history, low addiction or quitting history, and low addiction and quitting history, or being quit at least three months at follow-up). Beliefs in the harmfulness of SHS were factored into the home smoking rule variable as an intermediate level: no beliefs and no rules, beliefs, a smoke-free smoking home policy; almost no one with such a policy believed SHS was not harmful.

Table 8.7 Summary of results of studies examining the relationship between home smoking restrictions and *adult* smoking behaviour

Reference	Locality	Prevalence	Consumption	Quit attempt	Quit-any duration	Reduced relapse	Other
					Outcomes — Cessation		
Longitudinal							
Pierce et al., 1998b	California, USA						SIG-progress toward cessation
Pizacani et al., 2004	Oregon, USA			SIG	SIG	SIG	
Shields et al., 2005	Canada		SIG*		NS	SIG	
Borland et al., 2006a	Australia, Canada, UK,USA		SIG	NS	SIG		
Shields et al., 2007	Canada		SIG		SIG		
Messer et al., 2008a	USA		SIG		SIG		
Hyland et al., 2009	USA		NS**	SIG	SIG	SIG	
Cross-sectional							
Farkas et al., 1999	USA		SIG	SIG	SIG		
Gilpin et al., 1999	California, USA		SIG	SIG		SIG	SIG-intent to quit
Gilpin et al., 2000	USA	SIG	SIG				
Norman et al., 2000	California, USA		SIG	NS			SIG-desire to quit
Gilpin & Pierce, 2002b	California, USA		SIG				
Siahpush et al., 2003	Australia				SIG		
Shavers et al., 2006	USA	SIG	SIG	SIG			
Shopland et al., 2006	USA				SIG		
Gilpin et al., 2006	California, USA					SIG	
Lee & Kahende, 2007	USA				SIG		
Burns et al., 2007	Colorado, USA						SIG-duration of smoking
Ji et al., 2008	California, USA				SIG		
Shelley et al., 2008	New York City, USA		SIG	SIG			
Messer et al., 2008b	USA		SIG	SIG	SIG		
Tong et al., 2008	California, USA		SIG		SIG		
Pierce et al., 2009	USA		SIG		SIG		

SIG = significant difference in smoking behaviour indicated between smokers with and without home smoking restrictions. All significant differences were in the direction of reduced smoking (i.e. less consumption, more quitting) in homes with restrictions.
NS = No significant difference
No entry means that the outcome was not considered
*Cross-sectional analysis of baseline data
**SIG in model without baseline level of addiction

Analyses controlled for demographics. A smoke-free home was significantly associated with advancement along the quitting continuum (OR=3.4; 95% CI=1.9-5.9), but simply a belief in the harmfulness of SHS was not (OR=1.3; 95% CI=0.7-2.2). No smoking in the work area (OR=1.6; 95% CI=1.0-2.6) and having cessation assistance (OR=3.0; 95% CI=1.7-5.3) were also associated with progress; a work area policy less so than a smoke-free home policy. A further analysis showed that 41% of smokers with two or three of these factors progressed toward cessation, compared to 23% with just one and 13% with none. When the smoke-free home and workplace policies were established relative to the smoker making progress toward cessation was unknown.

The relationship between home smoking restrictions and relapse following a quit attempt, was examined using longitudinal data from a 1997 survey which identified smokers, their readiness to quit (pre-contemplation, contemplation, or preparation), and whether or not their home had no or partial restrictions or was completely smoke-free (Pizacani *et al.*, 2004). In 1999, a follow-up survey of 565 baseline smokers (52%) assessed quitting and duration of abstinence for those who had quit in the interim. Smokers with a smoke-free home were 2 times more likely (OR=2.0; 95% CI=1.0-3.9) to have made a quit attempt lasting a day or longer. This study showed that for smokers preparing to quit (in the next 30 days) at baseline, the presence of a smoke-free home both predicted a future quit attempt and prolonged the period of abstinence for that attempt,

compared to those with only partial or no restriction on smoking in the home; the odds were 4.4 (95% CI=1.1-18.7) of being off cigarettes at least a week when interviewed at follow-up. Relapse curves for these two groups were significantly different (p<0.02). For smokers not preparing to quit, but who nevertheless did make an attempt prior to follow-up, relapse curves for those with no or partial compared to a smoke-free policy were the same. While not formally analysed, baseline smoking intensity appeared to be related to having a smoke-free home versus partial or no smoking restrictions.

A series of Canadian longitudinal studies at two year intervals from 1994-95 to 2001-02 assessed, with combined data, the effects of both smoke-free homes and workplaces at baseline among daily smokers and continuous cessation initiated within two years prior to the follow-up period (Shields, 2005); follow-up exceeded 80%. Working in a smoke-free environment was not associated with quitting. Having a smoke-free home was related to indicators of addiction level, and this factor was significant bivariately in both men and women (men: OR=1.4; 95% CI=1.0-1.9, and women: OR=1.5; 95% CI=1.1-2.1). Yet in a multivariate analysis that controlled for demographics and addiction variables, it failed to reach statistical significance (men: OR=1.1; 95% CI=0.8-1.6, and women: OR=1.3; 95% CI=1.0-1.9). However, among former smokers at baseline, having a smoke-free home was significantly related to maintenance of abstinence multivariately for men (OR=0.6; 95% CI=0.4-0.9), but not for women (OR=1.0; 95% CI=0.6-

1.6). A cross-sectional analysis of 2003 data indicated that those living in a smoke-free environment smoked five fewer CPD (p<0.05). A combination of having both a smoke-free workplace and a smoke-free home was associated with an even greater difference in consumption, seven and six fewer CPD for men and women, respectively (p<0.05), compared to those working and living in environments where smoking is permitted.

A subsequent longitudinal analysis of these Canadian data (Shields, 2007) looked at the effect of newly imposed smoking restrictions both at work and in the home. Separate analyses were conducted for workplace and home restrictions over multiple survey waves from 1994 to 2005. Follow-up was 77% at the final wave analysed. The workplace analysis considered 1364 smokers age 15 years and older employed in one wave at a workplace where smoking was not restricted, and in a subsequent wave where it was restricted, and evaluated behaviour in the following (two years later) wave after the restriction was imposed. A similar combination of data from various survey waves identified 8463 smokers age 15 years and older subject to new smoking restrictions in the home. To evaluate the effect of newly imposed workplace restrictions, a multivariate analysis adjusted for cigarette consumption at baseline, sex, age, education, income, and occupation (white-collar, sales/service, and blue collar). Smokers working under a newly imposed smoke-free policy were 2.3 (95% CI=1.4-3.9) times more likely to be quit at follow-up (27%) than those working continuously where there was not a smoke-free policy (13%). The definition of quitting was report of smoking "not at all" at follow-up with no time criterion. Partial restrictions were not related to increased quitting. Daily smokers who did not quit but who worked under a new smoke-free policy reduced their cigarette consumption by 2.1 CPD; there was no change in consumption for those who continued to work in a workplace with no smoking restrictions. For the analysis of new home restrictions, the multivariate analysis substituted the presence of children for occupation and considered only a smoke-free home versus a home with no restrictions. Smokers living in a newly smoke-free home were 1.6 (95% CI=1.3-2.1) times more likely to be quit at the follow-up wave. Daily smokers who continued to smoke tended to decrease their consumption and averaged 2.0 CPD less at follow-up compared to 0.4 CPD less among those without new smoke-free home policies.

Another longitudinal study examined data from subsequent waves of the International Tobacco Control Four Country Survey (Borland et al., 2006a). The countries studied were Canada, the USA, the UK, and Australia; data were from 6754 respondents to the baseline survey in 2002, and the second wave conducted six to 10 months later (75% follow-up). At baseline, a smoke-free home was associated with both lower mean daily cigarette consumption and longer duration to the first cigarette after awakening in the morning. Implementing a smoke-free home policy between survey waves was associated with favorable

changes in both these factors (p<0.001). Compared to homes with no smoking restrictions, a smoke-free home was also associated with increased quit attempts (OR=1.32; 95% CI=1.11-1.57) and being abstinent for one month or longer at follow-up (OR=2.50; 95% CI=1.50-4.16), after adjusting for: demographic factors, the presence of smokers in the household, belief in the harmfulness of SHS, a social norm variable, and report of restrictions in other venues frequented (bars, restaurants, and workplaces). However, when an index of baseline addiction level and other predictors of cessation were included in the multivariate model, the smoke-free home effect for making a quit attempt was no longer significant. Yet, when duration of abstinence (at least a month) was analysed among those who made a quit attempt, even after controlling for addiction and all the other variables, having a smoke-free home, but not partial restrictions predicted the outcome (OR=2.07; 95% CI=1.20-3.56).

A recent further analysis of the Community Intervention Trial for Smoking Cessation (COMMIT) longitudinal data looked specifically at the effect of a smoke-free home policy at baseline related to changes in smoking behaviour (Hyland et al., 2009). There were 4963 smokers at baseline in 1988 who were interviewed again in 2001 and 2005. The latter two surveys asked about smoking restrictions in the participants' homes. The percentage of smokers in 2001 who reported a smoke-free home was 29%, and this increased to 38% by 2005. In logistic regression analyses that adjusted for age, sex, race/ethnicity, annual

household income (2001), education (1988), and number of cigarettes smoked (2001), smokers with a smoke-free home in 2001 were 1.7 (95% CI=1.4-2.2) times more likely to be quit at follow-up than those without such policies. If not quit in 2005, they were 1.5 (95% CI=1.3-1.9) times more likely to have made a serious attempt to quit in the interim. However, there was no significant effect for a smoke-free home policy on consumption in continuing smokers. Among those quit in 2001, having a smoke-free home helped them remain quit; they were only 0.6 times (95% CI=0.4-0.8) as likely to relapse as those without such a policy.

A final longitudinal study used data collected twice (one year apart) from the national Current Population Survey in the USA (Messer et al., 2008b). In this analysis of 3292 recent smokers, 28.4% had a smoke-free home at baseline in 2002, and among those who did not, 20% had adopted one by follow-up in 2003. The study examined cessation at follow-up, cessation for at least 90 days at follow-up, and cigarette consumption among continuing smokers. Multiple logistic regression analyses adjusted for age, sex, race/ethnicity, incomes below two times the poverty level, the presence of another smoker in the household, and cigarette consumption at baseline in 2002. Having a smoke-free home (versus all others) at baseline was predictive of increased quitting by follow-up: quit, OR=1.52; 95% CI=1.08-2.15, p<0.05, and quit 90+ days, OR=1.44; 95% CI=0.97-2.21, p<0.10. However, adoption of a smoke-free home by 2003 was highly predictive of increased quitting: quit, OR=3.89;

95% CI=2.55-5.87, and quit 90+days, OR=4.81; 95% CI=3.06-7.59. Among continuing smokers who adopted a smoke-free home, a multivariate analysis showed that consumption declined by 2.18 (95% CI=1.24-3.10) CPD compared to those who did not. Removal of a smoke-free home policy was associated with increased smoking compared to maintenance of a smoke-free home policy. It is possible that smokers adopted a smoke-free home simultaneously with their attempt to quit, and removed it when they relapsed. Nevertheless, adoption of a smoke-free home appeared to increase the chances of success markedly.

Cross-Sectional. A study which proposed an index of initial outcomes from tobacco control policies for US states included as components: the price of cigarettes, the percentage of indoor workers reporting smoke-free workplaces, and the percentage of the population reporting smoke-free homes (Gilpin *et al.*, 2000). Data concerning smoke-free homes and workplaces were from 237 733 self-respondents to the 1992-93 Current Population Survey (CPS); cigarette price data were from sales data reported to the Federal Trade Commission. The smoke-free home component correlated better among the US states (51, including the District of Columbia) with adult (r= -0.66, p<0.001) and youth smoking prevalence (r=-0.39, p<0.01) than the other two components. In fact, correlations for the composite index with these outcomes were r=-0.70 (p<0.0001) and -0.34 (p<0.05), suggesting that the other components of the index added little to explaining prevalence. However,

for per capita cigarette consumption, the correlation of adult smoking prevalence with the initial outcome index, r=-0.73 (p<0.0001), was only slightly higher than for cigarette prices, r=-0.71 (p<0.0001), and much higher than for smoke-free homes, r=-0.58 (p<0.0001), and smoke-free workplaces, r=-0.54, p<0.001. While these correlational results cannot demonstrate causality, they are suggestive that smoke-free homes are at least an indication of societal norms against smoking.

The relationship between work and home smoking restrictions and quitting behaviour was also analysed using the 1992-93 CPS data (n=48 584 smokers in the last year) (Farkas *et al.*, 1999). Variables analysed included making a quit attempt on at least one day or longer in the past year, cessation of at least six months when interviewed, and light smoking (<15 CPD). In multivariate logistic analyses that included age, sex, race/ethnicity, education, income, occupation, region, age of youngest child in household, and social factors (lives with a smoker, a former smoker, or a never smoker), compared to having no smoking restrictions, home smoking restrictions were significantly related to making a quit attempt (partial: OR=1.83; 95% CI=1.72-1.93, smoke-free: OR=3.86; 95% CI=3.57-4.18), cessation for at least six months (partial: OR=1.20; 95% CI=1.05-1.38, smoke-free: OR=1.65; 95% CI=1.43-1.91), and light smoking (partial: OR=1.81; 95% CI=1.69-1.95, smoke-free: OR=2.73; 95% CI=2.46-3.04). A partial home restriction was generally more related than a partial workplace

restriction (quit attempt: OR=1.14; 95% CI=1.05-1.24, six months cessation: OR=1.21; 95% CI=1.00-1.45, light smoking: OR=1.53; 95% CI=1.38-1.70), contrasted to no workplace smoking restrictions. In contrast to a completely smoke-free workplace, smoke-free work areas were not significantly related to the smoking behaviour outcomes examined.

Another analysis of CPS data from 1998-99 and 2001-02, examined the effect of workplace and home smoking restrictions on current smoking, cigarette consumption, and quit attempts in employed women (n=82 996) (Shavers *et al.*, 2006). Analyses were stratified by poverty level and race/ethnicity and adjusted for age, education, marital status, and occupation. Regardless of whether separate analyses considered women of each race/ethnicity or of similar poverty level, compared to having no restrictions, partial or no home smoking restrictions were associated with being a current smoker (adjusted odds ratios ranged from 11.1 to 28.8 for no restrictions, and from 3.8 to 11.2 for partial restrictions). The association was weaker among Native Americans (including Alaskan natives) than for other groups; it appeared strongest for African Americans. Workplace smoking restrictions showed little relation to current smoking. Among current smokers, having a smoke-free work area was significantly associated with less heavy smoking (20+ CPD) for some poverty groups but not others. Also, not having home restrictions was even more related (odds ratios ranged from 3.4 to 6.2 for completely smoke-free policy and from 1.4 to 2.9 for partial restrictions). Workplace smoking restrictions were not related to making a quit attempt, but no smoking restrictions in the home was significantly and inversely related to making a quit attempt in the last year (odds ratios ranged from 0.43 to 0.69).

Yet another study used data from the CPS to examine the determinants of smoking cessation among employed female daily smokers (one year before survey) age 25 years or older who did not live alone (Shopland et al., 2006). The sample sizes of women meeting these criteria were not reported, but the data were from the 1992-93 and 2001-02 CPS, which included a total of 128 024 employed women age 18 years and older. Smoking status one year prior to the survey was by retrospective recall. Two measures of cessation were considered: not smoking at all at the time of the survey, and quit for at least three months when interviewed. Factors examined for association with quitting included home smoking restrictions (no restrictions, partial restrictions, home smoke-free), age, education, race/ethnicity, workplace smoking restrictions (permitted versus not permitted), occupation, the presence of young children in the household (no children under 5 years versus children under 5 years), and household composition (multiple adults, no children, multiple adults and children, one adult and children). Separate analyses were performed for each quitting measure and for the 1992-93 data and the 2001-02 data. The percentage of all current smokers (employed females age 18 years and older) at the time of the survey reporting a smoke-free

home increased from 5.5% (95% CI=4.8-6.2) in 1992-93 to 22.0% (95% CI=20.4-23.5) in 2001-02. For both surveys and both measures of quitting, home smoking restrictions were the factors most strongly associated with cessation. In 1992-93, daily smokers a year previously were 7.77 (95% CI=5.91-10.21) times more likely to be quit, and those living under partial restrictions were 2.15 (95% CI=1.70-2.73) times more likely to be quit compared to those living where there was no restrictions. Similarly, in 2001-02, these adjusted odds ratios were 6.54 (95% CI=4.61-9.28) and 2.34 (95% CI=1.54-3.55), respectively. Only a few other factors were significant. There was no association with this outcome for smoke-free workplaces in either year. When cessation for at least three months was the dependent variable, again home smoking restrictions were highly related in both years: smoke-free, OR=7.41 (95% CI=5.55-9.90), and partial restrictions OR=2.18 (95% CI=1.63-2.92) in 1992-93; and smoke-free, OR=7.08 (95% CI=4.45-11.26) and partial restrictions OR=2.45 (95% CI=1.48-4.07) in 2001-2002. In 1992-93, a smoke-free workplace was directly related to cessation for at least three months (p<0.03).

Data on 8904 current smokers from the 1996 California Tobacco Survey were used to examine quit attempts in the last year, intent to quit in the next six months, light smoking (<15 CPD), smoking the first cigarette of the day within 30 minutes of awakening, and the duration of the longest quit attempt in the past year (Gilpin et al., 1999). The multivariate logistic regressions included

demographic factors, household composition (other smoker, children), belief in the harmfulness of SHS, and a family preference that the smoker not smoke. A belief in the harmfulness of SHS was significantly related to the three main dependent variables analysed (quit attempt, intention to quit, light smoking). Compared to no family preference and no restrictions, with a family preference that the smoker not smoke, a smoke-free home was related to all three outcomes (quit attempt: OR=3.9 (95% CI=3.0-5.2), intent: OR=5.8 (95% CI=3.8-8.2), light smoking: OR=2.2 (95% CI=1.2-3.0), and partial restrictions to making a quit attempt OR=2.7 (95% CI=2.0-3.6), and intent to quit: OR=3.7 (95% CI=2.7-5.1)), but not to being a light smoker: OR=1.1 (95% CI=0.8-1.5). Quitters living in smoke-free homes appeared to maintain their abstinence significantly longer than those with no or only partial home smoking restrictions; the latter two groups showed about the same relapse pattern. The percentage of light daily smokers delaying their first cigarette for at least 30 minutes after awakening was 89% in smoke-free homes and 82% in homes with no restrictions. For moderate to heavy smokers, these percentages were 64% and 47%, respectively. Smoke-free homes appeared to have a greater effect on moderate to heavy smokers than on light smokers.

Another analysis of data from the 1999 California Tobacco Survey focused on daily cigarette consumption (Gilpin & Pierce, 2002b). In a multivariate linear regression that adjusted for demographics, and included both having a smoke-free home and smoke-free workplace, both factors were significant (smoke-free homes, p<0.0001; smoke-free workplace, p<0.05). The estimated least-squares estimates for mean daily consumption for smokers living in smoke-free households was 8.0 CPD, compared to 11.1 CPD for those without smoke-free policies. The analogous results for workplaces were 9.4 versus 11.1 CPD. A further analysis computed the least-squares daily consumption means for smokers with no policies for a smoke-free home or workplace (13.9 CPD), a smoke-free workplace only (11.1 CPD), a smoke-free home only (9.4 CPD), and both types of these policies (7.5 CPD).

Data from the 1999 and 2002 California Tobacco Survey were combined to examine duration of abstinence for the most recent quit attempt in the past year (n=2640 quitters who smoked at least 15 CPD a year previously) for smoke-free home policies, in conjunction with having other smokers in the home, and the use of pharmaceutical aids (nicotine gum, patch, or bupropion) for smoking cessation (Gilpin et al., 2006). Cox proportional hazard analyses adjusted for age, sex, race/ethnicity, education, and daily cigarette consumption. There were significant interaction effects (less relapse) for a smoke-free home and no other smoker in the home (hazard ratio: 0.796 (95% CI=0.645-0.988)), and a smoke-free home and use of a pharmaceutical aid (hazard ratio: 0.774 (95% CI=0.622-0.963)). Abstinence duration was shorter if there was another smoker present in the household regardless of home smoking policy or pharmaceutical

aid use. Without a smoke-free home, pharmaceutical aids did not appear to prolong duration of abstinence. With a smoke-free home, and no other smoker in the home, pharmaceutical aids appeared to be most effective in prolonging abstinence. Because of small sample size, the results for aid use, when another smoker was present in a smoke-free home, were less clear, but aid users seemed to remain abstinent longer. It is possible that having a smoke-free home, or instituting one following a quit attempt, is an indication of the quitter's motivation to remain abstinent.

Another California survey from 1998 was used to examine 1315 smokers age 25 years and older for a relationship between smoke-free homes and daily cigarette consumption, days smoked in the past month, desire to quit, and making a quit attempt in the past year (Norman et al., 2000). Multivariate models adjusted for age, sex, education, race/ethnicity, and the presence of children in the home. A smoke-free home was related to lower cigarette consumption (p<0.01) and a desire to quit smoking (OR=2.9; 95% CI=1.8-4.9), but not to days smoked in the last month or making a quit attempt in the past year. Smokers living in a household with rules against smoking were about twice as likely (OR=2.29; 95% CI=1.22-4.29) to have reported hearing about community programs to discourage smoking and nearly three times (OR=3.18; 95% CI=1.34-7.57) as likely to report seeing and talking about anti-tobacco media spots.

A study of success in quitting (for at least one month) among recent quitters (attempts in the past

two years) considered a number of potential social/environmental influences, including home smoking rules (Siahpush et al., 2003). This study examined 2526 Australian smokers aged 14 years and older. In addition to demographics (sex, age, marital status, dependent child, education, occupation, and urban versus rural), it considered children in the home, belief in the harmfulness of SHS, having friends who smoke, smoking restrictions at work or school (none, some, total, not applicable), and alcohol consumption. In the adjusted model, having a smoke-free home increased the odds of cessation by 4.5 (95% CI=3.1-6.6) over having no restrictions. Workplace or school restrictions were unrelated to quitting success in this study.

A similar study contrasted unsuccessful quitters with those who had remained continuously abstinent for seven to 24 months (Lee & Kahende, 2007). Data were from 3990 quitters responding to the 2000 National Health Interview Survey. As a measure of smoking rules in the home, the survey asked how many times anyone had smoked anywhere in the home in the last week, and those answering zero were contrasted to all others. Those who worked in a smoke-free workplace were also contrasted to all others. The logistic regression analysis adjusted for age, education, marital status, race/ethnicity, number of lifetime quit attempts, and whether the smoker had ever switched to low tar/nicotine cigarettes. The adjusted odds ratio for no smoking in the home was 10.47 (95% CI=8.15-13.46) and for a smoke-free workplace it was 2.01 (95% CI=1.20-3.37).

Ever smokers of Korean descent (n=2830) were identified from a large telephone survey in California (Ji et al., 2005). Those quit for at least 90 days were contrasted to all others in a multivariate logistic regression analysis that included gender, education, family income, acculturation, number of smokers among family and friends, social network among family and friends, media influence, job satisfaction, health belief scale, health concern, body mass index, weight concern, exercise, family history of respiratory illness, and medical treatment for respiratory illness, as well as a variable for the extent of smoking restrictions in the home. This variable was coded into five categories: 1) no one allowed to smoke inside, 2) special guests allowed to smoke inside, 3) smoking allowed in certain areas, 4) smoking allowed anywhere, and 5) those not responding to the question. Compared to those with a smoke-free home, those with designated areas inside were less likely (OR= 0.17; 95% CI=0.12-0.24) to be former smokers, and those in homes where smoking was allowed anywhere were much less (OR=0.10; 95% CI=0.06-0.19) likely to have quit. Those with exceptions for special guests did not significantly differ in cessation propensity than those living in smoke-free homes, but those not responding to the home rule questions were only about half as likely to have quit (OR=0.53; 95% CI=0.36-0.78). Besides a smoke-free home, factors related to greater cessation included advanced acculturation, health concerns, a social network discouraging smoking, and a family history of respiratory illness.

The duration of smoking between Hispanic and non-Hispanic whites ever smokers (n=6100) interviewed in the 2001 Colorado Tobacco Attitudes and Behaviours Survey were compared (Burns et al., 2007). Former smokers were defined as being abstinent for at least three months when interviewed. Duration of smoking for continuing smokers was computed as the age when surveyed minus the age of initiation of regular smoking. For former smokers, it was the age when quit minus the age of initiation. Analyses controlled for present age, sex, marital status, language spoken in home, age of smoking initiation, education, poverty status, insurance status, and considered both home (none, partial, complete) and work area smoking restrictions (none or partial versus complete versus not applicable). A partial (hazard ratio: 2.39 (95% CI=1.94-2.94)) or complete (4.59 (95% CI=3.81-5.52)) smoke-free home was associated with shorter smoking durations (cessation). A smoke-free work area (1.48; 95% CI=1.19-1.84) was also important. Results were similar for Latinos and non-Hispanic whites, so the results reported above refer to the combined sample.

Chinese American male smokers (n=600), living in New York City, who took part in a city-wide population survey were the subject of a study conduced in 2002/03 (Shelley et al., 2008). Over one-third (37%) reported living in a smoke-free home, and another third (38%) reported partial restrictions. The authors examined cigarette consumption on weekdays and weekend days, as well as making a recent quit attempt. Those living in

smoke-free homes smoked 14.7 CPD on weekdays, with partial restrictions they smoked 17.2 CPD, and with no restrictions they smoked 19.9 CPD. Analogous data for weekend day consumption were: smoke-free 11.8 CPD, partial restrictions 14.7 CPD, and no restrictions 17.3 CPD. Quit attempt rates were 67.0%, 56.7%, and 45.0%, respectively, depending on level of restrictions. Multivariate analyses of cigarettes smoked adjusted for age, education, income, and marital status. Those with a smoke-free home smoked significantly fewer (p<0.01) cigarettes both on weekdays and weekend days than those with no restrictions. Partial restrictions were not significantly related to consumption. The odds ratio for making a recent quit attempt was 3.37 (95% CI=1.51-7.05) compared to no restrictions. Again, partial restrictions were not significantly related to quit attempts.

A study of 31 625 recent smokers (in the last year) examined a number of factors related to seriously trying to quit (any length quit attempt in the past year), quitting for one day or longer in the past year, and being quit for at least six months when surveyed (Messer et al., 2008a). Data were from the 2003 Tobacco Use Supplement to the Current Population Survey. Smoke-free homes and workplaces were evaluated along with a number of additional covariates including age, sex, race/ethnicity, education, smoking initiation at <15 years, smoking within 30 minutes of awakening, and use of a pharmaceutical aid. Having a smoke-free home was significantly related to all three outcomes: seriously trying (OR=1.21; 95% CI=1.12-1.30), 1+ day quit (OR=4.03; 95% CI=3.50-4.63), and 6+ months cessation (OR=4.13; 95% CI=3.25-5.26). A smoke-free workplace was not significantly related to any outcome, and use of a pharmaceutical aid was only significantly related to a 1+ day quit attempt (OR=1.25; 95% CI=1.04-1.49). Older smokers appeared less successful in quitting than younger ones, and further analyses showed that younger smokers smoked fewer CPD and were more likely to have smoke-free homes. The authors concluded that these characteristics might have contributed to their increased success in quitting.

A study from California examined the association between having a smoke-free home and being a former smoker (among ever smokers (n=767) – at least 100 cigarettes in lifetime) and being a light smoker (<10 CPD) among current smokers (n=352) in the Asian Population (Tong et al., 2008). A smoke-free home was categorised as smoking not allowed at all indoors versus all others. The multivariate logistic regression analyses adjusted for age, sex, Asian origin group, marital status, education, income, and years in the USA (<10 vs. all others including those born there), and coded an interaction term for years in the USA and having a smoke-free home. Longer-term residents were more likely (OR=14.19; 95% CI=4.46-45.12) to be former smokers and shorter-term residents were somewhat less but still significantly more likely (OR=2.25; 95% CI=1.79-5.90) to be former smokers if they lived in a smoke-free home compared to those not living in a smoke-free home. Among current smokers, longer-term residents were more likely (OR=5.37; 95% CI=2.79-

10.31) to be light smokers if they had a smoke-free home compared to if they did not. There was no significant difference for shorter-term residents (OR=1.19; 95% CI=0.33-4.23).

A recent study is particularly noteworthy in that it analyses cross-sectional Current Population Survey data spanning a full decade (1992/93, 1995/96, 1998/99, 2002/03), and included a total of 542 470 current smokers aged 18 to 64 years (Pierce et al., 2009). The authors examined trends in smoking prevalence, and the proportions of smokers who were moderate to heavy smokers (15+ CPC) and very light smokers (<5 CPD, including occasional smokers) within age groups (18-29, 30-44, and 45-64 years). They also examined trends in the prevalence of report of smoke-free workplaces and homes. The decline in smoking prevalence over the decade appeared to be entirely due to a decline in moderate to heavy smoking in the older age groups, but in the youngest group, the drop in prevalence was modest and there was an increase in the percentage of both very light smokers and in those smoking 5-15 CPD. Because of the increase in very light smoking among the 18-29 year old group, a multivariate analysis was conducted for this age group only, with very light smoking as the dependent variable. Independent variables included survey year, sex, education, income (above versus below two times the poverty level), a smoke-free workplace, and tobacco control policies ranking by tertile for state of residence as an indicator of social norms against smoking. Both a smoke-free home and a smoke-free workplace were significantly related

to increased light smoking: ORs were 2.81 (95% CI=2.60-3.04) and 1.28 (95% CI=1.18-1.38), respectively. Also significant was tertile of state tobacco control activity: ORs highest 1.68 (95% CI=1.53-1.85) and middle 1.26 (95% CI=1.15-1.38) versus lowest tertile. Education was directly and poverty status inversely significantly related to being a very light smoker. Of note is that survey year was not significant, but if the variable indicating a smoke-free home was eliminated from the model, year became highly significant; apparently, the increase in light smoking was mediated by the increase in smoke-free homes. There were increases in smoke-free homes documented in all age groups (also in all three tertiles of social norms against smoking), but the level was always higher in the younger age group in each survey year. In 2002/03, the percentages of smokers with a smoke-free home were 36.7%, 28.9%, and 21.7% in the 18-29, 30-44, 45-65 year old age groups, respectively.

Summary

In contrast to mandated smoking restrictions in public or workplaces, those in the home are "voluntary." There was very consistent evidence that smokers living in smoke-free homes smoke fewer CPD. However, this finding might simply reflect the fact that lighter smokers are more likely to agree to a smoke-free home, as they can more easily adapt to the inconvenience a smoke-free home presents than heavier smokers. Since less addicted smokers are able to quit more readily, it is not surprising that some longitudinal studies that controlled for smokers' baseline level of addiction failed to find as strong a relationship of home smoking restrictions to subsequent smoking cessation. Some quitters may institute a smoke-free home policy concurrently with a quit attempt or in anticipation of one, and there was generally consistent evidence that quitters living in smoke-free homes stay abstinent longer. Partial home smoking restrictions appeared less associated with smoking behaviour than completely smoke-free policy. In the studies that examined both workplace and home smoking restrictions, home smoking restrictions appeared to have a stronger association with smoking behaviour than did workplace restrictions.

Most of the studies in this section were from the USA. As other countries enact legislation to limit smoking in public and workplaces, restrictions will likely spread voluntarily to homes as well. Further research on the effect of such voluntary restrictions will be warranted.

Effects on youth

Why household smoking restrictions might affect youth smoking behaviour

A smoke-free home should reduce the opportunity for children to observe smoking in their immediate social environment. A behaviour that is frequently observed may come to be considered normal and acceptable, thus increasing the likelihood of adopting the behaviour. Restrictions on smoking in the home at the least express disapproval of exposing children, youth, or other nonsmokers to SHS, and in homes

where parents do not smoke it may reinforce the view that smoking is not an acceptable behaviour. Smoking parents who abide by such restrictions are modeling their conviction that their personal behaviour should not affect others deleteriously, and with appropriate framing, a smoke-free home may help convey the message that the parent does not wish the child to initiate smoking.

While it might be thought that smoking parents can do little to prevent their children from smoking, some studies indicate that there are things a parent can do to convey their desire that their child not smoke (Kandel & Wu, 1995; Jackson & Dickinson, 2003). A smoke-free home and other proactive socialisation measures against smoking (e.g. discussion of desire of the parent that the child not smoke, making clear the consequences for the child smoking, etc.) may partially counteract the effect of their own behaviour. In contrast, the absence of such socialisation measures may convey the message that smoking and SHS are not a concern, thus increasing the probability of the child or adolescent initiating smoking, even in homes where parents and other adults do not smoke.

Results for studies examining the effect of home smoking restrictions on youth smoking behaviour

Except for two (den Exter Blokland et al., 2006; Albers et al., 2008), the studies described below are all cross-sectional, with adolescent smoking status ascertained at the same time data on smoking restrictions and other possible determinants of

smoking were assessed. As such, they only can determine whether an association exists, and not whether growing up in a home with smoking restrictions lowers the probability of their smoking later (or whether adolescents unlikely to smoke have influenced whether their household restricts smoking). All these studies are summarised in Table 8.8 and described in detail in Appendix 7. All but two of the 19 studies reviewed analysed some measure of youth smoking status. Of these two, one looked at factors related to youth smoking (Conley Thomson et al., 2005), and the other at risk of early smoking initiation (Andreeva et al., 2007).

One of the first studies to examine adolescent smoking in households with and without smoking restrictions, mainly focused on self-reported SHS exposure (Biener et al., 1997). Secondary analyses of these 1606 Massachusetts 12-17 year olds, interviewed in 1993, found that adolescent smoking in the past 30 days was unrelated to the presence of home smoking restrictions.

A survey of central North Carolina 3rd and 5th graders (n=1352) examined early onset of smoking defined as any experimentation and readiness to smoke (intent to smoke when older, thinking cigarettes are easy to get, and whether they had almost smoked), and how these were related to anti-tobacco socialisation measures by their parents (as reported by the children) (Jackson & Henriksen, 1997). Preliminary analyses were stratified according to parental smoking status: 2 never-smokers, 1 or 2 former smokers (but both nonsmokers now), one parent

Table 8.8 Summary of results of studies examining the relationship between home smoking restrictions and *youth* smoking behaviour

Reference	Locality	Outcomes			
		Smoking Status	Consumption	Cessation	Other
Biener et al., 1997	Massachusetts, USA	NS			
Jackson & Henriksen, 1997	North Carolina, USA	SIG			
Rissel et al., 1997		SIG			
Henrikson & Jackson, 1998	California, USA	SIG			SIG-less intent to smoke
Wakefield et al., 2000a	USA	SIG			
Farkas et al., 2000	USA	SIG		SIG	
Proescholdbell et al., 2000	Arizona, USA	SIG		NS	
Komro et al., 2003	Minnesota, USA	NS			
Kodl & Mermelstein, 2004	USA	SIG			
Andersen et al., 2004	Washington, USA	SIG			SIG-lower perceived prevalence of adult smoking;
Thomson et al., 2005	Massachusetts, USA				SIG-greater perceived adult negative attitudes regarding smoking
den Exter Blokland et al., 2006	Utrecht, Netherlands	NS			
Clark et al., 2006	USA	SIG	SIG	SIG	
Szabo et al., 2006	Australia	SIG	SIG		
Fisher et al., 2007	USA	NS			
Andreeva et al., 2007	Ukraine				SIG-later age of first cigarette SIG- later age of daily smoking
Rodriguez et al., 2007	Pennsylvania, USA	NS			SIG-through peer smoking
Albers et al., 2008	Massachusetts, USA	SIG			
Rainio & Rimpela, 2008	Finland	SIG			

SIG = significant difference in smoking behaviour indicated between youth with and without home smoking restrictions. All significant differences were in the direction of reduced smoking (i.e. lower prevalence or status on the uptake continuum, lower consumption, more quitting) in homes with restrictions.
NS = No significant difference
No entry means that the outcome was not considered

a current smoker, and both parents current smokers. As would be expected, across groups there were differences in experimentation and readiness to smoke, with the children with parents who smoked showing the highest levels. While children with parents who were former smokers showed lower experimentation or readiness levels than with parents who were current smokers, they generally had higher levels than those with parents who had never smoked. The investigators conducted separate multivariate analyses of smoking experimentation in children in families with and without parental smokers that controlled for parental smoking status (never or former, one or two adults smoke). These analyses included variables for anti-smoking socialisation factors: expect parents would know if child smoked, expect negative consequences, parent has talked to them about their preference that they not smoke, and child would disregard anti-smoking message from parent. A lack of a smoke-free home was significantly related to early experimentation in homes without an adult current smoker (OR=1.5; 95% CI=1.2-1.83), and only marginally related in homes with one (OR=1.1; 95% CI=0.99-1.2).

Another survey of 3rd through 8th graders (n=937) was conducted in Northern California by the same authors (Henriksen & Jackson, 1998). Three schools that instructed predominantly in English were selected, yet 30% of the students responding were Hispanic. The study examined three measures of anti-smoking socialisation, including home smoking rules (permitted or not permitted), an index of students' report

of their parents warning them against smoking, and an index of students' expected punishment if they smoked. Dependent variables were intent to smoke and any experimentation. The indices were categorised for a multivariate analysis of respondents with complete data (n=870) into low, medium, and high groups. The analyses controlled for parental smoking status, but no interactions of this term and the anti-smoking socialisation variables were included. Children living where there were no restrictions on smoking were 1.77 (95% CI=1.19-2.64) times more likely to intend to smoke and 1.39 (95% CI=1.03-1.88) times more like to have tried smoking than children living in a smoke-free home. However, it is unknown whether these effects are mainly from the nonsmoking parental households (70% of sample).

The presence of home smoking restrictions was investigated, as reported by over 17 000 US high school students interviewed in 1996 (Wakefield et al., 2000a). Public smoking restrictions were determined from external sources, and the presence and degree of enforcement of a smoke-free school policy was garnered from students' report to their smoking status. Status was determined by successive levels on a five point smoking uptake continuum. Any smoking in the last 30 days was also analysed. Having home smoking restrictions, particularly a smoke-free home, was associated with a lower level on the smoking uptake continuum at every transition point: non-susceptible to susceptible (OR=0.64; 95% CI=0.52-0.76), susceptible to early experimenter (OR=0.69; 95%

CI=0.59-0.79), early experimenter to advanced experimenter (OR=0.71; 95% CI=0.60-0.82), and advanced experimenter to established smoker (OR=0.78; 95% CI=0.67-0.90), as well as reduced 30-day smoking prevalence (OR=0.79; 95% CI=0.67-0.91). A smoke-free home policy and partial home restrictions appeared to be associated with less smoking regardless of the presence of other smokers in the household, but no interaction between these variables was included in the models. Smoke-free policies were more strongly related than partial restrictions.

A non-random sample of 2573 10th and 11th grade students attending high schools with high Arabic and Vietnamese enrollment, examined various factors related to participants' self-reported smoking status (current vs. not current) (Rissel et al., 2000). Included in the logistic analyses, along with year in school, parental smoking, family closeness, sex, ethnic background, parental behaviours (strict vs. not strict, clear vs. not clear consequences), pocket money (<$20/week vs. more), out 0-2 evenings vs. 3+ per week with friends, positive school perceptions, positive teacher perceptions, positive peer perceptions, was students' report of whether or not their family had clear rules about smoking indoors. A 'yes' response was inversely related to current smoking (RR=0.67; 95% CI=0.49-0.90).

Data from the 1992-93 and 1995-96 US Current Population Surveys (n=17 185) allowed examination of the association between workplace and home smoking restrictions (partial or complete versus none) on the self-reported smoking status of over 17 000 15-17 year olds (Farkas et al.,

2000). Logistic regression analyses found that adolescents with smoke-free homes were only 0.74 (95% CI=0.62-0.88) times as likely to have ever smoked (at least 100 cigarettes in lifetime) compared to those living with no smoking restrictions. Having partial home smoking restrictions was unrelated to smoking experience. Those working in a completely smoke-free indoor environment were 0.68 (95% CI=0.51-0.90) times as likely to be ever smokers compared to those working where smoking was allowed. An analysis of ever smokers showed that having a smoke-free home was positively associated with being a former smoker (OR=1.80; 95% CI=1.23-2.65). This relationship was not significant for indoor workers in a smoke-free workplace. A further analysis suggested that the rate of adolescent current smoking in households with never smokers only, but with no smoking restrictions, approached that in households with at least one current smoker and partial restrictions or a completely smoke-free home. Perhaps in these settings the lack of a smoke-free home policy communicates implicitly the message that smoking is acceptable.

Tucson, Arizona middle and high school students (n=6686) surveyed in school answered questions about their smoking behaviour, that of their parents, their family structure, the students' perceptions of their parents' attitudes against smoking, and the home smoking policy for family members and for visitors (Proescholdbell et al., 2000). The investigators created a scale for the home policy that considered policies for smokers in the household and for visitors, if no adult household members were smokers. In separate multivariate logistic regression analyses of middle and high school students, those who had never tried smoking were contrasted with those who smoked just one cigarette as the dependent variable. The main effect for the home smoking policy scale indicated that the more restrictive the policy, the less likely the adolescent was to have tried smoking (p<0.001). There was a significant interaction for the parent being a current or former smoker with the smoking policy variable only for the high school students (p<0.01). Smoking policies in homes with parental smoking appeared less associated with older adolescent smoking experimentation. When current regular smokers (smoked at least one cigarette per month) were contrasted to those who had only tried one cigarette, the home policy scale was not significant. The authors concluded that home smoking policies may be more effective in preventing experimentation than regular smoking.

In 1998, investigators surveyed 1343 Minnesota children (8th, 9th, and 10th graders) and their parents to better understand the relationship between adolescent smoking (any in the last month) and home smoking restrictions (Komro et al., 2003). In the logistic regression, in addition to demographics, a number of potential parental influences that might directly impact adolescent smoking, besides home smoking restrictions, were considered. These included: scales of parental permissiveness of adult smoking, support for smoking regulations (bans and fines), estimates of smoking prevalence among adults and youth, variables assessing parent-child communication about rules and consequences of the child smoking, parental attitude towards punishment for child smoking, adult and other child smoking status in the home as reported by the parent and the child, as well as the extent to which cigarettes were present in the home. A bivariate relationship existed for less smoking with a smoke-free home, but was not evident in the multivariate analysis. The strongest association was for smoking by another child in the home, but most of the other covariates were also significant.

The longitudinal 'Growing up Today' study examined the relation between established (at least 100 cigarettes in lifetime) adolescent smoking and home smoking restrictions (Fisher et al., 2007). Participants (aged 12-18 years) chose one of the following three options as their home smoking rule: 1) People are allowed to smoke inside the house, 2) people are not allowed to smoke inside the house, and 3) there is no rule.

A smoke-free home (option 1) was contrasted to the others. The logistic regression adjusted for age, gender, peer smoking, possession of tobacco promotional items, and having at least one parent who smokes cigarettes. In a model without the variable for parental smoking, adolescent established smoking was inversely associated with a smoke-free home (OR=0.67; 95% CI=0.48-0.93), but the association was not significant when parental smoking was included (OR=0.94; 95% CI=0.65-1.35).

A longitudinal study of 600 families in Utrecht, Netherlands, with at least one child in the 7th grade, examined the effects of eight indicators of antismoking socialisation, including a scale score computed from six questions on smoking restrictions for adolescents and adults within the home (den Exter Blokland et al., 2006). Students responded to a questionnaire twice within the 2000-2001 school year. Adolescent smoking outcomes were: initiators (those who started smoking by the second wave of the study) and maintainers (those who reported smoking in both waves). Logistic analysis of each outcome variable adjusted for baseline communication, warnings, parental knowledge of child and child's friends smoking, parental psychological control, parental confidence in effecting child's smoking behaviour, availability of cigarettes in the home, parental norms about adolescent smoking, parental reaction to child's smoking, and parental smoking status. There was no significant effect for home rules for either the initiators or maintainers. In families with nonsmoking parents, there were significantly more rules about smoking than in homes where parents smoked.

The relationship was assessed between smoke-free home policies and youth perceptions about smoking: prevalence among youth, prevalence among adults, adult disapproval of adult smoking, and adult disapproval of youth smoking (Conley Thomson et al., 2005). It was noted that each of these perceptions has been associated with youth smoking; the first two directly and the second two inversely. Random telephone survey data from 3831 adolescents 12-17 years of age from Massachusetts were used. In bivariate analyses,

no smoking inside the home was significantly associated with each of these perceptions. In multivariate logistic regression analyses, no smoking in the home was significantly associated with lower perceived adult smoking prevalence (OR=2.1; 95% CI=1.7-2.5), but not to perceived adolescent smoking prevalence (OR=1.2; 0.94-1.5). This factor was also significantly associated with high perceived adult disapproval of adult (OR=2.0; 95% CI=1.6-2.5) and of youth smoking (OR=1.5; 95% CI=1.2-1.9). Additional analyses examining interaction effects, found that parental smoking modified the effect of no smoking in the home on perceived adult disapproval of teen smoking, strengthening the odds ratio for the home smoking term (OR=1.9; 95% CI=1.4-2.5). It was concluded that no smoking in the home may provide additional benefits regarding teens' perceptions protective of future smoking above their perceptions of disapproval of teen smoking by their parents.

Adolescent smoking status was assessed in pairs (n=345) of students (grades 6, 8, and 10) and parents as: 1) never users, not susceptible to smoking in the future; 2) never users, susceptible to smoking in the future; 3) former triers; 4) current experimenters; and 5) regular users (Kodl & Mermelstein, 2004). Parents' report of household smoking restrictions were dichotomised as: 1= no one may smoke in the home vs. 0=all others. The adjusted (grade, parental education, and parental smoking) mean percentage of smoke-free homes differed in some contrasts analysed; regular adolescent smokers vs. all others (p<0.05),

and never smokers nonsusceptible to smoking vs. those susceptible to smoking (p<0.05). Contrasts for current experimenters vs. never smokers susceptible to smoking, and for never smokers (susceptible and nonsusceptible) vs. all others were not statistically significant.

In a population-based cohort of 3555 adolescents and their parents, home smoking restrictions were assessed by parental response to whether or not they allow smoking within their home (Andersen et al., 2004). Response categories included: "No," "Rarely," "Sometimes," and "Usually," with the last three categories contrasted with the first one. Self-reported adolescent smoking was categorised as daily or monthly. Families with and without parental report of adult smokers were analysed separately, with the relative risk regression models adjusted for parents asking to sit in nonsmoking parts of restaurants and asking smokers not to smoke around them. In families with parental smokers, a smoke-free home tended to show reduced rates of adolescent daily, but not monthly, smoking (daily: RR=0.74; 95% CI=0.62-0.88, monthly: RR=1.02; 95% CI=0.89-1.17). For nonsmoking families, a smoke-free home was not statistically significant for either daily or monthly smoking.

An analysis similar to that of Farkas et al. (2000) was performed using data from the 1998-99 Current Population Survey (n=12 299) (Clark et al., 2006). They only considered home smoking restrictions and analysed persons aged 15-24 years. Consistent with Farkas et al. (2000), they found that complete, but not partial home smoking restrictions, were related to less ever smoking: adolescents (15-18 years) (OR=0.56; 95% CI=0.44-0.71) and young adults (19-24 years) (OR=0.56; 95% CI=0.45-0.70). This was also true for current smoking: adolescents (OR=0.51; 95% CI=0.40-0.67) and young adults (OR=0.45; 95% CI=0.36-0.58). An analysis of current versus former smokers among ever smokers also showed relatively fewer current smokers: adolescents (OR=0.64; 95% CI=0.41-1.00) and young adults (OR=0.33; 95% CI=0.21-0.53). The authors also examined self-reported daily cigarette consumption, contrasting higher levels (6-10 CPD and >10 CPD to 5 or fewer CPD) with polytomous logistic regression. Again, a smoke-free policy was associated with reduced daily cigarette consumption overall (15-24 years): 6-10 CPD (OR=0.40; 95% CI=0.28-0.59) and 10+ CPD (OR=0.51; 95% CI=0.34-0.77).

Another survey of 4125 students 12-17 years conducted in 2002 in Australia (Szabo *et al.*, 2006) examined the association of total (inside and outside the house) or partial home smoking restrictions (inside only) with smoking behaviour, considering both smoking in the family and among friends. This study, like the Proescholdbell *et al.* (2000) study, found that the lack of home smoking restrictions compared to total restrictive policy inside and outside, was associated with more smoking in the earlier stages of the smoking uptake continuum: susceptible versus nonsusceptible (OR=1.38; 95% CI=1.06-1.79), experimenter versus non-susceptible (OR=1.92; 95% CI=1.44-2.56), and experimenter versus susceptible (OR=1.39; 95% CI=1.08-1.79). For the

analysis of current smokers versus non-susceptible never smokers the odds were 1.30 (95% CI=0.92-1.86) and in the analysis for current versus experimenters they were 0.68 (95% CI=0.48-0.96), indicating paradoxically that current smokers were more likely to reside in smoke-free homes. The authors state that this association was due to inclusion of parental smoking status in the model. When interaction terms with parental smoking were included in the multivariate models, results indicated that smoke-free homes were only associated with being lower on the smoking continuum for households without smokers. As to be expected, smoking by friends was highly associated with smoking behaviour, but there were no significant interactions for this factor with home smoking policy. Likely, peer influences are operative whether or not there is a smoke-free home policy in place.

Data from a 2003 national survey of 6503 12, 14, 16 and 18 year olds in Finland assessed the level of home smoking restrictions (total, partial, none, the respondent could not say), as reported by the respondents with experimental or daily smoking (Rainio & Rimpela, 2008). Multivariate logistic analyses adjusted for the age and sex of the respondent, as well as parental smoking, parental education, urban residence, and parental permissiveness of child smoking. Compared to never smokers, the relationship of a lack of a smoke-free home was stronger for increased daily smoking (OR=14.3; 95% CI=8.6-23.7) than for increased experimental smoking (OR=2.02; 95% CI=1.2-3.4). For increased daily smoking, a smoke-free home

appeared to be more strongly related than partial restrictions (OR=2.9; 95% CI=2.3-3.6). For the group that could not say whether there were smoking restrictions in the home, the adjusted odds ratios were somewhat higher than for the partial restrictions, but lower than for a smoke-free policy. A separate analysis of daily smoking in families where both parents smoked produced an adjusted odds ratio of 1.5 (95% CI=0.7-3.0) for partial restrictions, 2.9 (95% CI=1.1-7.8) for no restrictions, and 2.8 (95% CI=1.2-6.5) for 'could not say' compared to a completely smoke-free policy. The authors conclude that a smoke-free home can help prevent smoking even in homes where both parents smoke, and that promoting smoke-free homes within the population is a promising tobacco control tool to prevent smoking among youth.

A Ukrainian study obtained data on 609 young people aged 15-29 years (Andreeva *et al.* 2007). The data included participants' reported age at first cigarette use and age of initiation of daily cigarette smoking. This study compared families with no smokers or with a completely smoke-free home vs. all others. Thus, this categorisation cannot evaluate the potential effect of nonsmoking households prohibiting smoking indoors. Separate survival analyses for males and females adjusted (if significant) for: age, education, town size, living in a city vs. village, number of people in household, income, exposure to tobacco smoke rarely vs. frequently, seeing outdoor tobacco advertising, tobacco-related knowledge low vs. high, receiving information about tobacco from magazines, and receiving tobacco information from friends. A smoke-free home was associated with reduced risk of earlier first cigarette, both in males (HR=0.78; 95% CI=0.61-0.99) and females (HR=0.39; 95% CI=0.28-0.53). Similarly, a smoke-free home was associated with reduced risk of early initiation of daily smoking (males: HR=0.64; 95% CI=0.49-0.84; females: HR=0.60; 95% CI=0.39-0.93).

A structural equation approach was used to analyse the association of a smoke-free home (household members allowed vs. not allowed to smoke in the home) with adolescent smoking in 163 Pennsylvanian 10th graders with a parental smoker (Rodriguez et al., 2007). This study only assessed the effect of a smoke-free home in families with a parental smoker. Adolescent smoking was determined from a question with a five-level ordered response: 0) did not smoke in the past month; 1) smoked one month ago or less; 2) smoke at least once a week; 3) smoke daily, but no more than 10 cigarettes per day; and 4) smoke 11 or more cigarettes per day. Results indicated that a smoke-free home was associated with having fewer peers who smoked, which in turn was associated with a lower level of smoking. Although the total (indirect plus direct) effect of indoor smoking restrictions was not significant, the indirect effect of adolescent smoking through peer smoking was (ß indirect= -0.569, z=-3.340, p=0.0008).

A longitudinal study (four years: 2001-02 to 2005-06) of 3834 Massachusetts youth (aged 12-17 at baseline), examined the effect of a smoke-free home on transition from never smoking to experimentation, and overall progression to established

(at least 100 cigarettes in lifetime) smoking (Albers et al., 2008). A smoke-free home at baseline was defined as visitors not being allowed to smoke inside the home if no adult smoker lived there, and if there was an adult smoker in the household, there was a complete ban on smoking inside. The analysis used a three level hierarchical linear model that analysed individual (two levels) and town level predictors of smoking transitions. Level one individual variables included baseline age and smoking status, presence of a close friend who smokes; level two predictors were gender, race/ethnicity, and household income; town level factors were percentage voting yes on Question 1, percent white, and percent youth. While progression to established smoker was not significantly related to not having a smoke-free home, there was greater significance among adolescents who lived with a smoker (OR=1.38; 95% CI=0.92-2.07) compared to those not living with a smoker (OR=1.08 ; 95% CI=0.61-1.93). The absence of a smoke-free home was associated with the transition from never smoking to early experimentation among youth who lived with nonsmokers (OR=1.89; 95% CI=1.30-2.70), but not for youth living with smokers (OR=0.88; 95% CI=0.73-1.37).

Summary

In 13 of the 19 studies reviewed, at least some evidence for an association between home smoking restrictions and adolescent smoking behaviour was present. One (Albers et al., 2008) of the two longitudinal studies (den Exter Blokland et al., 2006; Albers et al., 2008) showed a

significant relationship. The one that did not spanned only a short time interval, less than a full school year, and it is possible that there was not sufficient time for enough transitions to occur.

A single study (Clark et al., 2006) examined cigarette consumption, and found a significant association of a smoke-free home with lower consumption. Three studies examined cessation (Farkas et al., 2000; Clark et al., 2006; Szabo et al., 2006) and two involved older youth from the Current Population Surveys; both showed less current smoking among those who met the adult definition of an ever smoker (at least 100 cigarettes in lifetime). The other study that examined this outcome looked at current smoking among younger youth who had ever experimented and did not find an association (Szabo et al., 2006).

The studies differed in how they accounted for parental smoking. Six studies either included an interaction term for parental smoking and a smoke-free home, or analysed subjects in smoking and nonsmoking homes separately (Biener et al., 1997; Jackson & Henriksen, 1997; Farkas et al., 2000; Proescholdbell et al., 2000; Andersen et al., 2004; Albers et al., 2008). One study found no association in either type of home (Biener et al., 1997), four found a stronger association or an association only in families without adult smokers (Jackson & Henriksen 1997; Farkas et al., 2000; Albers et al., 2008; Proescholdbell et al., 2008), and one study showed an association only in families with adult smokers (Andersen et al., 2004). Nine studies included parental or adult smoking as a covariate in the multivariate analyses (Henriksen & Jackson, 1998; Rissel *et al.*, 2000; Wakefield *et al.*, 2000a; Komro *et al.*, 2003; Kodl & Mermelstein, 2004; Clark *et al.*, 2006; den Exter Blokland *et al.*, 2006; Fisher *et al.*, 2007; Raino & Rimpela, 2008), and in three of these this variable rendered home smoking rules nonsignificant (Komro *et al.*, 2003; den Exter Blokland *et al.*, 2006; Fisher *et al.*, 2007). Clearly these two factors are highly related and their relative prevalence in the sample might influence the results.

Four studies treated home smoking rules specifically as just one strategy parents could use, among others, to provide anti-smoking socialisation for their children (Jackson & Henriksen, 1997; Henriksen & Jackson, 1998, Kodl & Mermelstein, 2004; den Exter Blokland *et al.*, 2006), and only one (den Exter Blokland *et al.*, 2006) failed to find evidence that this might be a useful anti-tobacco socialisation strategy after accounting for others.

Some studies focused on the earlier stages of the smoking uptake process (Jackson & Henriksen, 1997; Henriksen & Jackson, 1998), some only on the later stages (Farkas *et al.*, 2000; Proescholdbell *et al.*, 2000; Clark *et al.*, 2006; Fisher *et al.*, 2007), and some included analyses for both (Wakefield *et al.,* 2000a; Kodl & Mermelstein, 2004; Andersen *et al.*, 2004; den Exter Blokland *et al.*, 2006; Szabo *et al.*, 2006; Andreeva *et al.*, 2007; Albers *et al.*, 2008; Raino & Rimpela, 2008). Of the 10 studies considering earlier stages, eight found an association, and seven of 12 of those considering the later stages did. The above summary

does not include those that focused on last 30-day smoking prevalence, since this measure includes both experimenters and regular smokers.

Taken together these results suggest that while a smoke-free home might be more effective in keeping adolescents from smoking if they live in homes without adult smokers, it is possible that this strategy might also apply to homes with adult smokers. A clear policy about no one smoking in the home ever by anyone might reinforce nonsmoking family norms against smoking, and be a strategy smoking parents can employ to convey to their child their desire that the child not smoke. A smoke-free home might be more likely to prevent experimentation than to prevent progression to established or regular smoking once an adolescent has experimented. There is a need for additional, larger longitudinal population studies of adolescents at each stage of the smoking uptake process to further explore whether the association between smoke-free homes and reduced adolescent smoking is in fact causal.

Chapter Summary

Where data are available, the prevalence of smokers with smoke-free home policies has shown a clear increase over time. Also, there is a shift from report of having partial restrictions to report of completely smoke-free homes. Smokers' reports of smoke-free homes may be a good indicator of population acceptance of the harmfulness of SHS in particular and tobacco control success in general.

Demographic characteristics consistently associated with smokers' reports of smoke-free homes include younger age, male sex, and higher education level. Also related to reports of smoke-free homes are the presence of nonsmokers, particularly children in the home, lower cigarette consumption (or addiction) level, and interest in quitting.

The proportion of children protected from SHS varies greatly by locality and is closely linked to parental smoking prevalence. Where data are available, generally in localities with tobacco control programs that include smoke-free policies, downward trends in children's SHS exposure rates in the home are apparent.

In families with smokers, the presence of smoke-free policies reduces children's exposure to SHS. Less extensive restrictions were not as effective, and in some cases were ineffective. Previous interventions with smokers to decrease SHS exposure in children have generally concentrated on getting parents to quit, and have produced disappointing results. Tobacco control efforts focused on the entire population may do more to reduce SHS exposure than efforts aimed directly at individual parents.

The studies of the effects of home smoking restrictions on smoking behaviour were consistently stronger than those for workplace policies (see Chapter 7). The longitudinal studies show reduced consumption and a more consistent effect on quitting. If a smoke-free home helps quitters remain abstinent longer – and several studies presented evidence that they do – such policies will have a positive impact on eventual increased successful cessation.

The preponderance of evidence to date suggests that fewer adolescent children of nonsmoking parents living in smoke-free homes initiate smoking compared to if the home is not smoke-free. A smoke-free home policy is a clear message from nonsmoking parents to their children that smoking is unacceptable. Whether such a message from a parent who smokes can influence their children not to smoke requires further research.

Conclusions

1. The level of exposure to SHS among children is related to parental smoking, but can be diminished by adoption of a smoke-free home policy.

2. In some localities, population-based strategies, such as public education campaigns on SHS in homes and laws prohibiting smoking in public and workplaces, appear to be more effective in ultimately reducing SHS exposure among children than individual-based programs targeted to parents.

3. When smoke-free public and workplace policies become more common, smokers appear increasingly willing to agree to a smoke-free home policy.

4. Home smoking restrictions lead to reduced consumption and greater quitting among adult smokers.

5. Insufficient evidence exists regarding the effect of smoke-free homes on youth smoking initiation.

6. A smoke-free policy, in which no one is allowed to smoke inside the house at any time under any circumstances, is more effective in reducing smoking than partial restrictions.

7. Home smoking restrictions appear to have a greater effect on smoking behaviour than restrictions on smoking in the workplace.

Recommendations

1. Monitor the prevalence of smoke-free homes among smokers in countries worldwide as a measure of changing population anti-tobacco norms and progress in tobacco control.

2. Conduct public education campaigns to encourage smokers to adopt smoke-free homes.

3. Recommendations to smokers to adopt a smoke-free home should be included in all efforts promoting cessation.

4. Further studies regarding the effect of smoke-free homes on youth initiation are required.

5. Further evidence of the effect of smoke-free homes on smoking behaviour in countries at different stages of the tobacco epidemic is needed.

Chapter 9
Summary

Health effects of exposure to SHS

This chapter describes the findings and conclusions of review groups that have conducted comprehensive assessments of the health effects of exposure to SHS. Over the four decades that research findings on SHS and health have been reported, increasingly stronger conclusions of reviewing groups have progressively motivated the development of protective policies. The rationale for such policies is solidly grounded in the conclusions of a number of authoritative groups that SHS exposure contributes to the causation of cancer, cardiovascular disease, and respiratory conditions.

The Working Group found a high degree of convergence of the research findings. In fact, since 1986, an increasing number of reports have added to an ever growing list of causal effects of SHS exposure. These reports have given exhaustive consideration to the epidemiological findings and the wide range of research supporting the plausibility of causal associations. They have also considered and rejected explanations other than causation for the associations observed in the epidemiological studies. Particular attention has been given to confounding by other risk factors and

to exposure misclassification, both of active smoking status and of exposure to SHS.

Conclusions

Exposure to SHS causes harm to health, including lung cancer and cardiovascular disease in adults, respiratory disease in adults and children, and Sudden Infant Death Syndrome (SIDS), as reported by numerous authoritative scientific review groups. As concluded by the US Surgeon General, there is no established risk-free level of SHS exposure. SHS exposure has both acute and chronic health effects; consequently, both immediate and longer-term benefits to public health can be anticipated from implementing the recommended smoke-free policies.

Evolution of smoke-free policies

The guidelines for the implementation of Article 8 of the WHO's Framework Convention on Tobacco Control (FCTC) provide public health officials and policymakers with a clear description of the elements of a smoke-free policy that offer effective

protection from SHS. An effective smoke-free policy should create 100% smoke-free spaces by law in all indoor public and workplaces, public transportation, and, as appropriate, other public places. The policy should emphasise that protection from exposure to SHS is a basic right, and that protection should be universal and ensure 100% smoke-free environments, as opposed to protecting only targeted populations or permitting smoking in restricted areas. An organised strategy for public education and enforcement is critical for successful implementation.

The historical development of smoke-free environments began in the mid-1970s and expanded in the 1990s. Beginning in the early 1980s, results of scientific studies and governmental and intergovernmental reports provided the information needed to advance smoke-free policies. However, there was no information on the ideal components of such a policy due to the lack of experience at that time. The early experience of multiple jurisdictions in the USA as well as in Australia and Canada provided case studies on the effectiveness of smoke-free policies.

In the 21st century, the number of countries passing 100% smoke-free legislation started to grow rapidly. In 2004, Ireland became the first country in the world to implement a 100% smoke-free policy in all indoor public and workplaces, including restaurants and bars.

Conclusions

As of January 2008, sixteen countries and dozens of sub-national jurisdictions have implemented model legislation. Passing a policy is only one part of the process of protecting a population from exposure to secondhand smoke; both public education and enforcement efforts are necessary when the smoke-free policy is implemented. The need for enforcement efforts usually decreases after the policy is established, as it typically becomes self-enforcing.

Economic impact and incidental effects

Smoke-free policies affect businesses in numerous ways, from improving the health and productivity of their employees to reducing their health and hazard insurance claims, cleaning of workplace environments, maintenance of designated smoking rooms, and potential litigation costs. Studies suggest that there are minimal short-term costs to businesses to implement comprehensive smoke-free policies. Existing evidence from developed countries indicates that smoke-free workplace policies have a net positive effect on businesses; the same is likely to be the case in developing countries. Establishing and maintaining designated indoor or outdoor smoking areas is more costly to implement than a completely smoke-free policy. There are minimal costs to governments related to enforcement and education about smoke-free policies.

Much of the debate over the economic impact of smoke-free policies, and as a result, much of the research, has focused on the hospitality sector. Methodologically sound research from developed countries consistently concludes that smoke-free policies do not have an adverse economic impact on the business activity of restaurants, bars, or establishments catering to tourists, with many studies finding a small positive effect of these policies. These studies include outcomes such as official reports of sales, changes in employment statistics, and the number of businesses opening and closing. Very limited evidence from South Africa, an upper middle-resource country, is consistent with these findings. It is likely that the same would be true in other developing countries; nevertheless, research confirming this would be useful as smoke-free policies are adopted in a growing number of countries. There are very few studies on the effects of smoke-free policies on various problem behaviours, including other substance use and its consequences, problem gambling, domestic violence, noise, and litter with findings inconclusive at this time.

Conclusions

Smoke-free policies do not cause a decline in the business activity of the restaurant and bar industry.

Attitudes and compliance

In developed countries, majority public support for smoke-free policies is typical for public and workplaces (including hospitality settings), and a range of other settings (e.g. schools and health care facilities). There is some suggestion that countries that use public education campaigns when enacting smoke-free laws achieve higher levels of support.

In developing countries, the Global Youth Tobacco Survey (GYTS) has identified majority student support for smoke-free policies in public places. Likewise, studies have shown majority adult support for smoke-free public and workplaces.

Trend data on attitudes indicate increasing support for smoke-free policies over time in nearly all settings. This also occurs after the implementation of smoke-free policies.

Smokers usually comply with smoke-free policies, but the level of compliance can vary widely. Non-compliance may be related to a lack of awareness or poor enforcement of the policy.

Studies in developed countries also indicate majority public support for smoke-free cars, parks, sports facilities, and transition areas, such as building entryways.

Conclusions

There is usually majority support for smoke-free public and workplaces. Public support among both smokers and nonsmokers for smoke-free policies increases following implementation of legislation. When smoke-free policies are implemented as described in the WHO FCTC guidelines, compliance is moderate to high.

Reductions in exposure to SHS and health effects

In the past, voluntary restrictions on smoking in the workplace have been an important vehicle for reducing exposure to SHS in many countries. However, such restrictions have uneven coverage, are generally not applied in some of the highest-exposure settings (such as bars and gaming venues), typically offer little protection for groups in the working population with the poorest health status, and therefore increase the likelihood of widening health inequalities. Comprehensive, mandatory restrictions do not have these shortcomings.

Studies of smoke-free legislation, that prohibits smoking in virtually all indoor workplaces, consistently demonstrate reduced exposure to SHS in high-risk settings by 80-90%. The residual exposures are likely caused by smoking around the boundaries of venues, including designated smoking areas on patios and verandas. As a result, indoor smoke-free workplace laws greatly reduce, but do not remove altogether, the potential for harm to health caused by SHS around bars, restaurants, and similar settings. Also, smoking in cars generates high levels of SHS.

The most comprehensive study to date indicates that legislation may reduce exposure to SHS population-wide by up to 40%. Several large, well-designed studies have found that comprehensive smoke-free policies

do not lead to increased exposure to SHS in the home. Another important feature of comprehensive legislation is its impact on inequalities; the largest absolute reductions in exposure to SHS in the workplace tend to occur among those groups that had the highest pre-legislation exposures.

Given the relatively recent introduction of comprehensive bans, there is only one study reporting on sustained changes in SHS exposure. More than 10 years of follow-up data from California show that the early reductions in SHS exposure have not been reversed.

There are short-term improvements in health linked to these restrictions on smoking. Workforce studies have reported reductions in acute respiratory illnesses after smoking bans, and early findings of substantial declines in hospital admissions for acute myocardial infarction have been replicated in numerous studies. The literature also indicates that wide-ranging bans on smoking in the workplace are followed by as much as a 10-20% reduction in hospital admissions for acute coronary events in the general population in the first year post-ban. At present, it is not possible to distinguish the contributions to the decline in hospital admissions of changes in smoking rates and prevalence, and those of reduced exposures to SHS. The precise magnitude of the reduction in admissions is uncertain, but will vary with the background incidence of heart disease, the prevalence of exposure to SHS preceding the ban, and the extent of the legislation and its implementation.

SHS increases the risk of lung cancer, but the time period between cessation of exposure and decrease in risk may be 10-20 years, making it difficult to link changes in disease rates with introduction of smoking restrictions. However, given the strength of the evidence linking SHS to increased risk of lung cancer, the reduction in exposure following smoke-free legislation is expected to ultimately be reflected in a decrease in the incidence of this particular disease.

Conclusions

Implementation of smoke-free policies leads to a substantial decline in exposure to SHS, reduces social inequalities in SHS exposure at work, appears to cause a decline in heart disease morbidity (the published data on this are consistent, but longer-term follow-up is required), and decreases respiratory symptoms in workers. Lung cancer incidence in nonsmokers can be expected to decline 10-20 years after smoke-free legislation is put into action. Thus far, data are not available documenting such declines, as most smoke-free legislation has only recently been implemented.

Effect on smoking behaviour

In areas where new smoke-free laws were part of multiple tobacco control efforts, there was clear and consistent evidence of a positive change in smoking behaviour from prior ongoing trends. However, if multiple tobacco control measures are instituted simultaneously, attribution of the change to a new law restricting smoking is not possible.

Studies that assessed smoking behaviour, before and after implementation of new laws restricting smoking in public and workplaces, were analytically weak and produced mixed results; some provided no statistical evaluation even though differences or trends appeared to be present.

Nearly all the studies correlating the extent and strength of laws restricting smoking with various aspects of smoking behaviour found the expected associations: localities with relatively stronger restrictions in more places, or that covered a greater proportion of the population, generally showed lower adult and youth prevalence rates and reduced cigarette consumption. Whether localities with strong anti-smoking norms were more likely to pass such regulations, or the regulations led to reduced smoking, is unknown.

At an individual level, studies of workers subject to smoke-free policies in the workplace indicate that these restrictions reduce smokers' cigarette consumption by 2-4 cigarettes per day. Whether or not the reduction in daily cigarette consumption is sufficient to make the smokers less addicted, and therefore more likely to quit in the future, is unknown, but some evidence suggests that the reduction in consumption in the short-term may lead to increased cessation in the long-term.

Population studies, even the cross-sectional ones, that adjusted for worker characteristics, including demographics and occupation, are likely minimally biased. Nearly all these studies found that smoke-free workplaces were more associated with decreased smoking among workers than settings that only implemented partial restrictions.

To date, there are limited data concerning the effect of a completely smoke-free campus for everyone (students and adults) on adolescent smoking behaviour. Not witnessing teachers smoking on campus may reinforce school-level anti-smoking norms and lead to reduced adolescent smoking initiation, but further research is required to explore this issue.

Conclusions

Smoke-free workplaces reduce cigarette consumption among continuing smokers and lead to increased successful cessation among smokers. Smoke-free policies appear to reduce tobacco use among youth. There is a greater decline in smoking when smoke-free policies are part of a comprehensive tobacco control program.

Home smoking restrictions

Where data are available, the prevalence of smokers who have implemented a smoke-free policy at home has shown a clear increase over time. Also, there is a shift from reports of households having partial restrictions to reports of completely smoke-free homes. This may be a good indicator of population acceptance of the harmfulness of SHS and tobacco control success.

Demographic characteristics consistently associated with reports by smokers of smoke-free homes include individuals of a younger age, male sex, and higher education level. Also, related to reports of smoke-free homes are the presence of nonsmokers, particularly children, lower cigarette consumption (or addiction) level, and interest in quitting.

The proportion of children protected from SHS varies greatly by locality and is closely linked to parental smoking prevalence. Where data are available, generally in localities with tobacco control programs that include smoke-free policies, downward trends in child SHS exposure rates in the home are apparent.

In families with smokers, the presence of smoke-free policies reduces children's exposure to SHS. Less extensive restrictions were not as effective, and in some cases were ineffective. Previous interventions with smokers, in an attempt to decrease their children's exposure to SHS, have generally concentrated on getting parents to quit, and have produced disappointing results. Tobacco control efforts focused on the entire population may do more to reduce SHS exposure than efforts aimed directly at individual parents.

The studies of the positive effects of home smoking restrictions on smoking behaviour were consistently stronger than those for workplace policies. Longitudinal studies show reduced consumption and a more consistent effect on quitting. If a smoke-free home helps quitters remain abstinent longer, and several studies presented evidence that they do, such policies will have a positive impact on eventual increased successful cessation.

The preponderance of cross-sectional evidence to date suggests that fewer adolescent children of non-smoking parents living in smoke-free homes initiate smoking compared to children from a home that is not smoke-free. A smoke-free home policy is a clear message from nonsmoking parents to their children that smoking is unacceptable. Whether such a message from a parent who smokes can influence their children not to smoke requires further research.

Conclusions

Smoke-free home policies reduce exposure of children to SHS, reduce adult smoking, and appear to reduce youth smoking.

Chapter 10
Evaluation

The Working Group evaluated the strength of the evidence for drawing the conclusions shown in the accompanying table, defined as follows:

Sufficient evidence:
An association has been observed in studies in which chance, bias, and confounding can be ruled out with reasonable confidence. The association is highly likely to be causal.

Strong evidence:
There is consistent evidence of an association, but evidence of causality is limited by the fact that chance, bias, or confounding have not been ruled out with reasonable confidence. However, explanations other than causality are unlikely.

Limited evidence:
There is some evidence of association, but alternative explanations are possible.

Evidence of no effect:
Methodologically sound studies consistently demonstrate the lack of an association.

Inadequate/no evidence:
There are no available methodologically sound studies showing an association.

In considering the evidence on the health consequences of secondhand smoke (SHS) (see Chapter 2):

• The Working Group agrees with other bodies: SHS causes harm to health, including lung cancer and cardiovascular disease in adults, respiratory disease in adults and children, and Sudden Infant Death Syndrome (SIDS) in infants.

• The Working Group agrees with the conclusion of the US Surgeon General: there is no established risk-free level of SHS exposure.

Evaluation of the weight of evidence

		Sufficient Evidence	Strong Evidence	Limited Evidence	Evidence of No Effect	Inadequate/ No Evidence
1	Smoke-free policies do not cause a decline in the business activity of the restaurant and bar industry (see Chapter 4).	X				
2	Implementation of smoke-free policies leads to a substantial decline in exposure to SHS (see Chapter 6).	X				
3	Implementation of smoke-free legislation reduces social inequalities in SHS exposure at work (see Chapter 6).		X			
4	Implementation of smoke-free legislation causes a decline in heart disease morbidity (see Chapter 6).		X			
5	Implementation of smoke-free legislation decreases respiratory symptoms in workers (see Chapter 6).	X				
6	Smoke-free workplaces reduce cigarette consumption among continuing smokers (see Chapter 7).	X				
7	Smoke-free workplaces lead to increased successful cessation among smokers (see Chapter 7).		X			
8	Smoke-free policies reduce tobacco use among youth (see Chapter 7).		X			
9	Smoke-free home policies reduce exposure of children to SHS (see Chapter 8).	X				
10	Smoke-free home policies reduce adult smoking (see Chapter 8).	X				
11	Smoke-free home policies reduce youth smoking (see Chapter 8).		X			

Based on the quality and volume of the evidence reviewed, the Working Group concluded that there is *sufficient evidence* **to support each of the following statements:**

1. There are an increasing number of governments enacting and implementing smoke-free policies that conform to the Guidelines for Article 8 of the WHO FCTC (see Chapter 3).

2. There is usually majority support for smoke-free workplaces and public places (see Chapter 5).

3. Public support among both smokers and non-smokers for smoke-free policies increases following implementation of legislation (see Chapter 5).

4. When implemented, as described in the WHO FCTC guidelines, compliance with smoke-free policies is moderate to high (see Chapter 5).

5. There is a greater decline in smoking when smoke-free policies are part of a comprehensive tobacco control program (see Chapter 7).

6. Smoking in cars generates high levels of SHS (see Chapter 6).

7. Lung cancer incidence in nonsmokers can be expected to decline over several decades after the enactment of smoke-free legislation. Data are not yet available, however, documenting such declines, as most smoke-free legislation has only recently been implemented (Chapter 6).

Chapter 11
Recommendations

Overall

Based on the body of evidence contemplated in this volume, the Working Group makes the following recommendations:

1. To protect public health it is essential that governments enact and implement smoke-free policies that, at a minimum, conform to the Guidelines for Article 8 of the WHO FCTC. This should be done as part of a comprehensive tobacco control strategy that implements all of the provisions called for by the WHO FCTC.

2. In addition to the above, governments should support well-designed public education campaigns to promote smoke-free homes.

3. A multi-national surveillance and monitoring system should be implemented to track exposure to secondhand smoke, attitudes towards smoke-free policies, implementation of and compliance with these policies, and tobacco use behaviour.

A research and evaluation programme is needed, especially in developing countries, to determine the impact of legislation on:

- inequalities in exposure to SHS
- health outcomes
- economic activity
- exposure to SHS in transition areas and outdoor venues
- smoking in cars
- tobacco use and other behaviours

Health effects of exposure to SHS

It is recommended that legislative bodies accept the current state of the evidence on the harm caused by SHS pending the upcoming IARC re-review of the evidence in a planned 2009 IARC monograph meeting.

Evolution of smoke-free policies

The global experience in tobacco control has produced valuable exemplars that can be used to further advance efforts to reduce exposure to SHS. Based on the review of smoke-free policies, the following recommendations should be considered:

1. The guidelines for implementation of Article 8 should be followed to provide guidance for national and sub-national governments to develop, enact, and implement smoke-free policies, which produce considerable health benefits for the population. The evidence shows that a growing number of governments have effectively implemented such policies.

2. Policymakers and public health advocates should learn from the experience of other locations that have fully implemented the guidelines, whether at the national or sub-national level, in developing and implementing smoke-free policies.

Economic impact and incidental effects

The results are mixed for the few studies that exist on the impact of smoke-free policies on gaming establishments; more research is needed on these venues.

Attitudes and compliance

Assessing attitudinal data among the general public, smokers, and any relevant population groups (e.g. hospitality workers) prior to the introduction of new smoke-free policies can be helpful in policy development.

1. If there is a shortage of recent representative data, then consideration should be given to undertaking representative

attitudinal surveys within the relevant jurisdiction (e.g. the Global Adult Tobacco Surveys [GATS]). For example, such data can inform public education campaigns, use of media advocacy, and the extent of signage and enforcement activities.

2. Once smoke-free laws are passed, further monitoring of attitudes and compliance is helpful in guiding implementation, enforcement, and future policy development.

3. Public health professionals should be prepared to respond to inaccurate or misleading information regarding the effect of smoke-free policies (see Chapter 4).

Reductions in exposure to SHS and health effects

1. There should be multi-country protocols for evaluating the effects of smoke-free policies on exposure to SHS and consequent health effects.

2. An international database should be developed to log the implementation of smoke-free policies, studies of the impacts of legislation on exposure to SHS, and assessments of health effects. Such a database should be the basis for monitoring the progress of smoke-free policies and their effectiveness, internationally.

Effect on smoking behaviour

1. Smoking restrictions for public or workplaces should prohibit smoking completely if they are to have an optimal impact on reducing smoking behaviour, as well as reducing exposure to SHS.

2. To have optimal effect, smoke-free policies should be part of comprehensive tobacco control programmes aimed at reducing the adverse health effects from tobacco use.

3. Since much of what is known regarding the effect of smoking restrictions on smoking behaviour is from developed countries,

further research on this topic is needed that involves multiple nations in different stages of the tobacco epidemic.

Home smoking restrictions

1. The prevalence of smoke-free homes among smokers in countries worldwide should be monitored as a measure of changing population anti-tobacco norms and progress in tobacco control.

2. Public education campaigns should be conducted to encourage smokers to adopt smoke-free homes.

3. Advice to smokers to adopt a smoke-free home should be included in all efforts promoting cessation.

4. Further studies regarding the effect of smoke-free homes on youth initiation are required.

5. Further evidence of the effect of smoke-free homes on smoking behaviour in countries at different stages of the tobacco epidemic is needed.

Appendix 1.
Overview of relative advantages and disadvantages of different secondhand smoke exposure assessment methods

Atmospheric measures

Current methods for assessing SHS exposure	Source	Validity assessment	Settings used	Advantages	Disadvantages	Examples of use in studies
Gas-phase						
	Airborne nicotine concentrations	Valid. *One study showed cotinine levels decreased in 35 hotel workers by 69% after a smoke-free law, while air nicotine levels decreased by 83%.	Indoor, outdoor	Specific to SHS	Costly; delay in results (gas chromatography required); recent exposure only	Phillips et al., 1996 LaKind et al., 1999 Maskarinec et al., 2000 Mulcahy et al., 2005* Gee et al., 2006 Ruprecht et al., 2006 Tominz et al., 2006 Barrientos-Gutierrez et al., 2007a,b Goodman et al., 2007 Bolte et al., 2008
	3-ethenylpyridine	Valid, but few studies report its use	Indoor, outdoor	Specific to SHS	Costly; delay in results	Kuusimäki et al., 2007 Bolte et al., 2008
	Carbon monoxide in air	Valid, but not specific to SHS	Indoor	Cheap	Not specific; recent exposure only	Klepeis et al., 1999 De Bruin et al., 2004 Rees & Connolly, 2006 Goodman et al., 2007 Waring & Siegel, 2007
	Volatile organic compounds (benzene, toluene, xylene)	Valid, but not specific to SHS	Indoor, outdoor	Educational (known carcinogens)	Costly; delay in results (gas chromatography required); recent exposure only	Daisey et al., 1998 McNabola et al., 2006 Goodman et al., 2007 Bolte et al., 2008
Solid-phase						
	Solanesol	Valid, but few studies report its use	Indoor	Specific to SHS	Costly	Jenkins et al., 2001
	Particulate matter	Valid. A Norwegian study showed a strong correlation between ambient particulate matter and air nicotine concentrations (r=0.83).	Indoor, outdoor	Cheap; real time results, educational (results can be shown to the public)	Not specific to tobacco smoke; recent exposure only	Henderson et al., 1989 Phillips et al., 1996 Hammond,1999 Gorini et al., 2004 Moshammer et al., 2004 Repace, 2004 Travers et al., 2004 Mulcahy et al., 2005 Nebot et al., 2005 Gasparrini et al., 2006 Gee et al., 2006 Maziak et al., 2008 Wipfli et al., 2008

	Method/Agent	Validity	Indoor, outdoor	Advantage	Limitation	References
Biomarkers						
	Polycyclic aromatic hydrocarbons	Valid. **A linear relationship between PAHs and $PM_{2.5}$ was observed in one study.	Indoor, outdoor	Educational	Costly; not specific to tobacco smoke; recent exposure only	Georgiadis et al., 2001a,b; Repace, 2004**; Bolte et al., 2008
	Cotinine, 4-Methylnitros-amino-1-(3-pyridyl)-1-butanol	Gold standard to which other assessments are measured		Specific to SHS	More expensive; recent exposure only	Jarvis et al., 2000; Ellingsen et al., 2006; Haw & Gruer, 2007; Goodman et al., 2007; Arheart et al., 2008; Maziak et al., 2008
	Hair nicotine	Similar validity to cotinine	Indoor	Up to last three month's exposure	Expensive; hair colour interference	Repace et al., 2006a; Barrientos-Gutierrez et al., 2007a; Wipfli et al., 2008; Maziak et al., 2008
Questionnaires						
Self-report surveys	Questionnaires (e.g. Global Adult Tobacco Survey)	Valid. Studies have shown large differences in indoor air pollution by type of smoking policy in workplaces, restaurants, bars, and homes.	Workplace, personal space, public place	Easy to asses; can use retrospectively	Misclassification	Matt et al., 1999; Jarvis et al., 2000; Chen et al., 2002; Pirkle et al., 2006; Haw & Gruer, 2007
Other indirect methods						
Observational compliance	Visual and/or olfactive assessment; cigarette butt count; ash tray presence; presence of smoke-free policy signs	Uncertain validity. Failure to observe smoking may not indicate compliance	Indoor, outdoor	Cheap; easy to implement in field	Misclassification; visual and olfactive measurements non-objective	Weber et al., 2003; Skeer et al., 2004

Appendix 2.
Measuring smoking behaviour

While the main purpose of clean-air legislation or policies is to protect smokers from SHS, Chapter 7 examines the evidence for these policies effecting smoking behaviour. Chapter 8 extends this theme to smoking policies within the home. Thus, it is important to understand the most generally used measures of smoking behaviour. Much of the data involving smoking behaviour for evaluation of clean-air policies are derived from population surveys that monitor health behaviours in general or tobacco-use behaviours in particular. Discussed below are the main measures that can vary in detail and issues related to their appropriateness and validity.

Smoking prevalence (adults). Standard survey questions addressing smoking status usually determine whether the respondent was an "ever" smoker. In the USA, the question "Have you smoked at least 100 cigarettes in your lifetime" is used for this purpose. In other countries, a question such as "Have you ever smoked daily for a period of six months?" is used. An affirmative response establishes the respondent as an ever smoker. The identified ever smokers are then asked a question about their current smoking status, such as "Do you now smoke cigarettes every day, some days, or not at all?" The response choice "some days" may identify persons who do not really consider themselves to be smokers, but who nevertheless smoke occasionally, perhaps only in social situations. In some localities, the proportion of smokers who identify themselves as "some days" smokers is not trivial and is growing, particularly among youth. Persons who say that they now smoke "not at all" are considered former smokers. Smoking prevalence is then defined as the percentage of current (daily and some-day) smokers in the survey sample, appropriately weighted to be representative of the population. The status data, and other features of smoking behaviour, are determined from self-reports. Research on the reliability of self-report data has compared the results both to biochemical markers and report of a significant other (Hatziandreu *et al.*, 1989; Gilpin *et al.*, 1994), and generally found good correspondence. However, as smokers become more subject to social norms against smoking, some may not answer accurately.

Quitting. Former smokers are usually asked when they quit smoking. If the former smoker quit a long time in the past, they may not remember the date, so for those unable to provide a date, a question with general time intervals can help establish whether cessation occurred recently or long ago. For instance, "What best describes how long ago you quit: within the past 3 months, 3 to 6 months ago, 6 to 12 months ago, 1-5 years ago, or more than five years ago." Intervals should be chosen to correspond to the timing of the evaluation survey with respect to implementation of new legislation. The quit ratio is defined as the percentage of ever smokers who are now quit, or quit for a given length of time or longer. Cessation for three months is a good early indicator of eventually successful cessation (Gilpin *et al.*, 1997). Some surveys also ask current smokers if they had tried to quit (usually for a day or longer) at least once in the previous year, and some try to establish how long the smoker abstained for the most recent or longest quit attempt in the past year. However, quit attempts of short duration are less likely to be recalled than those of longer duration (Gilpin & Pierce, 1994). A number of surveys ask current smokers about their intentions regarding quitting (i.e. within the next month, within the next 6 months, sometime but not within the next six months, and no intent to quit).

Self-reported cigarette consumption. Daily smokers are generally asked to estimate the average number of cigarettes they smoke a day, and some-day smokers are asked how many days they usually smoke per month, and on the days they do smoke, about how many cigarettes they consume. From their answers, an average daily or monthly consumption can be computed. Research has shown that smokers tend to round (likely down) to the nearest half-pack (U.S. Department of Health and Human Services, 1989). So if consumption is categorised for analysis, the categories should be chosen to include these boundaries. For example, in countries where cigarettes are sold in 20-cigarette packs, the categories <5, 5-14, 15-24, 25+ cigarettes per day might be used. It should also be noted that when smokers are asked to recall previous consumption levels, they tend to report higher levels than they do currently (Gilpin *et al.*, 2001). For this reason, it is problematical to ask smokers about their consumption prior to a new law and currently.

Population cigarette consumption. Such measures differ from self-reported cigarette consumption and are usually derived from data pertaining to cigarette sales volume. Some studies analyse total tobacco sales, or total sales of cigarettes, and others divide this figure by the number of adults (18+ years) in the population. Youth are generally not included since they only account for a small proportion of total sales (Cummings *et al.*, 1994).

Smoking initiation. The process of smoking initiation involves several transitions before a youth reaches the status of an adult smoker. This process can be interrupted at any point. The first transition occurs when the youth begins to consider the idea of smoking. This may occur before there is an articulated intent to smoke, and such "susceptibility to smoking" is generally established by lack of a strong denial of future smoking (Pierce *et al.*, 1996). For instance, an answer to the questions: "Do you think you will try a cigarette soon?" or "If your best friend offered you a cigarette, would you take it?" or "Do you think you will be smoking a year from now?" other than "definitely not" (i.e. "probably not," "probably yes," or "definitely yes"), suggests a susceptibility to smoking. These questions would be asked of youth who denied ever having tried a cigarette, or even having a puff on one. Versions of these questions could also be asked of those who have tried smoking, but not recently, as a measure of their likelihood of doing it again. Experimenters are generally defined as those who have tried a cigarette or smoked a whole cigarette. Becoming an established smoker can be defined using the adult criteria for being an ever smoker. Current smoking among youth is often defined as report of smoking on any day in the past month, but some studies use any day in the last week. Regular current smoking may be defined as smoking on every day in the last week or month.

Report of smoking restrictions. Population surveys also ask respondents about restrictions on smoking in their workplaces and/or at home. The proportion of smokers reporting restrictions is usually lower than that for nonsmokers (Gilpin *et al.*, 2000), either because smokers gravitate to work settings with fewer restrictions, live only with other smokers, or because they are in denial that restrictions actually are present either at work or home. Comparison of reports from smokers and nonsmokers within the same household are not in complete agreement (Mumford *et al.*, 2004), but if smokers act according to their perceptions, their report may be more valid.

Appendix 3.
Econometric studies relating scope and strength of laws restricting smoking to smoking behaviour

Reference Location	Population and design	Year	Assessment of law scope and strength	Smoking measures	Covariates, analysis	Results	Comments
Wasserman et al., 1991 USA	**Adults** >200 000 adult respondents to the National Health Interview Surveys **Teenagers** 1960 teen respondents to the National Health and Nutrition Examination Survey II (NHANESII)	NHIS 1970, 1974, 1979, 1980, 1983, 1985 NHANES-II 1976-1980	From reports published by the US Dept of Health and Human Services. Laws, regulation ordered categorical variable created as restrictions in: 1=private work places, 0.75=restaurants, 0.50=public places*, 0.25=< 4 public places, 0=none	Current smoking status Daily consumption among current smokers	Adult regression model included year, log cigarette price by year, income by year, family size, log family size, education, education by year, sex, age, birth cohort, sex by age, birth cohort by age, non-white race/ethnicity, and marital status. Teen regression model included year, log cigarette price by year, family size, log family size, family income, household head education, sex, age, non-white race/ ethnicity, and a variable for restrictions on sales of cigarettes to minors.	Regulation index significantly related to reduced adult reported cigarette consumption (p<0.05) but not to smoking status. Regulation index significantly related to less teen current smoking (p<0.01), but not to daily cigarette consumption among teens.	* If state had no restrictions on private places and restaurants but on at least in 4 different types of public places, then a score of 0.50 was assigned; if in less than 4, then a score of 0.25 was used.
Chaloupka, 1992 USA	Adult male and female respondents to NHANES II that surveyed approximately 28 000 people of all ages.	1976-1980	Same categories as for Wasserman et al., 1990 (extensive, moderate, basic, nominal), but binary variables used for each category instead of ordered categorical variable	Daily cigarette consumption	Separate regression model for males and females included current and past and next year's cigarette prices, past and next year consumption. Two analyses conducted for all respondents (nonsmokers coded zero CPD) and current smokers.	All respondents Males Extensive, NS Basic, p<0.01 Females Extensive, NS Basic, NS Current Smokers Males Extensive, NS Basic, p<0.01 Females Extensive, NS Basic< NS	The authors concluded that basic restrictions are unlikely to impede smoking further.
Chaloupka & Saffer, 1992	Summary data on 50 US states gathered from many sources	1970-1985	Same coding as Chaloupka et al., 1992, but only two binary variables used: extensive and basic: state wide rather than local laws coded	Per capita cigarette sales	Analysis included cigarette prices, tobacco production, three variables related to export and import of cigarettes (smuggling), income, percent of the population who were Mormons or Southern Baptists, the percentage of the population who voted, the percent divorced, and the percent unemployed.	Both restriction indicators significantly related to per capita cigarette sales, p<0.01.	The authors concluded that laws restricting smoking are more likely to be passed in states with higher cigarette prices, and that passing more smoking restrictions may not decrease cigarette sales.

Appendix 3.
Econometric studies relating scope and strength of laws restricting smoking to smoking behaviour

Reference Location	Population and design	Year	Assessment of law scope and strength	Smoking measures	Covariates, analysis	Results	Comments
Keeler et al., 1993 California, USA	Summary data from various sources	1980-1990	Regulation index that accounted for the percent of the state's population affected by regulation and the intensity of regulation for the population covered.	Per capita monthly cigarette sales	The time series regression analyses included the average of Arizona and Oregon taxes divided by the California tax, federal tax, per capita income, cigarette prices, state tax, and a time trend.	Without the time trend in the model, the regulation index was significantly and inversely related to per capita consumption (p<0.001). Including the time trend in the model, eliminated the effect for the regulation index.	The authors indicate that the time trend (increases in tobacco control activity) and the changes in consumption moved together over time and it was not possible to separate their effects.
Chaloupka & Grossman, 1996	110 717 8th, 10th, and 12th graders Monitoring the Future Surveys	1992, 1993, 1994	Five variables related to the fraction of the population covered by restrictions in private workplaces, retail stores, schools, or other public places	Any smoking in the past 30 days Measure of daily cigarette consumption among current smokers	Analyses adjusted for a number of individual level factors, as well as cigarette prices, restrictions on youth purchase of cigarettes, whether a portion of the cigarette tax was devoted to tobacco control, and whether there were any laws protecting the rights of smokers.	Smoking in past 30 days: Workplace, p<0.05 All four others, NS Consumption: Restaurants, schools, other public places, p<0.01 Other two, NS	
Chaloupka & Wechsler, 1997	16 560 college students from the Harvard College Alcohol Study	1993	Three binary variables for restrictions in restaurants, schools, other places. Ordered categorical variable similar to Wasserman, 1990	Any smoking in past 30 days Ordered categorical variable for cigarette consumption among current smokers (none, 1-9 CPD, 10-19 CPD, 20+ CPD)	Analyses adjusted for cigarette prices, age, sex, race/ethnicity, marital status, religiosity, parental education, on-campus residence, fraternity/ sorority membership, and employment, as well as college-level characteristics (co-ed, private, commuter, rural, with fraternity/sorority, and region).	Smoking in past 30 days: Restaurants, p<0.10 Schools, NS Other, NS Ordered categorical, NS Consumption: Restaurants, p<0.10 Schools, p<0.10 Other, NS Ordered categorical, NS	Authors suggested that restaurant smoking restrictions are a reflection of community level restrictions in general.
Lewit et al., 1997 Communities in USA and Canada	15 432 9th grade students from the Community Intervention Trial for Smoking Cessation communities (COMMIT)	1990 and 1992	Combination of three indices related to restrictions in private workplaces, restaurants, and other public places.	Any smoking in the past 30 days Among those who did not smoke in the past 30 days, intent to smoke in the future	Analyses controlled for a multitude of individual and community level characteristics, as well as other tobacco control policy variables including cigarette prices, school anti-tobacco classes,	Smoking in past 30 days: Combined index, NS School policy, p<0.01	

Reference Location	Population and design	Year	Assessment of law scope and strength	Smoking measures	Covariates, analysis	Results	Comments
Lewit et al., 1997 Communities in USA and Canada			The separate indices took into account the frequency of venue type and extent of the restrictions. There was also a variable for school smoking policy.		minimum age of purchase requirements, vending machine restrictions, restrictions of distribution of free samples and exposures to anti- and pro-tobacco media.	Intent to smoke: NS for all the restriction variables	
Tauras & Chaloupka, 1999a	See Tauras, 2005	See Tauras, 2005	Binary indicators (as for Tauras, 2005) but combined into ordinal categorical variable very similar to Wasserman, 1990	Current smoking status. Monthly cigarette consumption estimated from a categorical survey item to assess frequency of smoking	See Tauras, 2005	Current smoking, $p<0.01$ Monthly smoking, $P<0.01$	Authors commented that previous studies of cigarette price elasticity might have overestimated influence of cigarette prices by not accounting for the presence and strength of clean indoor air laws.
Tauras & Chaloupka, 1999b	See Tauras, 2005	See Tauras, 2005	Index as in Tauras & Chaloupka, 1999a, and other analyses with three separate indicator variables for private workplaces, restaurants, and all other places, and another analysis with the ordinal variable minus the workplace indicator and with another variable indicating a worker in a workplace with restrictions.	Smoking cessation	Separate analyses for males and females controlled for cigarette prices, white race, yearly income, age, religiosity, suburban, rural, work hours, marital status, household composition, education, current college attendance status, year, and region.	Males: NS for all the various codings of smoking restrictions. Females: only the variable indicating a worker in a workplace with restrictions was significantly related to increased cessation, $p<0.01$.	The authors also discussed that many previous researchers may have computed price elasticities of demand for cigarettes that were inflated, because they did not control for clean-indoor air laws. There is a correlation between these factors, and variance attributable to the clean indoor air laws was confounded with that for cigarette prices.

Appendix 3.
Econometric studies relating scope and strength of laws restricting smoking to smoking behaviour

Reference Location	Population and design	Year	Assessment of law scope and strength	Smoking measures	Covariates, analysis	Results	Comments
Tauras, 2005	Monitoring the Future longitudinal data on young adults--high school seniors followed over up to 8 years. Approximately 2400 students selected for cohort each year	1976-1993	Data on presence and magnitude of state clean indoor air laws from Centers for Disease Control-six binary variables (private workplaces, restaurants, health care facilities, government worksites, grocery stores, and other public places)	Transitions from non-daily to daily smoking Transition from light (1-5 CPD) to moderate (6-10 CPD) Transition from an average of 10 CPD to heavy smoking (20+ CPD)	Analyses adjusted for age, sex, income, college status, religiosity, marital status, household composition, region, and cigarette prices.	Transition non-daily to daily: all indicators NS Transition from light to moderate: Private worksite, $p<0.01$. Restaurants, $p<0.001$ Other public places, $p<0.01$ Transition from moderate to heavy daily smoking: all indicators NS	

*Public places included: public buses/trains, elevators, indoor recreational or cultural facilities, retail stores, schools, health care facilities, public meeting rooms, libraries, rest rooms, waiting rooms, jury rooms, halls and stairs, polling places, and prisons.
CPD=Cigarettes per day
NHIS = National Health Interview Surveys
NS = Not statistically significant

Appendix 4.
Other correlative studies relating scope and strength of laws restricting smoking to smoking behaviour

Study Location	Population and design	Year data gathered	Assessment of law scope and strength	Smoking measures	Covariates and analysis	Results	Comments
Emont et al., 1993 USA	State-specific data from the Current Population Survey, 50 states	1989	Same as for Chaloupka et al., 1992	Adults smoking prevalence Quit ratios (% of ever smokers now quit) Per capita cigarette sales	Analyses of 50 US states and District of Columbia (51 data points) Jonckheere test for ordered data relating increasing regulation categories to outcome variables.	Prevalence: p<0.001 Quit ratio: p<0.005 Consumption: p<0.0005	No individual or state level covariates included. Cigarette prices also correlated with all three outcomes.
Stephens et al., 1997 Canada	11 652 respondents to the General Social Survey	1991	Percentage of local population covered by a municipal bylaw restricting smoking	Current smoking status	Logistic regression analyses adjusted for age, sex, marital status, and education, as well as price, change in price, and some significant interactions.	Bylaw strength index was significantly related to being a nonsmoker (OR=1.21; 95% CI=1.08-1.36)	
Yurekli & Zhang, 2000 USA	State-specific data from multiple sources, 50 states	1970-1995	Index that considered the time people spend in various venues and restrictiveness for each year and for each state	Per capita cigarette consumption from sales data	Regression analyses of 50 US states and District of Columbia included many other state level factors: per capita disposable income, cigarette prices, cigarette tax, % with bachelor's degree, % of each race/ethnicity, % Morman, % unemployed, tourism expenditures, and variables related to smuggling.	The index for restrictions on smoking was significantly related to lower per capita consumption in all analyses, p<0.05	The main purpose of this study was to evaluate the effect of cigarette smuggling on cigarette tax revenue. From their final model the authors estimated that without such laws, total demand for cigarettes would have been 4.5% greater in 1995.
Moskowitz et al., 2000 California, USA	4680 employed current and recent former smokers from the 1990 California Tobacco Survey	1990	Local ordinance data from Americans for Nonsmokers' Rights and the California Smoke-Free Cities Project.	Having a worksite policy	The logistic regression analyses adjusted for age, sex, race/ethnicity, education, type of area, and workplace size.	Strong: (OR=1.61; 95% CI=1.29-2.15) cessation in the past six months Moderate: (OR=1.38; 95% CI=9.98-1.95) Weak: (OR=0.99; 95% CI=0.70-1.40) versus none	

Appendix 4.
Other correlative studies relating scope and strength of laws restricting smoking to smoking behaviour

Study Location	Population and design	Year data gathered	Assessment of law scope and strength	Smoking measures	Covariates and analysis	Results	Comments
Moskowitz et al., 2000 California, USA			Only ordinances pertaining to workplaces were considered and were coded as none, weak, moderate, and strong	Smoking cessation in the past six months		Strong: (OR=1.52; 95% CI=1.14-1.71) Moderate: (OR=1.35; 95% CI=0.94-1.95) Weak: (OR=1.38; 95% CI=0.95-2.00) versus none	
Wakefield et al., 2000a USA	Survey of 17 287 high school students from 202 schools	1996	A regulation index based on state laws effective in 1996 from records maintained by the Centers for Disease Control and Prevention were merged by school locale	Non-susceptible versus susceptible Susceptible versus early experimenter Early versus advanced experimenter Advanced experimenter versus established smoker (see text for definitions) Also, any smoking in past 30 days	Models included grade, sex, race/ethnicity, adult smokers in the home, sibling smokers, living in a smoke-free home, smoke-free school policy, and strength of enforcement of such policies. Separate logistic regression analyses of each successive pair of levels on the continuum.	Non-susceptible to susceptible: (OR=0.96; 95% CI=0.86-1.06) Susceptible to early experimenter: (OR=0.93; 95% CI=0.84-1.02) Early to advanced experimenter: (OR=0.92, 95% CI=0.83-1.00) Advanced experimenter to established smoker: (OR=0.90; 95% CI=0.81-0.98) Any smoking in the past 30 days: (OR=0.91; 95% CI=0.83-0.99)	
Stephens et al., 2001 Canada	14 355 respondents aged 25 years and older to the National Population Health Survey	1995, 1996	Federal government survey data used to create an index that summed a three level (0=no restrictions, 1=designated area, 2=smoke-free) variable for 12 locations.	Current smoking status	Men and women were analysed separately. The regression analyses (logistic for status and linear for consumption) included variables for a recent cigarette tax cut effective only in some localities, cigarette	Status : Women: Index- (OR=1.02; 95% CI=1.00-1.03) Enforcement and signage: NS	

Study Location	Population and design	Year data gathered	Assessment of law scope and strength	Smoking measures	Covariates and analysis	Results	Comments
Stephens et al., 2001 Canada			Also, there were variables for strength of enforcement and no-smoking signage requirements		prices, and expenditures for tobacco control.	Men: Index: NS Enforcement: (OR=1.21; 95% CI=1.00-1.46) Signage: (OR=1.25; 95% CI=1.01-1.55)	
				Daily cigarette consumption		Consumption Women: Index: p<0.05 Enforcement and signage: NS	
						Men: Index: NS Enforcement and signage: NS	
Viehbeck & McDonald, 2004 Canada	9249 current and former smokers responding to the Canadian Community Health Survey	2001	Similar communities matched according to strong or weak bylaw index score that accounted for comprehensiveness, enforcement level, and signage requirements	Being a former smoker	Mantel-Haenszel test compared pairs of communities. Logistic regression models included all the policy components of the scale used to match communities, but no other variables.	No pair of communities differed with respect to current-former smoking status. None of the policy components was significantly related to being a former smoker.	
McMullen et al., 2005 USA	State specific data from multiple surveys; 50 states analysed	1996-1999	Index of extensiveness of clean indoor air laws for nine venues including enforcement, and penalties as determined from the National Cancer Institute's Sate Cancer Legislative Database	Adult current smoking prevalence Youth (12-17 years) smoking prevalence Percentage of indoor workers working in a smoke-free workplace from data published by the American Non-smoker's Rights Foundation	Multivariate analyses of 50 US states and the District of Columbia adjusted for state poverty rates and cigarette excise taxes.	Adult current smoking prevalence: p<0.07 Youth smoking prevalence: p<0.01 Percentage of indoor workers in smoke-free workplace: p<0.01	

Appendix 4.
Other correlative studies relating scope and strength of laws restricting smoking to smoking behaviour

Study Location	Population and design	Year data gathered	Assessment of law scope and strength	Smoking measures	Covariates and analysis	Results	Comments
Siegel et al., 2005 Massachusetts, USA	Longitudinal population telephone survey of 2623 youth 12-17 years	Baseline: 2001-2002 Follow-up: 2003-2004	Ordered categorical variable for restaurant smoking restrictions: strong=no smoking allowed, medium=restricted to separately ventilated areas, weak=no restrictions or no separately ventilated area	Transition to established smoking (>100 cigarettes in lifetime) by follow-up	The logistic regression analyses controlled for a number of individual level characteristics including age, sex, race/ethnicity, baseline smoking experience, close friends who smoke, exposure to anti-smoking messages at school, smokers in the household, education of adult informant, and household income. Town level factors included %with college education, %voting in favor of increased cigarette tax, %white, %youth, number of restaurants in town, and population size.	Transition to established smoker for those with strong compared to week restaurant ordinances: (OR=0.39; 95% CI=0.24-0.66) Moderate ordinance compared to weak: (OR=1.06 ; 95% CI=0.70-1.62)	
Albers et al., 2007	1712 adult smokers in the same households as in Siegel et al., 2005	Baseline: 2001-2002 Follow-up: 2003-2004	Same coding as Siegel et al., 2005	Making a quit attempt ; Being quit at follow-up	In this study, hierarchical analyses adjusted for age, sex, race/ethnicity, education, household income, marital status, children <18 years in the household, and baseline level of addiction.	Quit attempt for those with quit attempt at baseline: (OR=3.12; 95% CI=1.51-6.44) those without a quit attempt at baseline: NS ; Being quit at follow-up: NS, regardless of baseline history	
Siegel et al., 2008 Massachusetts, USA	2217 of youth from Siegel et al., 2005 study followed-up again	Further follow-up in 2005-2006	Same coding as Siegel et al., 2005	Transitions from never smoker to experimenter ; Transition from experimentation to established smoker	The analyses used the same set of variables as for Siegel et al., 2005.	Transition from never to experimenter for strong versus weak ordinance: (OR=1.18; 95% CI=0.94-1.49) Transition from experimenter to established: (OR=0.53; 95% CI=0.33-0.86)	Living in a town with a strong ordinance appears to impede the transition from experimentation to becoming an established smoker.

Appendix 5.
Population studies examining the effect of workplace smoking policies on worker smoking behaviour

Reference Location	Population, design	Year	Worksite policy	Smoking behaviour measures	Covariates and analysis	Results	Comments
Longitudinal							
Patten et al., 1995 California, USA	1844 adult indoor workers	1990-1992 50% follow-up	Smoke-free work area in both years, in 1990 but not 1992, in 1992 but not 1990, and in neither year	Changes in smoking status Changes in cigarette consumption	Chi-square tests of changes in outcome variables among the four groups defined by the presence of a smoke-free work area. Also logistic regression of decrease in consumption by five CPD or by quitting adjusted for age, sex, race/ethnicity, and education.	The overall chi-square statistics of both outcomes were only marginally significant, p<0.10. Group comparisons showed substantial differences, but failed to reach statistical significance. Logistic regression showed that those working in a smoke-free work area in 1990 but not 1992 were significantly less likely to decrease consumption, p<0.05.	The group that had a smoke-free work area in 1990 but not in 1992 appeared to increase their daily cigarette consumption.
Glasgow et al., 1997 USA and Canada	8271 employed smokers from the Community Smoking Cessation Intervention Trial (COMMIT)	1988-1993 65.9% follow-up	Smoke-free worksite versus designated areas versus no restrictions in 1998	Quit attempt Cessation at follow-up Daily cigarette consumption	Regressions adjusted for sex, race/ethnicity, age, education, income, cigarette consumption, desire to quit, past quit attempts, and cessation services at worksite.	Quit attempt: Designated area OR=1.16 Smoke-free OR=1.27, p<0.05 Quit at follow-up: Designated area OR=1.0 Smoke-free OR=1.27, p<0.05 Consumption: Designated area coef=1.17 Smoke-free coef=-2.78, p<0.05	
Pierce et al., 1998c California, USA	1736 non-Hispanic smokers from the California Tobacco Survey over the age of 25 years	Baseline in 1990, follow-up in 1992 Follow-up rate not given	Smoke-free work area versus all other indoor workers versus everyone else assessed at follow-up	Advancement along a quitting continuum	The logistic regression included sex, age, race/ethnicity, education. Having a smoke-free home (and a belief that SHS is harmful), having assistance with cessation, and a smoke-free work area were also	All the programme-related variables were significantly related to increased progress toward quitting. The odds ratio for working in a smoke-free work area was OR=1.6; 95% CI=1.0-2.6	It was unknown when workplace policy was implemented (prior to baseline or during the follow-up period).

Appendix 5.
Population studies examining the effect of workplace smoking policies on worker smoking behaviour

Longitudinal

Reference Location	Population, design	Year	Worksite policy	Smoking behaviour measures	Covariates and analysis	Results	Comments
Pierce et al., 1998c California, USA					included as tobacco control programme-related variables.	Compared to other indoor workers not covered by a smoke-free work area.	
Biener & Nyman, 1999 USA	369 workers who smoked at baseline	1993-1996 66% follow-up	Smoke-free workplace in both years, in 1996 only, or in neither year. Reported exposure to secondhand smoke	Smoking "not at all" at follow-up	The logistic regression analysis adjusted for age, sex, education, smoking level at baseline, and intent to quit within 30 days	Cessation: (OR=2.0; 95% CI=0.7-6.0) Reduced or minimal exposure to SHS by 1996 predicted cessation: (OR=6.99; 95% CI=1.79-27.3)	The authors suggest that lack of enforcement as evidenced by exposure to SHS may account for the lack of a significant cessation effect.
Longo et al., 2001	1469 hospital workers and 920 workers in other venues who smoked pre-smoke-free policy implementation.	Pre-policy up to 1996 Follow-up rate not reported	Hospitals went smoke-free at various times to comply with mandated smoke-free policy by 1993	Quit ratios (smoking pre-policy, not smoking sometime after policy imposed)	Cox proportional hazards analysis adjusting for age, sex, education, employment group (blue collar, clerical, white collar), and accounted for different follow-up intervals.	Quitting was significantly higher (adjusted hazard ratio: 2.29 (95% CI=1.56-3.37)) among the hospital workers compared to the other workers.	A simple analysis of quit ratios suggested that they increased more over time for the hospital workers than for the other workers.
Bauer et al., 2005 Communities in USA and Canada	1967 indoor workers who smoked, also from COMMIT	1993-2001 53% follow-up	Workplace policy in both years, categorised by change: maintained no restrictions, partial in either year but not complete, complete in 2001 regardless of status in 1993	Quit attempt. Being quit 6+ months at follow-up Daily cigarette consumption	The regression analyses adjusted for age, sex, race/ethnicity, education, prior desire to quit, number of previous quit attempts, amount smoked and occupation.	Quit attempt: NS Cessation for 6+ months: Partial: (OR=1.73; 95% CI=0.96-3.11) Complete: (OR=1.92; 95% CI=1.11-3.32) Consumption declined significantly only for those with a completely smoke-free workplace by 2001, p<0.01.	There were very low reported levels of using smokeless tobacco in 2001, suggesting that workers did not switch to this form of tobacco from cigarettes because of workplace smoking restrictions.

Reference Location	Population, design	Year	Worksite policy	Smoking behaviour measures	Covariates and analysis	Results	Comments
Longitudinal							
Shields, 2005 Canada	14 207 in longitudinal sample, number of smokers, and number of quitters at baseline not reported. Respondent to National Population Health Survey	1995/95 2002/03 81% follow-up	Smoke-free workplace versus all other workers	Continuous cessation (duration not specified) initiated during the follow-up period, duration of abstinence for those quit at baseline	Separate logistic regression analyses conducted for men and women. The analyses adjusted for addiction level, age, chronic health conditions, body mass index, heavy drinking, psychological distress, low emotional support, chronic stress, age, education, income, and the presence of children > 5 years in the home.	A smoke-free workplace was unrelated to cessation in men: (OR=1.0; 95% CI=0.7- 1.4) and women:(OR=1.1; 95% CI=0.8-1.4)	
Shields, 2007 Canada	1364 indoor workers who smoked daily at baseline from Canadian Tobacco Use Monitoring Survey	Multiple survey waves from 1994-2005 combined 77% follow-up	Newly imposed smoke-free workplace versus new partial restrictions versus continuously working under no restrictions	Continuous abstinence (duration not specified) initiated during the follow-up period Change in daily consumption	Logistic regressions adjusted for sex, age, education, income, baseline cigarette consumption, and occupation Analysed by simple baseline versus follow-up comparison	A newly imposed smoke-free workplace was significantly related to being abstinent at follow-up compared to those continuously working under no restrictions: (OR=2.3; 95% CI=1.4-3.9) Between baseline and follow-up continuing smokers significantly reduced their CPD by 2.1 with a new smoke-free workplace	
Cross-sectional							
Brenner & Mielck, 1992	439 adult workers 21-65 years from Ministry of Youth, Family and Health Survey	1987	Smoking permitted at worksite or not	Quit Quit attempt Consumption among current smokers	Regressions for each sex separately adjusted for age, marital status, and education.	Quit: Permitted versus not Women: (OR=0.22; 95% CI=0.09-0.50) Men: (OR=0.80; 95% CI=0.44-1.45) Quit attempt: Prohibited versus not Women: (OR=2.08; 95% CI=0.98-4.40) Men: (OR= 2.15; 95% CI=1.18-3.91) Consumption: NS either sex	

279

Appendix 5.
Population studies examining the effect of workplace smoking policies on worker smoking behaviour

Reference Location	Population, design	Year	Worksite policy	Smoking behaviour measures	Covariates and analysis	Results	Comments
Cross-sectional							
Wakefield et al., 1992 Australia	1120 workers 15+ years N=231 smokers	1989	Smoke-free (31.9%), partial (33.2%), no restrictions (34.8%)	Difference between daily consumption on leisure and work days	Analysis of covariance adjusted for sex, cigarettes smoked on leisure days, occupation	Difference significant, Partial: -4.9 CPD Smoke-free: -5.2 CPD, compared to no restrictions, p<0.001	Results did not differ by occupational status.
Kinne et al., 1993 Washington, USA	1288 employed but not self-employed workers from Washington State Cancer Risk Behaviour Survey	1989-1990	Smoke-free versus partial restrictions versus no restrictions	Prevalence Consumption among current smokers	Males and females analysed separately. Multivariate analysis of consumption adjusted for time to first cigarette in morning, occupation, age, income, education, ethnicity, and urban residence.	Prevalence, simple comparison: Men, p<0.0001 Women, p=0.0021 Consumption: Men, p<0.0001 Women, NS	
Woodruff et al., 1993 California, USA	11 704 indoor workers from California Tobacco Survey	1990	Smoke-free versus work area restriction versus lesser restriction versus no restriction	Prevalence Consumption among current smokers Intent to quit Quit ratio	Regressions adjusted for age, education, Hispanic ethnicity, and sex. Supported univariate results reported in next column.	Prevalence: Smoke-free versus none, 13.7% versus 20.6%; p<0.001 Consumption: Smoke-free versus none, 296 versus 341 packs/year, p<0.001 Intent to quit: Smoke-free versus none, 31.8% versus 29.7%, p=0.014 Quit ratio: NS	Authors estimated that consumption now 21% less than if there were no restrictions. Would be 41% less if all workplaces were smoke-free, resulting in a loss of $406 million in annual sales to the tobacco industry.
Farkas et al., 1999 USA	48 584 current and recent former smokers (smoking one year previously) from the Current Population Survey	1992-1993	Less than smoke-free work area versus smoke-free work area but allowed in some common areas versus completely smoke-free workplace	Making a quit attempt of a day or longer in the past year Cessation of at least six months when interviewed Smoking <15 CPD (light smoker)	Logistic regression analysis adjusted for age, sex, race/ethnicity, education, income, occupation, region, age of youngest child in household, and smokers in household, and home smoking restrictions.	Quit attempt: Smoke-free versus none: (OR=1.14; 95% CI=1.05-1.24) Cessation six+ months: Smoke-free versus none: (OR=1.21; 95% CI=1.00-1.45) Smoking < 15 CPD Smoke-free versus none: (OR=1.53; 95% CI=1.38-1.70)	Lesser workplace restrictions not significantly related to any of the outcomes.

Reference Location	Year	Population, design	Worksite policy	Smoking behaviour measures	Covariates and analysis	Results	Comments
Cross-sectional							
Farrelly et al., 1999 USA	1992-1993	Nearly 100 000 non-self employed adult workers, including nearly 25 000 smokers from Current Population Survey	No restrictions versus partial work area/ common area restrictions versus smoke-free work area and partial common area restrictions versus completely smoke-free workplace	Prevalence Cigarette consumption among current smokers	The regression analyses adjusted for age, sex, race/ethnicity, education, marital status, number of persons in household, urban/rural status, state, income, hours worked per week, and type of industry or employment.	*Prevalence:* A smoke-free work area was 2.6 (95% CI=1.7-3.5) percentage points lower than no restrictions. Smoke-free 5.7 (95% CI=4.9-6.5) percentage points lower. *Consumption:* Smoke-free work area 1.5 (95% CI=1.1-1.90) CPD lower than no restrictions. Smoke-free 2.7 (95% CI=2.3-3.1) CPD lower.	Further analyses by demographic, and more importantly by industry subgroups, showed consistently lower pre-valence and CPD among workers in smoke-free workplaces compared to those with no restrictions. In groups with higher consumption the differences tended to be greater, suggesting a greater smoke-free workplace effect in workplaces with greater smoking levels.
Evans et al., 1999 USA	1991 and 1993	18 090 indoor workers from National Health Interview Surveys	Smoke-free work area versus restrictions in other indoor areas versus no restrictions	Prevalence of current smoking Cigarette consumption among current smokers	The regression analysis adjusted for age, age squared, family size, log income, region, education, race/ ethnicity, city size, marital status, cigarette tax, occupation, and year.	The primary analysis found prevalence to be 5.7% points lower among workers in a smoke-free workplace versus no restrictions, p<0.01. Consumption was 2.5 CPD less, p<0.01.	The extensive set of variables on health status and the workplace environment allowed investigation of whether such factors might account for different worker or workplace traits that might relate to smoking and level of workplace smoking restrictions. None were found.
Gilpin, et al., 2000 USA	1992-93	237 733 persons aged 15 years and older who were self-respondents to the Current Population Survey	Smoke-free workplace, smoke-free homes, and cigarette prices Also, an index combining these three factors	Adult and youth (15-24 years) smoking prevalence, and per capita cigarette consumption	The analyses were bivariate correlations among the 50 US states and the District of Columbia	Smoke-free workplaces were significantly correlated with all adult (25+ years) prevalence, r=-0.65, p<0.0001 and per capita cigarette consumption, r= 0.54, p<0.001, but not youth (15-24 years) prevalence, r= -0.26, p=NS	Analyses did not adjust for individual or state level factors that might be related to outcome measures.

Appendix 5.
Population studies examining the effect of workplace smoking policies on worker smoking behaviour

Cross-sectional

Reference Location	Population, design	Year	Worksite policy	Smoking behaviour measures	Covariates and analysis	Results	Comments
Gilpin &Pierce, 2002b California, USA	5677 current smokers from the California Tobacco Survey	1999	Smoke-free workplace versus all others	Daily cigarette consumption	A multivariate linear regression of daily cigarette consumption, adjusted for age, sex, race/ethnicity, education, belief in the harmfulness of SHS, having a smoke-free home, and a family preference that the smoker not smoke.	A smoke-free workplace was significantly associated with reduced consumption (p=0.0004). Adjusted CPD was 9.4±0.9 versus 11.1±1.0 for those in smoke-free workplaces compared to all others.	
Shavers et al., 2006 USA	82 966 employed women self-respondents to the Current Population Survey	1998/99 and 2001/02	No work place policy versus no work area policy versus smoke-free work area	Smoking prevalence	The analyses were stratified by poverty level and by race/ethnicity. Multivariate analyses adjusted for race/ethnicity (as appropriate), age, education, marital status, occupation, and home smoking restrictions.	Regardless of poverty status or race/ethnicity, a smoke-free work area was not significantly associated with lower smoking prevalence.	
				Heavy (>20 CPD) daily cigarette consumption among smokers		A smoke-free work area was inversely and significantly related to heavy smoking compared to no restrictions for some subgroups.	
				Making a quit attempt in past year		A smoke-free work area was not significantly related to making a quit attempt.	
Shopland et al., 2006 USA	128 024 employed female daily smokers a year previously who did not live alone responding to Current Population Survey	1992/93 and 2001/02	Smoke-free workplace versus all others	Cessation of any length	Logistic regression analyses adjusted for age, education, race/ethnicity, a child > 5 in household, household composition, home smoking restrictions, and occupation.	Cessation of any length not significant in either year, 1992-93 (OR=1.02; 95% CI=0.83-1.26), 2001-02 (OR=1.11; 95% CI=0.81-1.53)	The proportion of respondents reporting workplaces increased substantially between surveys.
				Cessation of at least 3 months when interviewed.		Cessation of at least 3 months in 1992-93 (OR=1.30; 95% CI=1.04-1.63), but not 2001-02 (OR=0.99; 95% CI=0.67-1.45)	

Cross-sectional

Reference Location	Population, design	Year	Worksite policy	Smoking behaviour measures	Covariates and analysis	Results	Comments
Morozumi & Li, 2006 Japan	1687 workers from household survey	2001	Smoke-free workplace versus separate designated areas versus no restrictions	Prevalence Consumption Cessation	Probit model adjusted for a multitude of demographic and other factors	Prevalence: smoke-free versus no restrictions, $p<0.05$ Consumption: smoke-free versus no restrictions, $p<0.05$ Cessation: smoke-free versus no restrictions, $p<0.05$	
Lee & Kahende, 2007 USA	3990 quitters in the past two years from the National Health Interview Survey	2000	Smoke-free workplace versus all others	Quit 7-24 months before the survey without a relapse (successful quitter) versus relapsed quitters in the past year	A logistic regression adjusted for age, education, marital status, race/ethnicity, the number of lifetime quit attempts, and whether the smoker had ever switched to low tar cigarettes.	A smoke-free workplace was significantly associated with successful cessation: OR=2.01 (95% CI=1.20-3.37)	
Burns et al., 2007 Colorado, USA	6100 ever smokers from the Colorado Tobacco Attitudes and Behaviour Survey	2001	Smoke-free work area versus other workers versus not applicable	Duration of smoking, with current smokers censored at time of survey	A Cox proportional hazard regression adjusted for age, sex, marital status, language spoken in home, age of smoking initiation, education, home smoking restrictions, poverty status, and insurance status.	Not having a smoke-free work area was significantly related to increased smoking duration. Hazard ratio: 1.48 (95% CI=1.19-1.84)	
Messer et al., 2008a USA	31 625 adult recent current smokers from the Current Population Survey	2001-2002	Seriously trying to quit Quit at least a day in the past year Quit for at least 6 months when interviewed	Smoke-free workplace versus all others (including those not employed)	A logistic regression analysis adjusted for sex, age, race /ethnicity, education, initiation < 15 years, delay of smoking for at least 30 minutes after awakening, home smoking restrictions, and use of a pharmaceutical aid.	A smoke-free workplace was not significantly related to any of the outcomes.	Results were similar for Latinos and non-Hispanic whites.

Appendix 5.
Population studies examining the effect of workplace smoking policies on worker smoking behaviour

Reference Location	Population, design	Year	Worksite policy	Smoking behaviour measures	Covariates and analysis	Results	Comments
Cross-sectional							
Pierce *et al.*, 2009 USA	542 470 current smokers aged 18-64 years in all the cross-sectional Current Population Surveys from 1992/93-2002/03	1992-2002	Very light (<5 CPD) smoking in those aged 18-29 years. The very light category includes occasional smokers (88% of group).	Smoke-free workplace versus all others (including those not employed)	Logistic analysis of very light smoking in 18-29 year old group, adjusted for survey year, sex, education, income versus below 2 times poverty threshold, smoke-free home, and tobacco control policies ranking by tertile for state of residence as an indicator of social norms against smoking.	A smoke-free workplace was significantly associated with greater very light smoking: (OR=1.28; 95% CI=1.18-1.38)	The authors selected the group aged 18-29 for the logistic regression analysis because of a marked increase in very light smoking in that group.

CPD = Cigarettes per day
SHS = Secondhand smoke

Appendix 6.
Studies examining the relationship between voluntary smoking policies in the home and *adult* smoking behaviour

Reference/ location	Population and design	Year of assessment	Household smoking restriction measure	Outcomes	Covariates and analysis	Results	Comments
Longitudinal studies							
Pierce *et al.*, 1998c California, USA	Adult (≥ 25 years) non-Hispanic smokers California Tobacco Survey N=1736	Baseline in 1990 and follow-up in 1992 Follow-up rate not reported	Work area restriction and smoke-free home assessed at follow-up. Those without a smoke-free home were further stratified according to whether they believed SHS to be harmful.	Advancement along a quitting continuum	Logistic regression, including terms for a smoke-free home (and a belief that SHS is harmful), and a smoke-free work area, and adjusted for having assistance with cessation (as tobacco control programme factors), sex, age, race/ethnicity, and education	Advancement on continuum Work area restriction: OR=1.6; 95% CI=1.0–2.6 Reference: all others Smoke-free home: OR=3.4; 95% CI=1.9–5.9 Reference: no rules/ belief Belief SHS is harmful: OR=1.3; 95% CI=0.7–2.2 Reference: no rules/ belief	It was unknown when workplace and home smoke-free policies were implemented (prior to baseline or during the follow-up period).
Pizacani *et al.*, 2004 Oregon, USA	Adult English speaking Oregonians Prospective cohort study (1133 subjects at baseline; 565 re-interviewed at follow-up)	Baseline survey in 1997 and follow-up in 1999 (median follow-up 21 months) Follow-up rate 51.5%	No restrictions versus partial restrictions versus smoke-free home	Any quit attempt and quit attempts according to duration of abstinence and stage of change Being in preparation stage versus all others	Logistic regression Cox proportional hazards regression analysis for duration of abstinence Adjustment for age, employment status, baseline cigarette consumption, and stage of change (preparation versus earlier stages)	Any quit attempt: OR=2.0; 95% CI=1.0–3.9 Pre- and contemplation: Quit at least 7 days: OR=0.9; 95% CI=0.4–2.3 Quit at least 90 days: OR=1.0; 95% CI=0.4–2.4 Being in preparation stage: Quit at least 7 days: OR=4.4; 95% CI= 1.1–18.7 Quit at least 90 days: OR=4.3; 95% CI=0.9–21.2	Although not formally analysed, smokers with smoke-free homes at baseline 35% smoked fewer than 15 CPD compared to only 11% with no such policy.

Appendix 6.
Studies examining the relationship between voluntary smoking policies in the home and *adult* smoking behaviour

Reference/ location	Population and design	Year of assessment	Household smoking restriction measure	Outcomes	Covariates and analysis	Results	Comments
Longitudinal studies							
Pizacani et al., 2004 Oregon, USA				Duration of abstinence according to stage of change		Duration of abstinence Pre- and contemplation: HR=0.3 (95% CI=0.8-2.0) Preparation: HR=0.5 (95% CI=0.2- 0.9)	
Shields, 2005 Canada	Adults ≥17 years National Population Health Survey 14 207 subjects in the longitudinal sample (number of smokers and number of quitters at baseline not reported)	1995/ 95 2002/ 03 Follow-up rate 81%	Smoke-free home versus all others Smoke-free workplace versus all others	Continuous cessation (duration not specified) initiated during the follow-up period Duration of abstinence for those quit at baseline	Logistic regression (separately for men and women) Adjustment for addiction level, age, chronic health conditions, body mass index, heavy drinking, psychological distress, low emotional support, chronic stress, age, education, income and the presence of children under 5 years in the home.	Quitting in a 2-year period Smoke-free workplace M: OR=0.9; 95% CI=0.7-1.4 W: OR=0.8; 95% CI=0.6-1.2 Smoke-free home M: OR=1.1; 95% CI=0.8-1.6 W: OR=1.3; 95% CI=1.0-.1.6 Relapse in a 2-year period Smoke-free home M: OR=0.6; 95% CI=0.4-0.9 W: OR=1.0; 95% CI=0.6-.1.6*	A smoke-free home was significant bivariately for women, but the addition of variables related to level of addiction diminished the effect. Lighter smoking and a new chronic condition were most related to quitting in both men and women. At baseline, the addiction level was lower among those living in smoke-free homes.
Borland et al., 2006a Canada, USA, UK, Australia	Adult (≥ 18 years) smokers The International Tobacco Control Four Country Survey N=6754	Baseline survey in 2002 and follow-up at 6-10 months Follow-up rate 75%	No restrictions versus partial versus smoke-free (S-F) home at baseline New smoke-free home during follow-up period	Making a quit attempt and quit for at least a month at follow-up Consumption in cig/day	Logistic regression adjusted for household composition, age of youngest child, number of five closest friends who smoke, belief that SHS causes lung cancer, reported smoking prohibitions in bars, restaurants, and in the workplace,	Quit attempt versus no restrictions S-F: OR=1.3; 95% CI=1.1-1.6 Part: OR=1.1; 95% CI=1.0-1.3 Quit one month or more versus no restrictions S-F: OR=2.5; 95% CI=1.5-4.2 Part: OR=1.0; 95% CI=0.0-1.6	Among continuing smokers with a smoke-free home at baseline, cigarette consumption declined and the time to first cigarette increased. The main purpose of the paper was to investigate the effects of a smoke-free home. The covariates for workplace policy,

Reference/ location	Population and design	Year of assessment	Household smoking restriction measure	Outcomes	Covariates and analysis	Results	Comments
Longitudinal studies							
Borland et al., 2006a Canada, USA, UK, Australia					attitude toward smoke-free workplaces	When additional covariates were included to account for baseline addiction level and intentions to quit, the smoke-free home effect was no longer significant for making a quit attempt, but it was significant for being quit at least a month at follow-up: OR=2.07; 95% CI=1.20-3.56 Mean CPD according to home restriction status: S-F : 13.6 Part. :16.5 None: 21.1 $p < 0.01$ for difference between means	or attitudes toward it, were not significantly related to making a quit attempt or being quit for at least a month at follow-up. Results for workplace restrictions for the other outcomes were not reported.
Shields, 2007 Canada	Population ≥ 15 years Canadian Tobacco Use Monitoring Survey 1364 employed smokers with no workplace restrictions and 8463 smokers not living in smoke-free homes at baseline	Multiple survey waves from 1994-2005 combined Follow-up rate 77%	Newly imposed (during follow-up period) smoke-free homes and workplaces	Continuous abstinence (duration not specified) initiated during the follow-up period. Daily consumption at follow-up among those smoking	Logistic regression adjusted for sex, age, education, income, baseline cigarette consumption, and occupation for the workplace analysis. Occupation was replaced by the presence of children in the home for the analysis of smoke-free homes.	Abstinence Smoke-free home: OR=2.3; 95% CI=1.4-3.9 Smoke-free workplace: OR=1.6; 95% CI=1.3-2.1 Mean daily consumption of cigarettes Home restrictions: Total: 9.2 CPD Partial: 15.0 CPD None:16.1 CPD Workplace restrictions: Total: 12.0 CPD Partial: 14.0 CPD None: 17.4 CPD	Baseline smoke-free policies were significantly associated cross-sectionally with the smoker being in a more advanced stage of change (action/ maintenance) with respect to smoking cessation Smoke-free home: OR=4.5; 95% CI=3.9-5.1 Smoke-free workplace: OR=1.3; 95% CI=1.1-1.6

Appendix 6.
Studies examining the relationship between voluntary smoking policies in the home and *adult* smoking behaviour

Reference/ location	Population and design	Year of assessment	Household smoking restriction measure	Outcomes	Covariates and analysis	Results	Comments
Longitudinal studies							
Messer *et al.*, 2008b	3292 recent smokers from the Current Population Survey	Baseline in 2002 and follow-up in 2003 Follow-up rate not reported	Smoke-free home in 2002 New smoke-free home policy in 2003	Quit at follow-up	Regression analyses adjusted for age, sex, race/ ethnicity, education, income below two times the poverty level, presence of another smoker in the household, and baseline consumption in 2002.	Smoke-free in 2002 Quit: OR=1.52; 95%CI=1.08-2.15 Quit 90+ days: OR=1.44; 95% CI=0.97-2.21 New Smoke-free in 2003 Quit: OR=3.89; 95% CI=2.55-5.97	
				Quit 90+ days at follow-up		Quit 90+ days: OR=4.81; 95% CI=3.06-7.59	
				Consumption among continuing smokers		Consumption decrease CPD: OR=2.18; 95% CI=1.24-3.10	
Hyland *et al.*, 2009 USA	COMMIT study Smokers at baseline N=4963	Baseline in 1998 and follow-up in 2001 and 2005 Follow-up of original cohort was 23% in 2005	Smoke-free home inside, determined in 2001 and 2005	Quit at follow-up (2005)	Logistic regression analyses adjusted for age, sex, race/ ethnicity, annual household income, education, and number of cigarettes smoked	Quit at follow-up (2005): OR=1.7; 95% CI=1.4-2.2	Cohort not representative of general population, but skewed towards older and heavier smokers.
				Quit attempt in interim		Quit attempt in interim: OR=1.5; 95% CI=1.3-1.9	
				Consumption among continuing smokers		Decrease of consumption among smokers: OR=1.2; 95% CI=0.9-1.4	
				Relapse among those who quit in 2001		Relapse among those who quit in 2001: OR= 0.6; 95% CI=0.4-0.8	

Cross-sectional studies

Reference/ location	Population and design	Year of assessment	Household smoking restriction measure	Outcomes	Covariates and analysis	Results	Comments
Farkas et al., 1999 USA	48 584 current and recent former smokers (smoking one year previously) from the Current Population Survey	1992/93	No restrictions, partial, smoke-free (S-F). Less than work area (WA), work area, completely smoke-free workplace	Making a quit attempt of a day or longer in the past year,	Logistic regression analysis adjusted for age, sex, race/ethnicity, education, income, occupation, region, age of youngest child in household, and smokers in household.	Quit attempt Home: S-F: OR=3.86; 95% CI=3.57-4.18 Part: OR=1.83; 95% CI=1.72-1.93 Work: S-F: OR=1.14; 95% CI=1.05-1.24 WA: OR=1.04; 95% CI=0.94-1.14	A smoke-free home was more related to the outcomes than a smoke-free workplace, and partial restrictions were less related than a smoke-free policy.
				Cessation of at least 6 months when interviewed,		Quit 6+ months Home: S-F: OR=1.65; 95% CI=1.43-1.91 Part: OR=1.20; 95%CI=1.05-1.38 Work: S-F: OR=1.21; 95% CI=1.0-1.45 WA: OR=0.93; 95% CI=0.73-1.18	
				Smoking <15 CPD (light smoker)		Light smoker (<15 CPD) Home: S-F: OR=2.73; 95% CI=2.46-3.04 Part: OR=1.81; 95% CI=1.69-1.95 Work S-F: OR=1.53; 95% CI=1.38-1.70 WA: OR=1.10; 95% CI=0.97-1.24	
Gilpin et al., 1999 California, USA	Adult (≥ 18 y) smoker population California Tobacco Survey n=8904	1996	Composite variable for family preference that the smoker not smoke, and having no restrictions, partial restrictions and smoke-free (S-F) home	Quit attempts in the last year	Logistic regression adjusted for age, sex, race/ethnicity, education, household composition (other smoker, child <18 years), and a belief that SHS is harmful. Kaplan-Meier analysis of relapse.	Quit attempt last year S-F: OR=3.9; 95% CI=3.0-5.2 Part: OR=2.7; 95% CI=2.0-3.6	Other results: A smoke-free home, but not partial restrictions, were associated with delay of the first cigarette after awakening, and with longer duration of abstinence.
				Intent to quit in the next six months		Intend to quit in 6 months S-F: OR=5.8; 95% CI=3.8-8.2 Part: OR=3.7; 95% CI=2.7-5.1	

Appendix 6.
Studies examining the relationship between voluntary smoking policies in the home and *adult* smoking behaviour

Reference/ location	Population and design	Year of assessment	Household smoking restriction measure	Outcomes	Covariates and analysis	Results	Comments
Cross-sectional studies							
Gilpin *et al.*, 1999 California, USA				Smoking <15 CPD		Smoking < 15 CPD S-F: OR=2.2; 95% CI=2.2*-3.0 Part: OR=1.1; 95% CI=1.2-3.0	In smoke-free homes, smokers who quit had a two-fold probability of being abstinent six months later as compared to those in homes with partial or no restrictions
Norman *et al.*, 2000	1315 current smokers aged 25+ years from Evaluation Survey	1998	Smoke-free home versus all others	Daily cigarette consumption Days smoked in past month Desire to quit Quit attempt in past year	Multiple linear or logistic regression analyses adjusted for age, sex, race/ethnicity, and presence of child in home.	Consumption: p<0.01 Days smoked in past month: NS Desire to quit: OR=2.9; 95% CI=1.8-4.9 NS	
Gilpin, *et al.*, 2000 USA	Ecological analysis based on data from population ≥15 years (for the 50 states and DC) Current Population Survey (3 surveys, Sept 1992, Jan 1993, and May 1993) N=237 733	1992-93	Smoke-free (S-F) home Smoke-free workplace, cigarette prices Composite index combining these three factors	Adult (≥ 25 years) and youth (15-24 years) smoking prevalence Per capita cigarette consumption	Simple correlations between tobacco control activity factors with smoking prevalence and cigarette consumption	Pearson's correlation coefficients *r* and (p-values) S-F Home: S-F home with: Adult prevalence -0.66 (p<0.0001) Youth prevalence -0.39 (p<0.01) Per capita cigarette consumption -0.58 (p<0.0001) S-F workplace with: Adult prevalence -0.65 (p<0.0001) Youth prevalence -0.26 (NS) Per capita cigarette consumption -0.54 (p<0.001)	Analyses did not adjust for individual or state level factors that might be related to outcome measures. The correlation between smoke-free workplaces and smoke-free homes was 0.76 (p<0.0001).

Reference/ location	Population and design	Year of assessment	Household smoking restriction measure	Outcomes	Covariates and analysis	Results	Comments
Cross-sectional studies							
Gilpin & Pierce, 2002b California, USA	5677 current smokers from the California Tobacco Survey	1999	Smoke-free home versus all others, smoke-free workplace versus all others	Daily cigarette consumption	A multivariate linear regression of daily cigarette consumption, adjusted for age, sex, race/ethnicity, education, belief in the harmfulness of SHS, and a family preference that smoker not smoke.	A smoke-free home was significantly and inversely associated with daily cigarette consumption, as was smoke-free workplace, but not as strongly. Daily consumption was only about half (7.5 versus 13.9 CPD) for smokers with both a smoke-free home and workplace compared to those with neither.	
Siahpush et al., 2003 Australia	Smokers aged ≥ 14 years who smoked or had quit in past 2 years Australian National Drug Strategy Household Survey N=2526	1998	Smoke-free versus all others	Quit for at least a month when surveyed	Logistic regression adjusted for sex, age, marital status, dependent child status, education, occupation, urban versus rural, children in the home, belief in the harmfulness of SHS, having friends who smoke, smoking restrictions at work or school, and alcohol consumption.	Quitting 1+ month: OR= 4.5; 95% CI=3.1-6.6	
Ji et al., 2005	2830 adult California residents of Korean descent who had ever smoked and were part of a large statewide telephone survey	Not reported	Five level variable: no one allowed to smoke inside, special guests allowed to smoke inside, smoking allowed in certain areas, smoking allowed anywhere, and nonresponse	Former smokers - ever (at least 100 cigarettes in lifetime) quit for at least 90 days when interviewed	Logistic regression analysis of cessation included gender, education, family income, acculturation, number of smokers among family and friends, social network among family and friends, media influence, job satisfaction, health belief scale, health concerns, body	Compared to a smoke-free home, those with designated areas inside were less likely (OR=0.17; 95% CI=0.12-0.24) to be a former smoker. Those in homes where smoking was allowed anywhere were much less likely to have quit (OR=0.10; 95% CI=0.06-0).	

Appendix 6.
Studies examining the relationship between voluntary smoking policies in the home and *adult* smoking behaviour

Reference/ location	Population and design	Year of assessment	Household smoking restriction measure	Outcomes	Covariates and analysis	Results	Comments
Cross-sectional studies							
Ji et al., 2005					mass index, weight concern, exercise, family history of respiratory illness, and medical treatment for respiratory illness.	Those with exceptions for special guests did not differ in cessation than those living in smoke-free homes. Those not responding to the home rule question were about half as likely to have quit (OR=0.53; 95% CI= 0.36–0.78).	
Shavers et al., 2006 USA	82 966 employed women self-respondents to the Current Population Survey	1998/99 and 2001/02	No work policy, no work area policy, no smoking in work area No restrictions, partial restrictions, and smoke-free home	Smoking prevalence Heavy (>20 CPD) daily cigarette consumption among current smokers Making a quit attempt in past year among current smokers	The analyses were stratified by poverty level and by race/ ethnicity. Multivariate analyses of each group adjusted for race/ethnicity (as appropriate), age, education, marital status and occupation.	*Prevalence:* Regardless of poverty status or race/ethnicity, work policies were unrelated, but home policies were significantly related to prevalence, smoke-free more than partial. *Heavy smoking:* Smoke-free work areas were inversely and significantly related to heavy smoking, but home restrictions were more strongly related. *Quit attempt:* A smoke-free home, but not a smoke-free work area was significantly and directly related to making a quit attempt.	

Cross-sectional studies

Reference/ location	Population and design	Year of assessment	Household smoking restriction measure	Outcomes	Covariates and analysis	Results	Comments
Gilpin *et al.*, 2006 California, USA	Adult moderate to heavy (15+ cig/day) daily smokers California Tobacco Surveys N=2640	Combined data from 1999 and 2002 surveys	Smoke-free home versus all others	Duration of abstinence for the most recent quit attempt in the last year	Cox proportional hazard analyses adjusted for age, sex, education, race/ethnicity, daily consumption, having another smoker in the household, use of pharmaceutical aids, and significant interactions between having a smoke-free home and no other smoker in the household, and a smoke-free home and using a pharmaceutical aid	Relapse Smoke-free home and no other smokers at home: HR=0.796; 95%CI=0.645-0.988 Smoke-free home and used pharmaceutical aid: HR=0.774; 95% CI=0.622-0.963	Pharmaceutical aids appear to prolong abstinence duration only when the home was smoke-free and regardless of whether or not there was another smoker in the household. Having a smoke-free home is likely an indication of the smoker's level of motivation to quit.
Shopland *et al.*, 2006 USA	Adult (≥ 18 years) females who were employed, daily smokers, and did not live alone Current Population Survey N=128 024	1992/93 and 2001/02	No restrictions, partial, and smoke-free home(S-F) Smoke-free workplace versus all others	Cessation of any length	Logistic regression analyses adjusted for age, education, race/ethnicity, a child < 5 years in household, household composition, and occupation.	Cessation of any length Home restrictions S-F: OR=7.77; 95% CI=5.91-10.21 in CPS 92-92 & OR=6.54; 95% CI=4.61-9.28 in CPS 01-02 Partial: OR=2.15; 95% CI=1.70-2.73 in CPS 92-93 & OR=2.34; 95% CI=1.54-3.55 in CPS 01-02 Work restrictions S-F: OR=1.02; 95% CI=0.83-1.26 in CPS 92-92 & OR=1.11; 95% CI=0.81-1.53 in CPS 01-02	The proportion of respondents reporting smoke-free homes and workplaces increased substantially between surveys.

Appendix 6.
Studies examining the relationship between voluntary smoking policies in the home and *adult* smoking behaviour

Reference/ location	Population and design	Year of assessment	Household smoking restriction measure	Outcomes	Covariates and analysis	Results	Comments
Cross-sectional studies							
Shopland et al., 2006 USA				Cessation of at least 3 months when interviewed		Cessation of ≥ 3 months Home restrictions S-F: OR=7.41; 95% CI=5.55-9.90 in CPS 92-92 & OR=7.08; 95% CI=4.45-11.26 in CPS 01-02 Partial: OR=2.18; 95% CI=1.63-2.92 in CPS 92-93 & OR=2.45; 95% CI=1.48-4.07 in CPS 01-02 Work restrictions S-F: OR=1.30; 95% CI=1.04-1.63 in CPS 92-92, but OR= 0.99; 95% CI=0.67-1.45 in CPS 01-02	
Lee & Kahende, 2007 USA	3990 quitters in the past 2 years from the National Health Interview Survey	2000	Indirect question "During the past week, how many days did anyone smoke cigarettes, cigars, or pipes anywhere inside your home?" Answer of zero contrasted with all others. Smoke-free workplace versus all others	Quit 7-24 months before the survey without a relapse (successful quitter) versus relapsed quitter in the past year	A logistic regression adjusted for age, education, marital status, race/ethnicity, the number of lifetime quit attempts, and whether the smoker had ever switched to low tar cigarettes.	Successfully quit: No one smokes in home: OR=10.47; 95% CI=8.15-13.46 Smoke-free workplace: OR=2.01; 95% CI=1.20-3.37	
Burns et al., 2007 Colorado, USA	6100 ever smokers from the Colorado Tobacco Attitudes and Behaviour Survey	2001	No restrictions, partial restrictions, smoke-free home Smoke-free work area versus other workers versus not applicable	Duration of smoking, current smokers censored at time of survey	A Cox proportional hazard regression adjusted for age, sex, marital status, language spoken in home, age of smoking initiation, education, poverty status, and insurance status.	Duration of smoking Home: Smoke-free: HR=4.59; 95% CI=3.81-5.52 Partial: HR=2.39; 95% CI= 1.94-2.94	Results were similar for Latinos and non-Hispanic whites

Reference/location	Population and design	Year of assessment	Household smoking restriction measure	Outcomes	Covariates and analysis	Results	Comments
Cross-sectional studies							
Burns et al., 2007 Colorado, USA						Workplace: HR=1.48; 95% CI=1.19-1.84	Study did not consider workplace restrictions.
Shelley et al., 2008 New York City, New York, USA	Adult (≥ 18 y) Chinese population in New York City Cross-sectional survey N=600 male current smokers	2002-03	No restrictions, partial home restrictions, and a smoke-free policy	Consumption on weekdays Consumption on weekend days	Mean values and multivariate (linear regression) of log CPD adjusted for marital status, education, age annual income, another smoker in the household, and awareness of the harmfulness of SHS. Logistic regression, same covariates as for consumption	Weekdays partial restrictions, 14.7 CPD Smoke-free, 17.2 CPD no restrictions, 19.9 CPD Multivariate: partial, NS smoke-free, p<0.05 Weekend days partial restrictions, 11.8 CPD smoke-free, 14.7 CPD no restrictions, 17.3 CPD Multivariate: Partial NS Smoke-free, p<0.05	
				Making a recent quit attempt		Quit attempt OR=3.37; 95% CI=1.51-7.05 versus no restrictions	
Messer et al., 2008a USA	31 625 adult recent current smokers from the Current Population Survey	2003	Seriously trying to quit Quit at least a day Quit for at least 6 months when surveyed	Smoke-free (S-F) home versus all others Smoke-free workplace versus all others	A logistic regression analysis adjusted for sex, age, race/ethnicity, education, initiation < 15 years, delay of smoking for at least 30 minutes after awakening, and use of a pharmaceutical aid.	Seriously trying to quit: S-F home: OR=1.21; 95% CI=1.12-1.30 S-F work: NS Quit 1+ days S-F home: OR=4.03; 95% CI=3.50-4.63 S-F work: NS Quit for 6+ months S-F home: OR=4.13; 95% CI=3.25-5.26 S-F work: NS	Younger smokers seemed more engaged in quitting, and appeared to be more successful. They tended to smoke fewer CPD and more had smoke-free homes. The authors suggest that these factors account for their increased success in quitting.

Appendix 6.
Studies examining the relationship between voluntary smoking policies in the home and *adult* smoking behaviour

Reference/ location	Population and design	Year of assessment	Household smoking restriction measure	Outcomes	Covariates and analysis	Results	Comments
Cross-Sectional Studies							
Tong et al., 2008 California, USA	767 current and former smokers from California Health Interview Survey	2003	Former smoker - 100 cigarettes in lifetime (ever) but not currently smoking Among current: Light smokers (<10 versus ≥10 CPD)	Smoke-free (S-F) home versus all others	Logistic regression adjusted for age, sex, Asian group, marital status, education, income, years in the USA (<10 versus all others including those born in the USA). Interaction term included for years in the USA and smoke-free home.	Longer-term residents more likely to be former smoker if have a S-F home OR=14.19; 95% CI=4.46-45.12 Shorter-term residents OR=2.25; 95% CI=1.79-5.90 Longer-term residents more likely to be light smokers if have a S-F home OR=5.37; 95% CI=2.79-10.31 Not significant for shorter-term residents OR=1.19; 95% CI=0.33-4.23	
Pierce et al., 2009 USA	542 470 current smokers aged 18-64 years in all the cross-sectional Current Population Surveys from 1992/93-2002/03	1992-2002	Very light (<5 CPD) smoking in those aged 18-29 years. The very light category includes occasional smokers (88% of group).	Smoke-free home versus all others Smoke-free workplace versus all others (including those not employed)	Logistic analysis of very light smoking in 18-29 year old group, adjusted for survey year, sex, education, income above versus below two times the poverty threshold, having a smoke-free workplace, and tobacco control policies ranking by tertile for state of residence as an indicator of social norms against smoking.	Very light smoking: Smoke-free versus others Home: OR=2.81; 95% CI=2.60-3.04 Work: OR=1.28; 95% CI=1.18-1.38 Also significant was tertile of state tobacco control activity: Highest: OR=1.68; 95% CI=1.53-1.85 Middle: OR=1.26; 95% CI= 1.15-1.38 versus lowest tertile	The authors selected the group aged 18-29 for the logistic regression analysis because of a marked increase in very light smoking in that group. Survey year was not significant, but when the variable for a smoke-free home was eliminated from the model, survey year became highly significant indicating the increase in light smoking was mediated by the increase in smoke-free homes.

Appendix 7.
Studies examining the relationship between voluntary smoking policies in the home and *youth* smoking behaviour

Study location	Population and design	Year of assessment	Household smoking restriction measure	Smoking measures	Covariates and analysis	Results	Comments
Biener et al., 1997 Massachusetts, USA	Population survey of 1606 adolescents 12-17 years	1993	No restrictions, allowed in designated areas, smoke-free	Any smoking in past 30 days	Age, sex, household adult education status	Regardless of whether or not there was an adult smoker in the household, the analyses failed to detect a significant relationship between home smoking restrictions and adolescent smoking.	The main purpose of this study was to assess adolescent exposure to SHS. Separate logistic regression analyses were conducted for those in households with and without adult smokers.
Jackson & Henriksen 1997 Central and North Carolina, USA	School survey of 1352 3rd and 5th graders	Not reported	Smoking allowed indoors versus not allowed	Any experimentation Readiness to smoke	Multivariate analyses of experimentation stratified by parental smoking status: at least one current smoker. Parental smoking status (former, never, 1 current, both current) and several anti-smoking socialisation measures.	No parent smokes: Smoking not allowed: OR=1.50; 95% CI=1.20-1.83 Parent smokes: Smoking not allowed: OR=1.10; 95% CI=0.99-1.20 Readiness to smoke was only evaluated bivariately, and was associated with parental smoking but not home smoking restrictions.	Separate analyses conducted for children with and without parents who smoke.
Henriksen & Jackson, 1998 Northern California, USA	School survey of 937 3rd-8th graders receiving English language instruction	Not reported	Smoke-free home versus all others	Any experimentation Intent to smoke	Multivariate analysis included three types of anti-smoking socialisation: home rules, parental warnings against smoking, expectations regarding punishment for smoking, and controlled for parental smoking status.	Increased experimentation: Others versus smoke-free OR=1.39, 95% CI=1.03-1.88 Increased Intent to smoke: Others versus smoke-free OR=1.77, 95% CI=1.19-2.64	No interaction term was examined for parental smoking status and a smoke-free home.
Wakefield et al., 2000a USA	School survey of 17 287 high school students	1996	No restrictions, only guests can smoke, allowed only in certain areas, smoke-free (S-F)	Non-susceptible versus susceptible versus early experimenter versus advanced experimenter versus established smoker	Grade, sex, race/ethnicity, adult smokers in the home, sibling smokers, smoke-free school policy and strength of enforcement,	Reduced transition from: Non-susc versus susc: S-F: OR=0.64; 95%CI=0.52-0.76 Part: OR=0.83; 95% CI=0.74-0.92*	No interaction term was examined for parental smoking status and a smoke-free home.

Appendix 7.
Studies examining the relationship between voluntary smoking policies in the home and *youth* smoking behaviour

Study location	Population and design	Year of assessment	Household smoking restriction measure	Smoking measures	Covariates and analysis	Results	Comments
Wakefield et al., 2000a USA					and an index on smoking restrictions in public places from an external source. Separate logistic regression analyses of each successive pair of levels on the continuum.	Susc. versus early exp: S-F: OR=0.69; 95% CI=0.59-0.79 Part: OR=0.83; 95% CI=0.74-0.92* Early versus advanced exp: S-F: OR=0.71; 95% CI=0.60-0.82 Part: OR=0.83; 95% CI=0.74-0.92* Advanced exp versus estab: S-F: OR=0.78; 95% CI=0.67-0.90 Part: OR=0.83; 95% CI=0.74-0.92*	*author commented on the effect being the same
				Any smoking in past 30 days		Smoking in past 30 days: S-F: OR=0.79; 95% CI=0.67-0.91 Part: OR=0.85; 95% CI=0.74-0.95	
Rissel et al., 2000 Sydney, NSW, Australia	2573 students in grades 10 and 11 attending high schools with high Arabic and Vietnamese enrollment	1998	Family had clear rules about not smoking inside the home (yes versus no)	Self-defined current smoking	Logistic regression adjusted for year in school, parental smoking, family closeness, sex, ethnic background, parental behaviours (strict versus not strict, clear versus not clear consequences), pocket money (<$20/ week versus more), out 0-2 evenings versus 3+ per week with friends, positive school perceptions, positive teacher perceptions, positive peer perceptions	Students in families with clear rules about not smoking in the home were less likely to be current smokers (OR=0.67; 95% CI=0.49-0.90) than those without clear rules.	

Study location	Population and design	Year of assessment	Household smoking restriction measure	Smoking measures	Covariates and analysis	Results	Comments
Proescholdbell et al., 2000 Tucson, Arizona	School survey of 6686 middle and high school students	Not reported	Scale incorporating both resident and visitor rules regarding smoking in the home	Smoked one cigarette versus never smoked Smoked one cigarette versus current regular (at least one cigarette a month)	Grade, sex, ethnicity, home structure (e.g. single parent, biological parent), parent smoking, parent smoking attitude, various interactions. Separate logistic regressions for middle and high school students	Smoked a cigarette versus never: Middle school: OR=1.32; 95% CI=1.12-1.56 High school: OR=1.25; 95% CI=1.10-1.41 Smoked but not current versus current regular: Middle school: NS High school: NS	An interaction was present for the home smoking rule scale and parental smoking status for high school students only, indicating a larger effect in households without smoking parents.
Komro et al., 2003 Minnesota	School and parent survey of 1343 parent-child pairs among 8th, 9th and 10th graders	1998	Allowed, exceptions, smoke-free (S-F) home	Any smoking in the past 30 days	Grade, parental variables (education, marital status, attitudes, norms and perceptions about adult smoking), rules and consequences about adolescent smoking, adult and child smokers in home, and access to cigarettes in the home.	When analyzed bivariately, a smoke-free home policy (but not partial restrictions) was significantly associated with less smoking in the past 30 days. S-F: OR=1.83; 95% CI=1.40-2.40 Part: OR=1.09; 95% CI=0.69-1.70 But in the multivariate analysis it was not (odds ratios not presented).	No interaction term was examined for parental smoking status and a smoke-free home.
Kodl & Mermelstein, 2004 USA	245 6th, 8th, and 10th grader survey respondents with a parent who responded to survey	Not reported	No one may smoke in the home versus all others	Smoking level: nonsusceptible never smoker, susceptible never smoker, former trier, current experimenter, regular user	Multivariate analysis of covariance of child smoking status adjusting for parental smoking status, parental education status, and including multiple variables for parental efficacy and monitoring, beliefs, family relations.	Model for adolescent smoking level indicated that a smoke-free home was highly related to lower level of adolescent smoking (p<0.001). Contrasts analyzed indicated a significant difference in adjusted mean rule level between regular users and all others (p<0.05) and between nonsusceptible and susceptible never smokers (p<0.05).	

Appendix 7.
Studies examining the relationship between voluntary smoking policies in the home and *youth* smoking behaviour

Study location	Population and design	Year of assessment	Household smoking restriction measure	Smoking measures	Covariates and analysis	Results	Comments
Andersen *et al.*, 2004 Washington, USA	3555 12th graders in the Hutchinson Smoking Prevention Project from whom a parent survey was available	Not reported	Not allowed versus allowed rarely, sometimes, or usually	Smoke monthly and smoke daily	Separate relative risk regression models for students with and without smokers in their families, adjusted for parents asking to sit in nonsmoking parts of restaurants and asking smokers not to smoke around them.	In the multivariate analysis, for families with smokers (RR=0.88; 95% CI=0.74-1.06) for daily smoking. Monthly smoking not significant. The results in nonsmoking families did not approach statistical significance.	
Clark *et al.*, 2006 USA	Population survey of 12 299 youth 15-24 years	1998-99	No restrictions, partial restrictions, completely smoke-free (S-F) home	Ever smoke (at least 100 cigarettes in lifetime) Current versus never Current versus former among ever smokers Consumption among current smokers	Age, sex, household income, race/ethnicity, smoking status of other household members. Overall and separate logistic regression analyses conducted for adolescents (15-18 years) and young adults (19-24 years).	Reduced ever versus never: S-F: OR=0.56; 95% CI=0.45-0.70 Part: OR=0.99; 95% CI=0.78-1.26 Reduced current versus never: S-F: OR=0.45; 95% CI=0.36-0.58 Part: OR=0.88; 95% CI=0.68-1.14 Less current among ever S-F: OR=0.33; 95% CI=0.21-0.53 Part: OR=0.46; 95% CI=0.29-0.73 Consumption > 10 CPD: S-F: OR=0.42; 95% CI=0.24-0.71 Part: OR=0.87; 95% CI=0.51-1.48	No interaction term was examined for parental smoking status and a smoke-free home. The results were generally similar for adolescents and young adults.
den Exter Blokland *et al.*, 2006 Utrecht, Netherlands	600 7th graders with a parent respondent	Two successive survey waves during the 2000-01 school year	Six questions on the existence of home smoking rules for both adults and adolescents combined into a single scale. Details	Initiators - had not smoked at wave one, but had by wave two.	Logistic analysis of each status variable adjusted for baseline communication, warnings, parental knowledge of child and child's friends	The home rule scale was not significant for either initiation or maintenance of smoking.	

Study location	Population and design	Year of assessment	Household smoking restriction measure	Smoking measures	Covariates and analysis	Results	Comments
den Exter Blokland et al., 2006 Utrecht, Netherlands			not provided.	Maintainers - smoked at both times.	smoking, parental psychological control, parental confidence in effecting child's smoking behaviour, availability of cigarettes in home, parental norms about adolescent smoking, parental reaction to child's smoking, and parental smoking status.		
Thomson et al., 2006 Massachusetts	Population survey of 3831 adolescents 12-17 years	2000-01	Smokers smoke inside of home versus smoke-free	Perceived prevalence of adult and adolescent smoking Perceived adult negative attitudes about social acceptability of adult and adolescent smoking	Age, sex, ethnicity, household income, adult education, household composition (1 versus >1 adult), peer smoking, parental smoking, perceived parental disapproval of smoking, and percentage of town voting on measure to restrict smoking	Perceived prevalence no smoke-free home versus smoke-free home Adult: OR=2.0; 95% CI=1.5-2.6 Adol: OR=1.2; 95% CI=0.94-1.50 Perceived adult negative attitudes of smoking no smoke-free home versus smoke-free home: Adult: OR=2.0; 95% CI=1.6-2.5 Adol: OR=1.5; 95% CI=1.2-1.9	Interaction was present for home smoking rule scale and parental smoking status for high school students only, indicating larger effect in households without smoking parents. Both perceived prevalence and acceptability of smoking have been related to future smoking among adolescents in multiple previous studies.
Szabo et al., 2006 Victoria, Australia	School survey of 4125 secondary students	2002	Permitted in some or all areas, prohibited inside, prohibited both inside and outside the home	Smoking uptake stage Non-susceptible never smoker versus susceptible never smoker	Age, sex, school type. Polytomous logistic regressions contrasted each higher stage to non-susceptible never smokers, experimenters versus susceptibles, and current smokers versus experimenters.	Increased transition compared to total smoking prohibitions inside and outside the home: Non-susceptible versus susceptible never: Not inside: OR=1.21; 95% CI=0.97-1.51 Partial: OR=1.38; 95% CI=1.06-1.79	Further models with interactions for smoking policy and parental smoking showed that policies were not associated with smoking uptake stage when parents smoked.

Appendix 7.
Studies examining the relationship between voluntary smoking policies in the home and *youth* smoking behaviour

Study location	Population and design	Year of assessment	Household smoking restriction measure	Smoking measures	Covariates and analysis	Results	Comments
Szabo *et al.*, 2006 Victoria, Australia				Susceptible never versus experimenter		Susceptible never versus experimenter: Not inside: OR=1.49; 95% CI=1.19-1.88 Partial: OR=1.92; 95% CI=1.44-2.56	
				Current smoker		Current versus not current: Not inside: OR=1.03; 95% CI=0.77-1.37 Partial: OR=1.30; 95% CI=0.92-1.86	
Fisher *et al.*, 2007 USA	10 593 adolescents in the "Growing up Today" study aged 12-18 years who were children of women in the Nurse's Health Study	1999	Not allowed versus allowed or no policy	Established smokers (>100 cigarettes in lifetime)	Logistic regression adjusted for age, gender, peer smoking, possession of tobacco promotional items, and having at least one parent who smokes cigarettes.	In a model including all covariates, except parental smoking, a smoke-free home was significantly associated with less established smoking (OR=0.67; 95% CI= 0.48-0.93), but in the full model, parental smoking was highly significant (OR=1.81; 95% CI=1.40-2.35) and a smoke-free home was not (OR=0.94; 95% CI= 0.65-1.35).	
Andreeva *et al.*, 2007 Ukraine	609 persons aged 15-29 years interviewed at home in a national survey	2005	No smokers in family or smoke-free home versus all others	Age of first cigarette	Separate survival analyses for males and females adjusted (if significant) for age, education, town size, living in a city versus village, number of people in household, income, exposure to tobacco smoke rarely versus	No smokers in the family or a smoke-free home was related to reduced risk of earlier smoking: Age of first cigarette : Males: HR=0.78; 95% CI=0.61-0.99 Females: HR=0.39; 95% CI=0.28-0.94	

Study location	Population and design	Year of assessment	Household smoking restriction measure	Smoking measures	Covariates and analysis	Results	Comments
Andreeva et al., 2007 Ukraine				Age of initiation of daily smoking	frequently, seeing outdoor tobacco advertising, tobacco-related knowledge low versus high, receiving information about tobacco from magazines, receiving tobacco information from friends	Age of daily smoking : Males: HR=0.64; 95% CI=0.49-0.84 Females: HR=0.60; 95% CI=0.39-0.93	
Rodriguez et al., 2007 Pennsylvania, USA	163 10th grade students with a household member who smokes	2006	Household members allowed versus not allowed to smoke in the home	Smoking level: 0=not in past month; 1=in last month; 2=at least once a week; 3=daily, but <11 CPD; and 4=daily, 11 or more CPD	Structural equation modeling with peer smoking, lifetime alcohol use and gender included with the home rule variable	No direct effect of smoke-free home on smoking level, but model showed an effect through peer smoking (p=0.0008). Having a smoke-free home was associated with having fewer peers who smoked, which in turn was associated with lower smoking level.	
Rainio & Rimpela, 2008 Finland	Population survey of 6503 12-, 14-, 16- and 18-year olds	2005	No restrictions (NR), partial, smoke-free, or respondent could not say (CNS)	Never smokers versus experimenters Daily/weekly current smokers versus all others	Multivariate logistic regression analyses adjusted for age, sex, parental smoking, family structure, parental education, urban residence, and parental permissiveness toward child smoking.	Increased compared to those with a smoke-free home: Never versus experimenters NR: OR=2.02; 95% CI=1.2-3.4 Part: OR=1.33; 95% CI=1.1-1.6 CNS: OR=1.68; 95% CI=1.3-2.2 Daily/weekly versus all others: NR: OR=14.3; 95% CI=8.6-23.7 Part: OR=2.9; 95% CI=2.3-3.6 CNS: OR=4.4; 95% CI=3.3-5.9	No interaction term was examined for parental smoking status and a smoke-free home.

Appendix 7.
Studies examining the relationship between voluntary smoking policies in the home and *youth* smoking behaviour

Study location	Population and design	Year of assessment	Household smoking restriction measure	Smoking measures	Covariates and analysis	Results	Comments
Albers *et al.*, 2008 Massachusetts, USA	3824 adolescents 12-17 years in baseline population survey	2001-02 to 2005-06	At baseline, visitors not allowed to smoke inside the home, and if an adult smoker lived in the household, there was a complete ban on smoking inside	At final follow-up, had transitioned to established smoking	Separate hierarchical regression analyses of each transition conducted for adolescents living and not living with smokers. Variables in the models included age, baseline smoking status, presence of a close friend who smokes, gender, race/ethnicity, household income, and town level factors (percentage voting yes on Question 1, percent white, percent youth).	Progression to established smoker was not significantly related to not having a smoke-free home, but tended to greater significance among adolescents who lived with a smoker (OR=1.38; 95% CI=0.92-2.07) compared to those not living with a smoker (OR=1.08; 95% CI= 0.61-1.93).	
				At final follow-up had transitioned from nonsmoker to experimentation		Not having a smoke-free home was significant for the transition from nonsmoking to experimentation only for those who lived with nonsmokers (OR=1.89; 95% CI= 1.30-2.74). For those living with smokers (OR=0.88; 95% CI=0.73-1.37)	

References

Adams S, Cotti C (2008). Drunk driving after the passage of smoking bans in bars. *J Public Econ*, 92(5-6):1288-1305.

Adda J, Cornaglia F (2005). The effects of taxes and bans on passive smoking. University College London, Institute for Fiscal Studies. Department of Economics. Centre for microdata and methods and practice (CEMMAP) Working Paper 20/05 *(http://cemmap.ifs.org.uk/wps/cwp2005.pdf)*.

Akhtar PC, Currie DB, Currie CE, et al. (2007). Changes in child exposure to environmental tobacco smoke (CHETS) study after implementation of smoke-free legislation in Scotland: national cross sectional survey. *Br Med J*, 335(7619):545-549.

Al-Delaimy W, Fraser T, Woodward A (2001a). Nicotine in hair of bar and restaurant workers. *N Z Med J*, 114(1127):80-83.

Al-Delaimy WK (2002). Hair as a biomarker for exposure to tobacco smoke. *Tob Control*, 11(3):176-182.

Al-Delaimy WK, Crane J, Woodward A (2001b). Passive smoking in children: effect of avoidance strategies, at home as measured by hair nicotine levels. *Arch Environ Health*, 56(2):117-122.

Al-Delaimy WK, Mahoney GN, Speizer FE, et al. (2002a). Toenail nicotine levels as a biomarker of tobacco smoke exposure. *Cancer Epidemiol Biomarkers Prev*, 11(11):1400-1404.

Al-Delaimy WK, Crane J, Woodward A (2002b). Is the hair nicotine level a more accurate biomarker of environmental tobacco smoke exposure than urine cotinine? *J Epidemiol Community Health*, 56(1):66-71.

Al-Delaimy WK, Cho E, Chen WY, et al. (2004). A prospective study of smoking and risk of breast cancer in young adult women. *Cancer Epidemiol Biomarkers Prev*, 13(3):398-404.

Al-Delaimy WK, Pierce J, Messer K, et al. (2007). The California Tobacco Control Program's effect on adult smokers: (2) Daily cigarette consumption levels. *Tob Control*, 16(2):91-95.

Al-Delaimy WK, White MM, Trinidad DR, et al. (2008). The California Tobacco Program: can we maintain the progress? Results from the California Tobacco Survey, 1990-2005. Sacramento, CA, California Department of Public Health *(http://ssdc.ucsd.edu/tobacco/)*.

Alamar B, Glantz S (2004). Smoke-free ordinances increase restaurant profit and value. *Contemp Econ Policy*, 22(4):520-525.

Alamar B, Glantz S (2007). Effect of smoke-free bar laws on bar value and profits. *Am J Public Health*, 97(8):1401-1402.

Alberg AJ, Kouzis A, Genkinger JM, et al. (2007). A prospective cohort study of bladder cancer risk in relation to active cigarette smoking and household exposure to secondhand cigarette smoke. *Am J Epidemiol*, 165(6):660-666.

Albers AB, Siegel M, Cheng DM, et al. (2007). Effect of smoking regulations in local restaurants on smokers' anti-smoking attitudes and quitting behaviours. *Tob Control*, 16(2):101-106.

Albers AB, Biener L, Siegel M, et al. (2008). Household smoking bans and adolescent antismoking attitudes and smoking initiation: findings from a longitudinal study of a Massachusetts youth cohort. *Am J Public Health*, 98(10):1886-1893.

Allred EN, Bleecker E, Chaitman B, et al. (1989). Short-term effects of carbon monoxide exposure on the exercise performance of subjects with coronary artery disease. *N Engl J Med*, 321(21):1426-1432.

Allwright S, Paul G, Greiner B, et al. (2005). Legislation for smoke-free workplaces and health of bar workers in Ireland: before and after study. *Br Med J*, 331(7525):1117-1120.

Alpert HR, Carpenter CM, Travers MJ, et al. (2007). Environmental and economic evaluation of the Massachusetts smoke-free workplace law. *J Community Health*, 32(4):269-281.

American Society of Heating, Refrigerating, and Air-Conditioning Engineers (2005). Environmental tobacco smoke. Atlanta, GA, American Society of Heating Refrigerating and Air-Conditioning Engineers *(http://www.ashrae.org/doclib/20058211239_347.pdf)*.

American Nonsmokers' Rights Foundation (2009). 100% smokefree correctional facilities. Berkeley, CA *(http://no-smoke.org/pdf/100smokefreeprisons.pdf)*.

Andersen MR, Leroux B, Bricker J, et al. (2004). Antismoking parenting practices are associated with reduced rates of adolescent smoking. *Arch Pediatr Adolesc Med*, 158(4):348-352.

Anderson HR, Cook DG (1997). Passive smoking and sudden infant death syndrome: review of the epidemiological evidence. *Thorax*, 52(11):1003-1009.

Andreeva TI, Krasovsky KS, Semenova DS (2007). Correlates of smoking initiation among young adults in Ukraine: a cross-sectional study. *BMC Public Health*, 7:106.

Arcus J, Boey S, Bradshaw R, et al. (2007). SMOKES 2007 - Smoking outdoors in a kids environment: a pilot study: evaluating the Upper Hutt City Council smokefree parks policy. Wellington, New Zealand, University of Otago *(http://www.smokefreecouncils.org.nz/fileadmin/clients/cancer_society/pdf/The_SMOKE_study_2007_report__FINAL.pdf)*.

Arheart KL, Lee D, Dietz N, et al. (2008). Declining trends in serum cotinine levels in US worker groups: the power of policy. *J Occup Environ Med*, 50(1):57-63.

Ashley MJ, Ferrence R (1998). Reducing children's exposure to environmental tobacco smoke in homes: issues and strategies. *Tob Control*, 7(1):61-65.

Ashley MJ, Cohen J, Ferrence R, et al. (1998). Smoking in the home: changing attitudes and current practices. *Am J Public Health*, 88(5):797-800.

Auerbach O, Petrik TG, Stout AP, et al. (1956). The anatomical approach to the study of smoking and bronchogenic carcinoma; a preliminary report of forty-one cases. *Cancer*, 9(1):76-83.

Auerbach O, Forman JB, Gere JB, et al. (1957). Changes in the bronchial epithelium in relation to smoking and cancer of the lung; a report of progress. *N Engl J Med*, 256(3):97-104.

Australian National Research Council (NRC) (1986). *Environmental tobacco smoke: measuring exposures and assessing health effects.* Washington, DC, National Academy Press *(http://books.nap.edu/catalog. php?record_id=943).*

Author Unknown (1961).The great debate [editorial]. *N Engl J Med,* 264:1266.

Aveyard P, Markham W, Cheng K (2004). A methodological and substantive review of the evidence that schools cause pupils to smoke. *Soc Sci Med,* 58(11):2253-2265.

Baker JA, Odunuga OO, Rodabaugh KJ, *et al.* (2006). Active and passive smoking and risk of ovarian cancer. *Int J Gynecol Cancer,* 16(Suppl 1):211-218.

Bakoula CG, Kafritsa Y, Kavadias G, *et al.* (1997). Factors modifying exposure to environmental tobacco smoke in children (Athens, Greece). *Cancer Causes Control,* 8(1):73-76.

Barnett TA, Gauvin L, Lambert M, *et al.* (2007). The influence of school smoking policies on student tobacco use. *Arch Pediatr Adolesc Med,* 161(9):842-848.

Barnoya J, Glantz S (2005). Cardiovascular effects of secondhand smoke: nearly as large as smoking. *Circulation,* 111(20):2684-2698.

Barnoya J, Mendoza-Montano C, Navas-Acien A (2007). Secondhand smoke exposure in public places in Guatemala: comparison with other Latin American countries. *Cancer Epidemiol Biomarkers Prev,* 16(12):2730-2735.

Barone-Adesi F, Vizzini L, Merletti F, *et al.* (2006). Short-term effects of Italian smoking regulation on rates of hospital admission for acute myocardial infarction. *Eur Heart J,* 27(20):2468-2472.

Barrientos-Gutierrez T, Reynales-Shigematsu L, Vila-Tang E, *et al.* (2007a). [Environmental tobacco smoke exposure in homes of Mexico City: analysis of environmental samples and children and women hair]. *Salud Publica Mex,* 49(Suppl 2):S224-S232.

Barrientos-Gutierrez T, Valdes-Salgado R, Reynales-Shigematsu L, *et al.* (2007b). [Involuntary exposure to tobacco smoke in public places in Mexico City] *Salud Publica Mex,* 49(Suppl 2):S205-S212.

Bartecchi C, Alsever R, Nevin-Woods C, *et al.* (2006). Reduction in the incidence of acute myocardial infarction associated with a citywide smoking ordinance. *Circulation,* 114(14):1490-1496.

Baska T, Sovinova H, Nemeth A, *et al.* (2007). Environmental tobacco smoke of youngsters in Czech Republic, Hungary, Poland and Slovakia--findings from the Global Youth Tobacco Survey (GYTS). *Int J Public Health,* 52(1):62-66.

Bates MN, Fawcett J, Dickson S, *et al.* (2002). Exposure of hospitality workers to environmental tobacco smoke. *Tob Control,* 11(2):125-129.

Bauer JE,, Hyland A, *et al.* (2005). A longitudinal assessment of the impact of smoke-free worksite policies on tobacco use. *Am J Public Health,* 95(6):1024-1029.

Behan DF, Eriksen M, Lin Y (2005). Economic effects of environmental tobacco smoke. Society of Actuaries *(http://www.soa.org/ research/life/research-economic-effect.aspx).*

Bello S, Soto M, Michalland S, *et al.* (2004). Encuesta nacional de tabaquismo en funcionarios de salud. *Rev Med Chile,* 132(2):223-232.

Bennett WP, Alavanja MC, Blomeke B, *et al.* (1999). Environmental tobacco smoke, genetic susceptibility, and risk of lung cancer in never-smoking women. *J Natl Cancer Inst,* 91(23):2009-2014.

Benowitz NL (1999). Biomarkers of environmental tobacco smoke exposure. *Environ Health Perspect,* 107(Suppl 2):349-355.

Berg CJ, Cox L, Nazir N, *et al.* (2006). Correlates of home smoking restrictions among rural smokers. *Nicotine Tob Res,* 8(3):353-360.

Berman S (2003). Caring for parents vs caring for children: is there a difference? *Arch Pediatr Adolesc Med,* 157(3):221-222.

Berman BA, Wong GC, Bastani R, *et al.* (2003). Household smoking behavior and ETS exposure among children with asthma in low-income, minority households. *Addict Behav,* 28(1):111-128.

Best JA, Hakstian AR (1978). A situation-specific model for smoking behavior. *Addict Behav,* 3(2):79-92.

Bewley BR, Johnson M, Banks M (1979). Teachers' smoking. *J Epidemiol Community Health,* 33(3):219-222.

Biener L, Nyman AL (1999). Effect of workplace smoking policies on smoking cessation: results of a longitudinal study. *J Occup Environ Med,* 41(12):1121-1127.

Biener L, Cullen D, Di Z, *et al.* (1997). Household smoking restrictions and adolescents' exposure to environmental tobacco smoke. *Prev Med,* 26(3):358-363.

Biener L, Harris J, Hamilton W (2000). Impact of the Massachusetts tobacco control programme: population based trend analysis. *Br Med J,* 321(7257):351-354.

Biener L, Garrett C, Skeer M, *et al.* (2007). The effects on smokers of Boston's smoke-free bar ordinance: a longitudinal analysis of changes in compliance, patronage, policy support, and smoking at home. *J Public Health Manag Pract,* 13(6):630-636.

Bird Y, Moraros J, Olsen L, *et al.* (2007). Smoking practices, risk perception of smoking, and environmental tobacco smoke exposure among 6th-grade students in Ciudad Juarez, Mexico. *Nicotine Tob Res,* 9(2):195-203.

Bjerregaard BK, Raaschou-Nielsen O, Sorensen M, *et al.* (2006). Tobacco smoke and bladder cancer--in the European prospective investigation into cancer and nutrition. *Int J Cancer,* 119(10):2412-2416.

Blackburn C, Spencer N, Bonas S, *et al.* (2003). Effect of strategies to reduce exposure of infants to environmental tobacco smoke in the home: cross sectional survey. *Br Med J,* 327(7409):257.

Blecher EH (2006). The effects of the tobacco products control amendment Act of 1999 on restaurant revenues in South Africa: A panel data approach. *S Afr J Econ,* 74(1):123-130.

Bloch M, Shopland D (2000). Outdoor smoking bans: more than meets the eye. *Tob Control,* 9(1):99.

Bolte G, Heitmann D, Kiranoglu M, *et al.* (2008). Exposure to environmental tobacco smoke in German restaurants, pubs and discotheques. *J Expo Sci Environ Epidemiol,* 18(3):262-271.

Bonita R, Duncan J, Truelsen T, *et al.* (1999). Passive smoking as well as active smoking increases the risk of acute stroke. *Tob Control,* 8(2):156-160.

Borland R, Pierce JP, Burns DM, *et al.* (1992). Protection from environmental tobacco smoke in California. The case for a smoke-free workplace [see comment]. *JAMA,* 268(6):749-752.

Borland R, Cappiello M, Owen N (1997). Leaving work to smoke. *Addiction,* 92(10):1361-1368.

Borland R, Mullins R, Trotter L, *et al.* (1999). Trends in environmental tobacco smoke restrictions in the home in Victoria, Australia. *Tob Control,* 8(3):266-271.

Borland R, Yong H, Cummings K, *et al.* (2006a). Determinants and consequences of smoke-free homes: findings from the International Tobacco Control (ITC) four country survey. *Tob Control,* 15(Suppl 3):iii42-iii50.

Borland R, Yong H, Siahpush M, *et al.* (2006b). Support for and reported compliance with smoke-free restaurants and bars by smokers in four countries: findings from the International Tobacco Control (ITC) four country survey. *Tob Control,* 15(Suppl 3):iii34-iii41.

Bourns B, Malcomson A (2001). Economic impact analysis of the non-smoking by law on the hospitality industry in Ottawa. KPMG *(http://www.tobaccoscam.ucsf.edu/pdf/087-OttawaKPMG.pdf).*

Boyle P, Levin B (2008). *World Cancer Report 2008.* Lyon, International Agency for Research on Cancer.

Brandt AM (2007). *The cigarette century: the rise, fall, and deadly persistence of the product that defined America.* New York, NY, Basic Books.

Braverman MT, Aarø LE, Hetland J (2008). Changes in smoking among restaurant and bar employees following Norway's comprehensive smoking ban. *Health Promot Int,* 23(1):5-15.

Brenner H, Mielck A (1992). Smoking prohibition in the workplace and smoking cessation in the Federal Republic of Germany. *Prev Med,* 21(2):252-261.

Brown DC, Pereira L, Garner JB (1982). Cancer of the cervix and the smoking husband. *Can Fam Physician,* 28:499-502.

Brownell KD, Glynn TJ, Glasgow R, *et al.* (1986). Interventions to prevent relapse. *Health Psychol,* 5 (Suppl):53-68.

Brownson RC, Eriksen MP, Davis R, *et al.* (1997). Environmental tobacco smoke: health effects and policies to reduce exposure. *Annu Rev Public Health,* 18:163-185.

Buckley JD, Harris RW, Doll R, *et al.* (1981). Case-control study of the husbands of women with dysplasia or carcinoma of the cervix uteri. *Lancet,* 2(8254):1010-1015.

Burch JD, Rohan TE, Howe GR, *et al.* (1989). Risk of bladder cancer by source and type of tobacco exposure: a case-control study. *Int J Cancer,* 44(4):622-628.

Burns DM, Lee L, Gilpin E, *et al.* (1996). Cigarette smoking behaviour in the United States. In: *Changes in cigarette-related disease risks and their implication for prevention and control.* Smoking and Tobacco Control Monograph 8. Bethesda, MD, U.S. Department of Health and Human Services, National Institutes of Health, National Cancer Institute. NIH Pub. No. 974213; 13-112.

Burns EK, Levinson A, Lezotte D, *et al.* (2007). Differences in smoking duration between Latinos and Anglos. Nicotine *Tob Res,* 9(7):731-737.

Butler T, Richmond R, Belcher J, *et al.* (2007). Should smoking be banned in prisons? *Tob Control,* 16(5):291-293.

California Department of Health Services (2006). California tobacco control update 2006: the social norm change approach. Sacramento, California, California Department of Health Services *(http://www.dhs.ca.gov/tobacco/).*

California Department of Public Health (2007). Tobacco control section *(http://www.cdph.ca.gov/programs/Tobacco/Pages/default.aspx).*

California Environmental Protection Agency (Cal EPA) (1997). Health effects of exposure to environmental tobacco smoke, California Environmental Protection Agency, Office of Environmental Health Hazard Assessment *(http://www.oehha.org/air/environmental_tobacco/finalets.html).*

California Environmental Protection Agency: Air Resources Board (2005). Proposed identification of environmental tobacco smoke as a toxic air contaminant. Tobacco control. Surveys and program evaluations from outside UCSF. Sacramento, CA, California Environmental Protection Agency. *(http://repositories.cdlib.org/context/tc/article/1194/type/pdf/viewcontent/)*

Cameron L, Williams J (2001). Cannabis, alcohol and cigarettes: substitutes or complements? *Econ Rec,* 77(236):19-34.

Cameron M, Wakefield M, Trotter L, *et al.* (2003). Exposure to secondhand smoke at work: a survey of members of the Australian Liquor, Hospitality and Miscellaneous Workers Union. *Aust N Z J Public Health,* 27(5):496-501.

Carmella SG, Han S, Fristad A, *et al.* (2003). Analysis of total 4-(methylnitrosamino)-1-(3-pyridyl)-1-butanol (NNAL) in human urine. *Cancer Epidemiol Biomarkers Prev,* 12(11 Pt 1):1257-1261.

Celermajer DS, Adams M, Clarkson P, *et al.* (1996). Passive smoking and impaired endothelium-dependent arterial dilatation in healthy young adults. *N Engl J Med,* 334(3):150-154.

Centers for Disease Control and Prevention (1999). Decline in cigarette consumption following implementation of a comprehensive tobacco prevention and education program-Oregon, 1996-1998. *MMWR Morb Mortal Wkly Rep,* 48(7):140-143.

Centers for Disease Control and Prevention (2005a). Annual smoking-attributable mortality, years of potential life lost, and productivity losses--United States, 1997-2001. *MMWR Morb Mortal Wkly Rep,* 54(25):628.

Centers for Disease Control and Prevention (2005b). Tobacco use among students aged 13-15 years--Philippines, 2000 and 2003. *MMWR Morb Mortal Wkly Rep,* 54(4):94-97.

Centers for Disease Control and Prevention (2006a). State-specific prevalence of current cigarette smoking among adults and secondhand smoke rules and policies in homes and workplaces--United States, 2005. *MMWR Morb Mortal Wkly Rep,* 55(42):1148-1151.

Centers for Disease Control and Prevention (2006b). Tobacco use among students aged 13-15 years--Kurdistan Region, Iraq, 2005. *MMWR Morb Mortal Wkly Rep,* 55(20):556-559.

Centers for Disease Control and Prevention (2007a). State-specific prevalence of smoke-free home rules-United States, 1992-2003. *MMWR Morb Mortal Wkly Rep,* 56(20):501-504.

Centers for Disease Control and Prevention (2007b). Reduced secondhand smoke exposure after implementation of a comprehensive statewide smoking ban-New York, June 26, 2003-June 30, 2004. *MMWR Morb Mortal Wkly Rep*, 56(28):705-708.

Centers for Disease Control and Prevention (2007c). Decline in smoking prevalence -New York City, 2002-2006. *MMWR Morb Mortal Wkly Rep*, 56(24):604-608.

Centers for Disease Control and Prevention (2008). Global Youth Tobacco Surveillance, 2000-2007. *MMWR Morb Mortal Wkly Rep*, 57(SS-1):1-32.

Cesaroni G, Forastiere F, Agabiti N, *et al.* (2008). Effect of the Italian smoking ban on population rates of acute coronary events. *Circulation*, 117(9):1183-1188.

Chaloupka FJ (1992). Clean indoor air laws, addiction and cigarette smoking. *Appl Econ*, 24:193-205.

Chaloupka FJ, Saffer H (1992). Clean indoor air laws and the demand for cigarettes. *Contemporary Policy Issues*, 72-83.

Chaloupka FJ, Grossman M (1996). Price, tobacco control policies and youth smoking. National Bureau of Economic Research. NBER Working Paper Series. Working Paper #5740 *(http://www.nber.org/)*.

Chaloupka FJ, Wechsler H (1997). Price, tobacco control policies and smoking among young adults. *J Health Econ*, 16(3):359-373.

Chaloupka F, Warner K (2000). The economics of smoking. In: Cuyler A, Newhouse J, eds. *The handbook of health economics*. New York, Elsevier Science: 29;1539-1627.

Chaloupka FJ, Pacula RL, Farrelly MC, *et al.* (1999). Do higher cigarette prices encourage youth to use marijuana? Cambridge, MA, National Bureau of Economic Research.

Chang JS, Selvin S, Metayer C, *et al.* (2006). Parental smoking and the risk of childhood leukemia. *Am J Epidemiol*, 163(12):1091-1100.

Chapman S (2000). Banning smoking outdoors is seldom ethically justifiable. *Tob Control*, 9(1):95-97.

Chapman S (2007). *Public health advocacy and tobacco control: Making smoking history*. Oxford, Blackwell Publishing.

Chapman S, Borland R, Scollo M, *et al.* (1999). The impact of smoke-free workplaces on declining cigarette consumption in Australia and the United States. *Am J Public Health*, 89(7):1018-1023.

Charlton A, While D (1994). Smoking prevalence among 16-19-year-olds related to staff and student smoking policies in sixth forms and further education. *Health Educ J*, 53(1):28-39.

Chen R, Tavendale R, Tunstall-Pedoe H (2002). Measurement of passive smoking in adults: self-reported questionnaire or serum cotinine? *J Cancer Epidemiol Prev*, 7(2):85-95.

Chen YC, Su HJ, Guo YL, *et al.* (2005). Interaction between environmental tobacco smoke and arsenic methylation ability on the risk of bladder cancer. *Cancer Causes Control*, 16(2):75-81.

Cheng YJ, Hildesheim A, Hsu M, *et al.* (1999). Cigarette smoking, alcohol consumption and risk of nasopharyngeal carcinoma in Taiwan. *Cancer Causes Control*, 10(3):201-207.

Chuang JC, Callahan PJ, Lyu CW, *et al.* (1999). Polycyclic aromatic hydrocarbon exposures of children in low-income families. *J Expo Anal Environ Epidemiol*, 9(2):85-98.

Clark PI, Schooley MW, Pierce B, *et al.* (2006). Impact of home smoking rules on smoking patterns among adolescents and young adults. *Prev Chronic Dis*, 3(2):1-13.

Clarke V, White V, Hill D (1994). School structural and policy variables associated with student smoking. *Tob Control*, 3:339-346.

Claxton LD, Morin RS, Hughes TJ, *et al.* (1989). A genotoxic assessment of environmental tobacco smoke using bacterial bioassays. *Mutat Res*, 222(2):81-99.

Coghlin J, Hammond S, Gann P (1989). Development of epidemiologic tools for measuring environmental tobacco smoke exposure. *Am J Epidemiol*, 130(4):696-704.

Cogliano VJ, Baan R, Straif K, *et al.* (2004). The science and practice of carcinogen identification and evaluation. *Environ Health Perspect*, 112(13):1269-1274.

Coker AL, Rosenberg AJ, McCann MF, *et al.* (1992). Active and passive cigarette smoke exposure and cervical intraepithelial neoplasia. *Cancer Epidemiol Biomarkers Prev*, 1(5):349-356.

Coker AL, Bond S, Williams A, *et al.* (2002). Active and passive smoking, high-risk human papillomaviruses and cervical neoplasia. *Cancer Detect Prev*, 26(2):121-128.

Collins DJ, Lapsley HM (1996). *The social costs of drug abuse in Australia in 1988 and 1992*. Canberra, Australia, Australian Government Publishing Service *(http://www.health.gov.au/internet/main/publishing.nsf/Content/health-pubhlth-publicat-document-mono30-cnt.htm/)*.

Collins DJ, Lapsley HM (2002). *Counting the cost: estimates of the social costs of drug abuse in Australia in 1998-9*. National Drug Strategy Monograph Series (No 49). Canberra, Australia, Australian Government Publishing Service.

Collins DJ, Lapsley HM (2008). *The costs of tobacco, alcohol and illicit drug abuse to Australian society in 2004/2005*. National Drug Strategy Monograph Series (No 64). Canberra, Australia, Australian Government Publishing Service.

Conference Board of Canada (1997). Smoking and the bottom line: the costs of smoking in the workplace. Ottawa, Health Canada *(http://www.hc-sc.gc.ca/hl-vs/pubs/tobac-tabac/bottomline-bilan/index-eng.php)*.

Conley Thomson C, Siegel M, Winickoff J, *et al.* (2005). Household smoking bans and adolescents' perceived prevalence of smoking and social acceptability of smoking. *Prev Med*, 41(2):349-356.

Connolly GN, Carpenter C, Hillel R, *et al.* (2005). Evaluation of the Massachusetts smoke-free workplace law. San Francisco, CA, University of California *(http://repositories.cdlib.org/context/tc/article/1180/type/pdf/viewcontent/)*.

Connolly GN, Carpenter CM, Travers M, *et al.* (2006). How smoke-free laws improve air quality: a global study of Irish pubs. Harvard School of Public Health Division of Public Health Practice, Roswell Park Cancer Institute Department of Health Behavior, Health Service Executive-West Environmental Health Department, Research Institute for a Tobacco Free Society, Office of Tobacco Control *(http://www.tobaccofreeair.org/downloads/Irishstudy_3.13.3_final5.pdf)*.

Coppotelli HC, Orleans CT (1985). Partner support and other determinants of smoking cessation maintenance among women. *J Consult Clin Psychol*, 53(4):455-460.

Corti B, Holman C, Donovan R, et al. (1997). Warning: attending a sport, racing or arts venue may be beneficial to your health. Aust N Z J Public Health, 21(4 Spec No):371-376.

Coultas DB, Peake GT, Samet JM (1989). Questionnaire assessment of lifetime and recent exposure to environmental tobacco smoke. Am J Epidemiol, 130(2):338-347.

Cowling DW, Bond P (2005). Smoke-free laws and bar revenues in California--the last call. Health Econ, 14(12):1273-1281.

Crawford FG, Mayer J, Santella RM, et al. (1994). Biomarkers of environmental tobacco smoke in preschool children and their mothers. J Natl Cancer Inst, 86(18):1398-1402.

Cremieux P, Ouellette P (2001). Actual and perceived impacts of tobacco regulation on restaurants and firms. Tob Control, 10:33-37.

Cummings KM, Markello SJ, Mahoney MC, et al. (1989). Measurement of lifetime exposure to passive smoke. Am J Epidemiol, 130(1):122-132.

Cummings KM, Pechacek T, Shopland D (1994). The illegal sale of cigarettes to U.S. minors: estimates by state. Am J Public Health, 84(2):300-302.

Daisey JM, Mahanama KR, Hodgson AT (1998). Toxic volatile organic compounds in simulated environmental tobacco smoke: emission factors for exposure assessment. J Expo Anal Environ Epidemiol, 8(3):313-334.

Darling H, Reeder A (2003). Smoke-free schools? Results of a secondary school smoking policies survey 2002. N Z Med J, 116(1180):U560.

Darling H, Reeder A, Waa A (2006). Implementation of the smoke-free environments act (2003 Amendments) in New Zealand primary schools. Aust N Z J Public Health, 30(1):87.

De Bruin YB, Carrer P, Jantunen M, et al. (2004). Personal carbon monoxide exposure levels: contribution of local sources to exposures and microenvironment concentrations in Milan. J Expo Anal Environ Epidemiol, 14(4):312-322.

Dearlove JV, Bialous SA, Glantz SA (2002). Tobacco industry manipulation of the hospitality industry to maintain smoking in public places. Tob Control, 11(2):94-104.

Dee TS (1999). The complementarity of teen smoking and drinking. J Health Econ, 18(6):769-793.

Deloitte & Touche LLP (2003). The impact of non-smoking ordinances on restaurant financial performance. Washington, DC, Deloitte & Touche LLP.

DeMarini DM (2004). Genotoxicity of tobacco smoke and tobacco smoke condensate: a review. Mutat Res, 567(2-3):447-474.

den Exter Blokland EA, Hale WW, III, Meeus W, et al. (2006). Parental anti-smoking socialization. Associations between parental anti-smoking socialization practices and early adolescent smoking initiation. Eur Addict Res, 12(1):25-32.

DerSimonian R, Laird N (1986). Meta-analysis in clinical trials. Control Clin Trials, 7(3):177-188.

Diez-Roux AV, Nieto F, Comstock G, et al. (1995). The relationship of active and passive smoking to carotid atherosclerosis 12-14 years later. Prev Med, 24(1):48-55.

Dinno A, Glantz S (2007). Clean indoor air laws immediately reduce heart attacks. Prev Med, 45(1):9-11.

Doll R, Hill AB (1950). Smoking and carcinoma of the lung; preliminary report. Br Med J, 2(4682):739-748.

Doll R, Hill AB (1954). The mortality of doctors in relation to their smoking habits; a preliminary report. Br Med J, 1(4877):1451-1455.

Doll R, Peto R (1978). Cigarette smoking and bronchial carcinoma: dose and time relationships among regular smokers and lifelong non-smokers. J Epidemiol Community Health, 32(4):303-313.

Donnan GA, McNeil J, Adena M, et al. (1989). Smoking as a risk factor for cerebral ischaemia. Lancet, 2(8664):643-647.

Drobes DJ, Tiffany ST (1997). Induction of smoking urge through imaginal and in vivo procedures: physiological and self-report manifestations. J Abnorm Psychol, 106(1):15-25.

Dubois G (2005). [Prevention of air pollution by indoor tobacco smoke in France]. Bull Acad Natl Med, 189(5):803-812.

Dunnick JK, Elwell MR, Huff J, et al. (1995). Chemically induced mammary gland cancer in the National Toxicology Program's carcinogenesis bioassay. Carcinogenesis, 16(2):173-179.

Eadie D, Heim D, Macaskill S, et al. (2008). A qualitative analysis of compliance with smoke-free legislation in community bars in Scotland: implications for public health. Addiction, 103(6):1019-1026.

Eagan TM, Hetland J, Aaro LE (2006). Decline in respiratory symptoms in service workers five months after a public smoking ban. Tob Control, 15(3):242-246.

Eaton DK, Kann L, Kinchen S, et al. (2006). Youth risk behavior surveillance--United States, 2005. MMWR Surveill Summ, 55(5):1-108.

Edwards R, Bullen C, O'Dea D, et al. (2007). After the smoke has cleared: evaluation of the impact of a new smokefree law (A report commissioned by the New Zealand Ministry of Health). Tob Control, 1-10.

Edwards R, Thomson G, Wilson N, et al. (2008). After the smoke has cleared: evaluation of the impact of a new national smoke-free law in New Zealand. Tob Control, 17(1):e2.

Eisner MD, Smith AK, Blanc PD (1998). Bartenders' respiratory health after establishment of smoke-free bars and taverns. JAMA, 280(22):1909-1914.

el-Bayoumy K, Chae YH, Upadhyaya P, et al. (1995). Comparative tumorigenicity of benzo[a]pyrene, 1-nitropyrene and 2-amino-1-methyl-6-phenylimidazo[4,5-b]pyridine administered by gavage to female CD rats. Carcinogenesis, 16(2):431-434.

Ellingsen DG, Fladseth G, Daae H, et al. (2006). Airborne exposure and biological monitoring of bar and restaurant workers before and after the introduction of a smoking ban. J Environ Monit, 8(3):362-368.

Emaus A, Lochen M, Hoifodt R (2001). [Application of tobacco smoking regulations in restaurants in Tromso 1998]. Tidsskr Nor Laegeforen, 121(4):410-412.

Emmanuel SC, Phe A, Chen A (1988). The impact of the anti-smoking campaign in Singapore. Singapore Med J, 29(3):233-239.

Emmons KM, Hammond S, Fava J, et al. (2001). A randomized trial to reduce passive smoke exposure in low-income households with young children. Pediatrics, 108(1):18-24.

Emont SL, Choi WS, Novotny TE, et al. (1993). Clean indoor air legislation, taxation, and smoking behavior in the United States: an ecological analysis. Tob Control, 2:13-17.

Engelen M, Farrelly M, Hyland A (2006). The health and economic consequences of New York's Clean Indoor Air Act. Albany, NY, New York State Department of Health *(http://www.health.state.ny.us/prevention/tobacco_control/)*.

Enstrom JE (1979). Rising lung cancer mortality among nonsmokers. *J Natl Cancer Inst*, 62(4):755-760.

Enstrom JE, Kabat GC (2003). Environmental tobacco smoke and tobacco related mortality in a prospective study of Californians, 1960-98. *Br Med J*, 326(7398):1057-1061.

Environics Research Group (2001). *Public support for international efforts to control tobacco: A survey in five countries*. Toronto, Canada, Environics Research Group.

Eriksen MP, Gottlieb NH (1998). A review of the health impact of smoking control at the workplace. *Am J Health Promot*, 13(2):83-104.

Eriksen MP, Chaloupka FJ (2007). The economic Impact of Clean Indoor Air Laws. *CA Cancer J Clin*, 57:367-378.

Escobedo LG, Peddicord JP (1996). Smoking prevalence in US birth cohorts: the influence of gender and education. *Am J Public Health*, 86(2):231-236.

Escoffery C, Kegler M, Butler S (2008). Formative research on creating smoke-free homes in rural communities. *Health Educ Res*,1-11.

European Commission (2007). Attitudes of Europeans toward tobacco [Special Eurobarometer 272c], European Commission *(http://ec.europa.eu/health/ph_publication/eb_health_en.pdf)*.

Evans WN, Farrelly MC, Montgomery E (1999). Do workplace smoking bans reduce smoking? *Am Econ Rev*, 89:728-747.

Ezra D (1994). Sticks and stones can break my bones, but tobacco smoke can kill me: can we protect children from parents that smoke? *Saint Louis Univ Public Health Law Rev*, 13:547-590.

Fagerstrom KO, Schneider NG (1989). Measuring nicotine dependence: a review of the Fagerstrom Tolerance Questionnaire. *J Behav Med*, 12(2):159-182.

Fang J, Gan DK, Zheng SH, et al. (2006). [A case-control study of the risk factors for lung cancer among Chinese women who have never smoked]. *Wei Sheng Yan Jiu*, 35(4):464-467.

Farkas AJ, Pierce JP, Zhu SH, et al. (1996). Addiction versus stages of change models in predicting smoking cessation. *Addiction*, 91(9):1271-1280.

Farkas AJ, Gilpin EA, Distefan JM, et al. (1999). The effects of household and workplace smoking restrictions on quitting behaviours. *Tob Control*, 8(3):261-265.

Farkas AJ, Gilpin EA, White MM, et al. (2000). Association between household and workplace smoking restrictions and adolescent smoking. *JAMA*, 284(6):717-722.

Farrelly MC, Evans WN, Sfekas AE (1999). The impact of workplace smoking bans: results from a national survey. *Tob Control*, 8(3):272-277.

Farrelly MC, Bray J, Zarkin G, et al. (2001). The joint demand for cigarettes and marijuana: evidence from the national household surveys on drug abuse. *J Health Econ*, 20(1):51-68.

Farrelly MC, Niederdeppe J, Yarsevich J (2003). Youth tobacco prevention mass media campaigns: past, present, and future directions. *Tob Control*, 12(Suppl 1):i35-i47.

Farrelly MC, Nonnemaker J, Chou R, et al. (2005). Changes in hospitality workers' exposure to secondhand smoke following the implementation of New York's smoke-free law. *Tob Control*, 14(4):236-241.

Federico B, Costa G, Kunst A (2007). Educational inequalities in initiation, cessation, and prevalence of smoking among 3 Italian birth cohorts. *Am J Public Health*, 97(5):838-845.

Fernandez E, Fu M, Martinez C, et al. (2008). Secondhand smoke in hospitals of Catalonia (Spain) before and after a comprehensive ban on smoking at the national level. *Prev Med*, 47(6):624-628.

Fernandez E, Fu M, Pascual J, et al. (2009). Impact of the Spanish smoking law on exposure to second-hand smoke and respiratory health in hospitality workers: a prospective cohort study. *PLoS ONE*, 4(1):e4244.

Fernando D, Fowles J, Woodward A, et al. (2007). Legislation reduces exposure to second-hand tobacco smoke in New Zealand bars by about 90%. *Tob Control*, 16(4):235-238.

Feyerabend C, Russell MA (1980). Assay of nicotine in biological materials: sources of contamination and their elimination. *J Pharm Pharmacol*, 32(3):178-181.

Fichtenberg CM, Glantz SA (2002). Effect of smoke-free workplaces on smoking behaviour: systematic review. *Br Med J*, 325(7357):188-191.

Fidan F, Guven H, Eminoglu O, et al. (2005). Turkish coffeehouse kahvehane is an important tobacco smoke exposure area in Turkey. *J Toxicol Environ Health A*, 68(16):1371-1377.

Fielding JE (1991). Smoking control at the workplace. *Annu Rev Public Health*, 12:209-234.

Filippini G, Maisonneuve P, McCredie M, et al. (2002). Relation of childhood brain tumors to exposure of parents and children to tobacco smoke: the SEARCH international case-control study. Surveillance of Environmental Aspects Related to Cancer in Humans. *Int J Cancer*, 100(2):206-213.

Fisher LB, Winickoff JP, Camargo CA Jr, et al. (2007). Household smoking restrictions and adolescent smoking. *Am J Health Promot*, 22(1):15-21.

Flanders WD, Lally CA, Zhu BP, et al. (2003). Lung cancer mortality in relation to age, duration of smoking, and daily cigarette consumption: results from Cancer Prevention Study II. *Cancer Res*, 63(19):6556-6562.

Flight Attendants Medical Research Institute (1991). *(http://www.famri.org/intro/)*.

Fong GT, Hyland A, Borland R, et al. (2006). Reductions in tobacco smoke pollution and increases in support for smoke-free public places following the implementation of comprehensive smoke-free workplace legislation in the Republic of Ireland: findings from the ITC Ireland/UK Survey. *Tob Control*, 15(Suppl 3):iii51-iii58.

Fontham ET, Correa P, Reynolds P, et al. (1994). Environmental tobacco smoke and lung cancer in nonsmoking women. A multicenter study. *JAMA*, 271(22):1752-1759.

Ford L (2008). Thank you for smoking -- in a hut. *Chicago Tribune*.

Franco-Marina F. (2008). Personal communication to E. Khaykin and J. Samet.

Franco-Marina F, Villalba-Caloca J, Corcho-Berdugo A (2006). Role of active and passive smoking on lung cancer etiology in Mexico City. *Salud Publica Mex*, 48(Suppl 1):S75-S82.

Frieden TR, Mostashari F, Kerker B, et al. (2005). Adult tobacco use levels after intensive tobacco control measures: New York City, 2002-2003. *Am J Public Health,* 95(6):1016-1023.

Friend K, Levy D (2002). Reductions in smoking prevalence and cigarette consumption associated with mass-media campaigns. *Health Educ Res,* 17(1):85-98.

Friis RH, Safer AM (2005). Analysis of responses of Long Beach, California residents to the smoke-free bars law. *Public Health,* 119(12):1116-1121.

Fukuda K, Shibata A (1990). Exposure-response relationships between woodworking, smoking or passive smoking, and squamous cell neoplasms of the maxillary sinus. *Cancer Causes Control,* 1(2):165-168.

Galan I, Mata N, Estrada C, et al. (2007). Impact of the "tobacco control law" on exposure to environmental tobacco smoke in Spain. *BMC Public Health,* 7(147):224.

Galeone D, Laurendi G, Vasselli S, et al. (2006). Preliminary effects of Italy's ban on smoking in enclosed public places. *Tob Control,* 15(2):143.

Gallet GA, Eastman HS (2007). The impact of smoking bans on alcohol demand. *Soc Sci J,* 44(4):664-676.

Gallicchio L, Kouzis A, Genkinger J, et al. (2006). Active cigarette smoking, household passive smoke exposure, and the risk of developing pancreatic cancer. *Prev Med,* 42(3):200-205.

Gallus S, Pacifici R, Colombo P, et al. (2006). Prevalence of smoking and attitude towards smoking regulation in Italy, 2004. *Eur J Cancer Prev,* 15(1):77-81.

Gallus S, Zuccaro P, Colombo P, et al. (2007). Smoking in Italy 2005-2006: effects of a comprehensive National Tobacco Regulation. *Prev Med,* 45(2-3):198-201.

Gammon MD, Eng SM, Teitelbaum SL, et al. (2004). Environmental tobacco smoke and breast cancer incidence. *Environ Res,* 96(2):176-185.

Garfinkel L (1981). Time trends in lung cancer mortality among nonsmokers and a note on passive smoking. *J Natl Cancer Inst,* 66(6):1061-1066.

Garland C, Barrett-Connor E, Suarez L, et al. (1985). Effects of passive smoking on ischemic heart disease mortality of nonsmokers. A prospective study. *Am J Epidemiol,* 121(5):645-650.

Garvey AJ, Bliss RE, Hitchcock JL, et al. (1992). Predictors of smoking relapse among self-quitters: a report from the Normative Aging Study. *Addict Behav,* 17(4):367-377.

Gasparrini A, Gorini G, Marcolina D, et al. (2006). [Second-hand smoke exposure in Florence and Belluno before and after the Italian smoke-free legislation]. *Epidemiol Prev,* 30(6):348-351.

Gee IL, Watson A, Carrington J, et al. (2006). Second-hand smoke levels in UK pubs and bars: do the English Public Health White Paper proposals go far enough? *J Public Health (Oxf),* 28(1):17-23.

Gehrman CA, Hovell MF (2003). Protecting children from environmental tobacco smoke (ETS) exposure: a critical review. *Nicotine Tob Res,* 5(3):289-301.

Georgiadis P, Stoikidou M, Topinka J, et al. (2001a). Personal exposures to PM(2.5) and polycyclic aromatic hydrocarbons and their relationship to environmental tobacco smoke at two locations in Greece. *J Expo Anal Environ Epidemiol,* 11(3):169-183.

Georgiadis P, Topinka J, Stoikidou M, et al. (2001b). Biomarkers of genotoxicity of air pollution (the AULIS project): bulky DNA adducts in subjects with moderate to low exposures to airborne polycyclic aromatic hydrocarbons and their relationship to environmental tobacco smoke and other parameters. *Carcinogenesis,* 22(9):1447-1457.

Giles-Corti B, Clarkson J, Donovan R, et al. (2001). Creating smoke-free environments in recreational settings. *Health Educ Behav,* 28(3):341-351.

Gillespie J, Milne K, Wilson N (2005). Secondhand smoke in New Zealand homes and cars: exposure, attitudes, and behaviours in 2004. *N Z Med J,* 118(1227):U1782.

Gilpin E, Pierce J (1994). Measuring smoking cessation: problems with recall in the 1990 California Tobacco Survey. *Cancer Epidemiol Biomarkers Prev,* 3(7):613-617.

Gilpin EA, Pierce JP (2002a). Demographic differences in patterns in the incidence of smoking cessation: United States 1950-1990. *Ann Epidemiol,* 12(3):141-150.

Gilpin EA, Pierce J (2002b). The California tobacco control program and potential harm reduction through reduced cigarette consumption in continuing smokers. *Nicotine Tob Res,* 4(Suppl 2):S157-S166.

Gilpin EA, Pierce J, Cavin S, et al. (1994). Estimates of population smoking prevalence: self vs proxy reports of smoking status. *Am J Public Health,* 84(10):1576-1579.

Gilpin EA, Pierce JP, Farkas AJ (1997). Duration of smoking abstinence and success in quitting. *J Natl Cancer Inst,* 89(8):572-576.

Gilpin EA, White MM, Farkas AJ, et al. (1999). Home smoking restrictions: which smokers have them and how they are associated with smoking behavior. *Nicotine Tob Res,* 1(2):153-162.

Gilpin EA, Stillman F, Hartman A, et al. (2000). Index for US state tobacco control initial outcomes. *Am J Epidemiol,* 152(8):727-738.

Gilpin EA, Emery S, Farkas A, et al. (2001). *The California tobacco control program: a decade of progress. Results from the California Tobacco Survey, 1990-1999.* La Jolla, CA, University of California, San Diego (http://ssdc.ucsd.edu/).

Gilpin EA, Farkas A, Emery S, et al. (2002). Clean indoor air: advances in California, 1990-1999. *Am J Public Health,* 92(5):785-791.

Gilpin EA, White M, White V, et al. (2003). *Tobacco control successes in California: A focus on young people, results from the California Tobacco surveys, 1990-2002.* La Jolla, CA; University of California, San Diego (http://libraries.ucsd.edu/ssds/pub/CTS/cpc00007/2002FINAL_RPT.pdf).

Gilpin EA, Lee L, Pierce J, et al. (2004). Support for protection from secondhand smoke: California 2002. *Tob Control,* 13(1):96.

Gilpin EA, Messer K, Pierce JP (2006). Population effectiveness of pharmaceutical aids for smoking cessation: what is associated with increased success? *Nicotine Tob Res,* 8(5):661-669.

Glantz SA (2007). Commentary: Assessing the effects of the Scottish Smokefree Law--the placebo effect and the importance of obtaining unbiased data. *Int J Epidemiol,* 36(1):155-156.

Glantz SA, Smith LRA (1994). The effect of ordinances requiring smoke-free restaurants on restaurant sales. *Am J Public Health,* 84(7):1081-1085.

Glantz SA, Parmley WW (1995). Passive smoking and heart disease. Mechanisms and risk. *JAMA*, 273(13):1047-1053.

Glantz SA, Smith LRA (1997). The effect of ordinances requiring smoke-free restaurants and bars on revenues: A follow up. *Am J Public Health*, 87(10):1687-1693.

Glantz SA, Charlesworth A (1999). Tourism and hotel revenues before and after passage of smoke-free restaurant ordinances. *JAMA*, 281(20):1911-1918.

Glantz SA, Balbach ED (2000). *Tobacco war: inside the California battles.* Berkeley, CA, University of California Press *(http:// escholarship.cdlib.org/ucpress/tobacco-war. xml).*

Glantz SA, Wilson-Loots R (2003). No association of smoke-free ordinances with profits from bingo and charitable games in Massachusetts. *Tob Control*, 12:411-413.

Glantz SA, Alamar B (2005). Correction for Mandel L, Alamar BC, Glantz SA: Smoke-free law did not affect revenue from gaming in Delaware. *Tob Control*, 14:360.

Glantz SA, Barnes DE, Bero L, et al. (1995). Looking through a keyhole at the tobacco industry. The Brown and Williamson documents. *JAMA*, 274(3):219-224.

Glaser SL, Keegan TH, Clarke CA, et al. (2004). Smoking and Hodgkin lymphoma risk in women United States. *Cancer Causes Control*, 15(4):387-397.

Glasgow RE, Cummings KM, Hyland A (1997). Relationship of worksite smoking policy to changes in employee tobacco use: findings from COMMIT. Community Intervention Trial for Smoking Cessation. *Tob Control*, 6(Suppl 2):S44-S48.

Glasgow RE, Boles S, Lichtenstein E, et al. (2004). Adoption, reach, and implementation of a novel smoking control program: analysis of a public utility-research organization partnership. *Nicotine Tob Res*, 6(2):269-274.

Goldstein AO, Sobel RA (1998). Environmental tobacco smoke regulations have not hurt restaurant sales in North Carolina. *N C Med J*, 59(5):284-287.

Gonzales M, Malcoe L, Kegler M, et al. (2006). Prevalence and predictors of home and automobile smoking bans and child environmental tobacco smoke exposure: a cross-sectional study of U.S.- and Mexico-born Hispanic women with young children. *BMC Public Health*, 6:265.

Goodman MT, Tung KH (2003). Active and passive tobacco smoking and the risk of borderline and invasive ovarian cancer (United States). *Cancer Causes Control*, 14(6):569-577.

Goodman P, Agnew M, McCaffrey M, et al. (2007). Effects of the Irish smoking ban on respiratory health of bar workers and air quality in Dublin pubs. *Am J Respir Crit Care Med*, 175:840-845.

Gorini G, Fondelli M, Lopez M, et al. (2004). [Environmental tobacco smoke exposure in public places in Florence, Italy]. *Epidemiol Prev*, 28(2):94-99.

Gower KB, Burns DM, Shanks TG, et al. (2000). Workplace smoking restrictions, rules about smoking in the home, and attitudes toward smoking restrictions in public places. In: Shopland DR, Hobart R, Burns DM, et al., eds., *State and local legislative action to reduce tobacco use.* Bethesda, MD, U.S. Department of Health and Human Services, National Institutes of Health, National Cancer Institute. Smoking and Tobacco Control Monograph No. 11; 187-340.

Greenberg RA, Strecher V, Bauman K, et al. (1994). Evaluation of a home-based intervention program to reduce infant passive smoking and lower respiratory illness. *J Behav Med*, 17(3):273-290.

Griesbach D, Inchley J, Currie C (2002). More than words? The status and impact of smoking policies in Scottish schools. *Health Promot Int*, 17(1):31-41.

Groner JA, Ahijevych K, Grossman LK, et al. (2000). The impact of a brief intervention on maternal smoking behavior. *Pediatrics*, 105(1 Pt 3):267-271.

Groner JA, Hoshaw-Woodard S, Koren G, et al. (2005). Screening for children's exposure to environmental tobacco smoke in a pediatric primary care setting. *Arch Pediatr Adolesc Med*, 159(5):450-455.

GTSS Collaborative Group (2006). A cross country comparison of exposure to secondhand smoke among youth. *Tob Control*, 15(Suppl 2): ii4-ii19.

Gupta R, Dwyer J (2001). Focus groups with smokers to develop a smoke-free home campaign. *Am J Health Behav*, 25(6):564-571.

Hackshaw A (2003). Passive smoking: paper does not diminish conclusion of previous reports. *Br Med J*, 327(7413):501-502.

Hackshaw AK, Law MR, Wald NJ (1997). The accumulated evidence on lung cancer and environmental tobacco smoke. *Br Med J*, 315(7114):980-988.

Hahn E, Rayens M, York N, et al. (2006). Effects of a smoke-free law on hair nicotine and respiratory symptoms of restaurant and bar workers. *J Occup Environ Med*, 48(9):906-913.

Hallamore C (2006). *Smoking and the bottom line: updating the costs of smoking in the workplace.* Ontario, Canada, Conference Board of Canada *(http://www.conferenceboard. ca/documents.asp?rnext=1754).*

Halterman JS, Fagnano M, Conn K, et al. (2006). Do parents of urban children with persistent asthma ban smoking in their homes and cars? *Ambul Pediatr*, 6(2):115-119.

Hamajima N, Hirose K, Tajima K, et al. (2002). Alcohol, tobacco and breast cancer--collaborative reanalysis of individual data from 53 epidemiological studies, including 58,515 women with breast cancer and 95,067 women without the disease. *Br J Cancer*, 87(11):1234-1245.

Hammond D, McDonald P, Fong G, et al. (2004). The impact of cigarette warning labels and smoke-free bylaws on smoking cessation: evidence from former smokers. *Can J Public Health*, 95(3):201-204.

Hammond D, Fong G, Zanna M, et al. (2006). Tobacco denormalization and industry beliefs among smokers from four countries. *Am J Prev Med*, 31(3):225-232.

Hammond EC, Horn D (1954). The relationship between human smoking habits and death rates. *JAMA*, 155:1316-1328.

Hammond SK (1999). Exposure of U.S. workers to environmental tobacco smoke. *Environ Health Perspect*, 107(Suppl 2):329-340.

Hammond SK, Emmons KM (2005). Inmate exposure to secondhand smoke in correctional facilities and the impact of smoking restrictions. *J Expo Anal Environ Epidemiol*, 15(3):205-211.

Harakeh Z, Scholte R, de Vries H, et al. (2005). Parental rules and communication: their association with adolescent smoking. Addiction, 100(6):862-870.

Hassan MM, Abbruzzese J, Bondy M, et al. (2007). Passive smoking and the use of noncigarette tobacco products in association with risk for pancreatic cancer: a case-control study. Cancer, 109(12):2547-2556.

Hatsukami DK, Le C, Zhang Y, et al. (2006). Toxicant exposure in cigarette reducers versus light smokers. Cancer Epidemiol Biomarkers Prev, 15(12):2355-2358.

Hatziandreu EJ, Pierce J, Fiore M, et al. (1989). The reliability of self-reported cigarette consumption in the United States. Am J Public Health, 79(8):1020-1023.

Haw SJ, Gruer L (2007). Changes in exposure of adult non-smokers to secondhand smoke after implementation of smoke-free legislation in Scotland: national cross sectional survey. Br Med J (Clin Res Ed), 335(7619):549-552.

Haw SJ, Gruer L, Amos A, et al. (2006). Legislation on smoking in enclosed public places in Scotland: how will we evaluate the impact? J Public Health (Oxf), 28(1):24-30.

Health Canada (2006). Canadian Tobacco Use Monitoring Survey (CTUMS) 2006. Ottawa, Health Canada (http://www.hc-sc.gc.ca/hl-vs/tobac-tabac/research-recherche/stat/ctums-esutc_2006_e.html).

Healton CG, Vallone D, Martyak J, et al. (2007). Using social marketing to increase the prevalence of voluntary smoking bans in the home and car. (Austin TX. SYM7C). Austin, TX, Society for Research on Nicotine and Tobacco.

Hecht SS (2002). Human urinary carcinogen metabolites: biomarkers for investigating tobacco and cancer. Carcinogenesis, 23(6):907-922.

Hecht SS (2003). Tobacco carcinogens, their biomarkers and tobacco-induced cancer. Nat Rev Cancer, 3(10):733-744.

Hecht SS, Hoffmann D (1988). Tobacco-specific nitrosamines, an important group of carcinogens in tobacco and tobacco smoke. Carcinogenesis, 9(6):875-884.

Hedley AJ, Mcghee S, Repace J, et al. (2006). Risks for heart disease and lung cancer from passive smoking by workers in the catering industry. Toxicol Sci, 90(2):539-548.

Helakorpi S, Martelin T, Torppa J, et al. (2004). Did Finland's tobacco control act of 1976 have an impact on ever smoking? An examination based on male and female cohort trends. J Epidemiol Community Health, 58(8):649-654.

Helakorpi S, Martelin T, Torppa J, et al. (2008). Impact of the 1976 tobacco control act in Finland on the proportion of ever daily smokers by socioeconomic status. Prev Med, (4):340-345.

Helgason AR, Lund KE (2001). Environmental tobacco smoke exposure of young children--attitudes and health-risk awareness in the Nordic countries. Nicotine Tob Res, 3(4):341-345.

Hellberg D, Valentin J, Nilsson S (1986). Smoking and cervical intraepithelial neoplasia. An association independent of sexual and other risk factors? Acta Obstet Gynecol Scand, 65(6):625-631.

Heloma A, Jaakkola M (2003). Four-year follow-up of smoke exposure, attitudes and smoking behaviour following enactment of Finland's national smoke-free work-place law. Addiction, 98(8):1111-1117.

Heloma A, Jaakkola M, Kahkonen E, et al. (2001). The short-term impact of national smoke-free workplace legislation on passive smoking and tobacco use. Am J Public Health, 91(9):1416-1418.

Henderson FW, Reid HF, Morris R, et al. (1989). Home air nicotine levels and urinary cotinine excretion in preschool children. Am Rev Respir Dis, 140(1):197-201.

Henriksen L, Jackson C (1998). Anti-smoking socialization: relationship to parent and child smoking status. Health Commun, 10(1):87-101.

Hernandez-Mezquita M, Barrueco M, Jimenez-Ruiz C, et al. (2000). [Extent of law compliance and anti-smoking teaching at Spanish schools]. Rev Esp Salud Pública, 74(5-6):537-547.

Hetland J, Aaro L (2005). [Smoking status, attitudes towards and reported compliance with the ban on smoking at hospitality venues - a prospective panel study]. Oslo, Norway, Statens Institutt for Rusmiddelforskning. Report No. 2 (http://www.sirus.no/files/pub/201SIRUSskrifter0205.pdf).

Hill AB (1965). The environment and disease: association or causation? Proc R Soc Med, 58:295-300.

Hill D, Borland R (1991). Adults' accounts of onset of regular smoking: influences of school, work, and other settings. Public Health Rep, 106(2):181-185.

Hill SE, Blakely T, Kawachi I, et al. (2007). Mortality among lifelong nonsmokers exposed to secondhand smoke at home: cohort data and sensitivity analyses. Am J Epidemiol, 165(5):530-540.

Hinds WC (1982). Aerosol technology: properties, behavior, and measurement of airborne particles. New York, John Wiley & Sons.

Hirayama T (1981). Non-smoking wives of heavy smokers have a higher risk of lung cancer: a study from Japan. Br Med J (Clin Res Ed), 282(6259):183-185.

Hirayama T (1984). Cancer mortality in nonsmoking women with smoking husbands based on a large-scale cohort study in Japan. Prev Med, 13(6):680-690.

Hirayama T (1985). Passive smoking--a new target of epidemiology. Tokai J Exp Clin Med, 10(4):287-293.

Hirose K, Tajima K, Hamajima N, et al. (1995). A large-scale, hospital-based case-control study of risk factors of breast cancer according to menopausal status. Jpn J Cancer Res, 86(2):146-154.

Hirose K, Tajima K, Hamajima N, et al. (1996). Subsite (cervix/endometrium)-specific risk and protective factors in uterus cancer. Jpn J Cancer Res, 87(9):1001-1009.

Holm AL, Davis RM (2004). Clearing the airways: advocacy and regulation for smoke-free airlines. Tob Control, 13(Suppl 1):i30-i36.

Hopkins DP, Briss PA, Ricard CJ, et al. (2001). Reviews of evidence regarding interventions to reduce tobacco use and exposure to environmental tobacco smoke. Am J Prev Med, 20(2 Suppl):16-66.

Horwitz MB, Hindi-Alexander M, Wagner TJ (1985). Psychosocial mediators of abstinence, relapse, and continued smoking: a one-year follow-up of a minimal intervention. Addict Behav, 10(1):29-39.

Hovell MF, Zakarian J, Matt G, et al. (2000). Effect of counseling mothers on their children's exposure to environmental tobacco smoke: randomised controlled trial. Br Med J, 321(7257):337-342.

Hovell MF, Meltzer S, Wahlgren D, et al. (2002). Asthma management and environmental tobacco smoke exposure reduction in Latino children: a controlled trial. Pediatrics, 110(5):946-956.

Howard G, Burke G, Szklo M, et al. (1994). Active and passive smoking are associated with increased carotid wall thickness. The atherosclerosis risk in communities study. Arch Intern Med, 154(11):1277-1282.

Howard G, Wagenknecht L, Burke G, et al. (1998). Cigarette smoking and progression of atherosclerosis: the Atherosclerosis Risk in Communities (ARIC) study. JAMA, 279(2):119-124.

Howell F (2004). Ireland's workplaces, going smoke free. Br Med J, 328(7444):847-848.

Hu J, Mao Y, Ugnat AM (2000). Parental cigarette smoking, hard liquor consumption and the risk of childhood brain tumors--a case-control study in northeast China. Acta Oncol, 39(8):979-984.

Hughes SC, Corcos IA, Hofstetter CR, et al. (2008). Children's exposure to secondhand smoke at home in Seoul, Korea. Asian Pac J Cancer Prev, 9(3):491-495.

Hurley SF, McNeil JJ, Donnan GA, et al. (1996). Tobacco smoking and alcohol consumption as risk factors for glioma: a case-control study in Melbourne, Australia. J Epidemiol Community Health, 50(4):442-446.

Hyland A, Cummings K (1999). Restaurateur reports of the economic impact of the New York City Smoke-free Air Act. J Public Health Manag Pract, 5(1):37-42.

Hyland A, Cummings K, Nauenberg E (1999). Analysis of taxable sales receipts: was New York City's Smoke-free Air Act bad for business? J Public Health Manag Pract, 5(1):14-21.

Hyland A, Travers M, Dresler C, et al. (2008a). A 32-country comparison of tobacco smoke derived particle levels in indoor public places. Tob Control, 17(3):159-165.

Hyland A, Higbee C, Hassan L, et al. (2008b). Does smoke-free Ireland have more smoking inside the home and less in pubs than the United Kingdom? Findings from the International Tobacco Control Policy Evaluation Project. Eur J Public Health, 18(1):63-65.

Hyland A, Higbee C, Travers MJ, et al. (2009). Smoke-free homes and smoking cessation and relapse in a longitudinal population of adults. Nicotine Tob Res,.

IARC (1986). IARC Monographs on the Evaluation of Carcinogenic Risks to Humans, Vol. 38, Tobacco Smoke and Involuntary Smoking. Lyon, IARC Press.

IARC (2004). IARC Monographs on the Evaluation of Carcinogenic Risks to Humans, Vol. 83, Tobacco Smoke and Involuntary Smoking. Lyon, International Agency for Research on Cancer.

IARC (2008). IARC Handbooks of Cancer Prevention, Tobacco Control, Vol. 12: Methods for Evaluating Tobacco Control Policies. Lyon, International Agency for Research on Cancer.

Institute of Medicine (2001). Clearing the smoke: assessing the science base for tobacco harm reduction. Washington DC, National Academy Press.

Invernizzi G, Ruprecht A, Mazza R, et al. (2002). [Real-time measurement of indoor particulate matter originating from environmental tobacco smoke: a pilot study]. Epidemiol Prev, 26(1):30-34.

Jaakkola MS, Jaakkola JJ (1997). Assessment of exposure to environmental tobacco smoke. Eur Respir J, 10(10):2384-2397.

Jackson C, Henriksen L (1997). Do as I say: parent smoking, antismoking socialization, and smoking onset among children. Addict Behav, 22(1):107-114.

Jackson C, Dickinson D (2003). Can parents who smoke socialise their children against smoking? Results from the smoke-free kids intervention trial. Tob Control, 12(1):52-59.

Jarvis MJ, Goddard E, Higgins V, et al. (2000). Children's exposure to passive smoking in England since the 1980s: cotinine evidence from population surveys. Br Med J, 321(7257):343-345.

Javitz HS, Zbikowski S, Swan G, et al. (2006). Financial burden of tobacco use: an employer's perspective. Clin Occup Environ Med, 5(1):9-29, vii.

Jee SH, Ohrr H, Kim IS (1999). Effects of husbands' smoking on the incidence of lung cancer in Korean women. Int J Epidemiol, 28(5):824-828.

Jenkins RA, Maskarinec M, Counts R, et al. (2001). Environmental tobacco smoke in an unrestricted smoking workplace: area and personal exposure monitoring. J Expo Anal Environ Epidemiol, 11(5):369-380.

Jha P, Chaloupka F (1999). Curbing the epidemic. Washington, DC, The World Bank (http://www1.worldbank.org/tobacco/book/html/cover2a.html).

Ji M, Hofstetter C, Hovell M, et al. (2005). Smoking cessation patterns and predictors among adult Californians of Korean descent. Nicotine Tob Res, 7(1):59-69.

Jiang X, Yuan JM, Skipper PL, et al. (2007). Environmental tobacco smoke and bladder cancer risk in never smokers of Los Angeles County. Cancer Res, 67(15):7540-7545.

Johansson A, Hermansson G, Ludvigsson J (2004). How should parents protect their children from environmental tobacco-smoke exposure in the home? Pediatrics, 113(4):e291-e295.

Johnson KC (2005). Accumulating evidence on passive and active smoking and breast cancer risk. Int J Cancer, 117(4):619-628.

Johnsson T, Tuomi T, Riuttala H, et al. (2006). Environmental tobacco smoke in Finnish restaurants and bars before and after smoking restrictions were introduced. Ann Occup Hyg, 50(4):331-341.

Jones K, Wakefield M, Turnball D (1999). Attitudes and experiences of restaurateurs regarding smoking bans in Adelaide, South Australia. Tob Control, 8(1):62-66.

Joseph AM, Knapp JM, Nichol KL, et al. (1995). Determinants of compliance with a national smoke-free hospital standard. JAMA, 274(6):491-494.

Junker MH, Danuser B, Monn C, et al. (2001). Acute sensory responses of nonsmokers at very low environmental tobacco smoke concentrations in controlled laboratory settings. Environ Health Perspect, 109(10):1045-1052.

Juster HR, Loomis BR, Hinman TM, et al. (2007). Declines in hospital admissions for acute myocardial infarction in New York State after implementation of a comprehensive smoking ban. Am J Public Health, 97(11):2035-2039.

Kaiserman MJ (1997). The cost of smoking in Canada, 1991. Chronic Dis Can, 18(1):13-19.

Kallio K, Jokinen E, Raitakari O, et al. (2007). Tobacco smoke exposure is associated with attenuated endothelial function in 11-year-old healthy children. Circulation, 115(25):3205-3212.

Kandel DB, Wu P (1995). The contributions of mothers and fathers to the inter-generational transmission of cigarette smoking in adolescence. J Res Adolesc, 5:225-252.

Kang JM, Jiang Y, Lin XG, *et al.* (2007). [Study on the level of tobacco-generated smoke in several restaurants and bars in Beijing, China]. *Zhonghua liu xing bing xue za zhi,* 28(8):738-741.

Keeler TE, Hu T, Barnett P, *et al.* (1993). Taxation, regulation, and addiction: a demand function for cigarettes based on time-series evidence. *J Health Econ,* 12(1):1-18.

Kegler MC, Malcoe LH (2002). Smoking restrictions in the home and car among rural Native American and white families with young children. *Prev Med,* 35(4):334-342.

Kegler MC, Escoffery C, Groff A, *et al.* (2007). A qualitative study of how families decide to adopt household smoking restrictions. *Fam Community Health,* 30(4):328-341.

Kegler MC, Escoffery C, Butler S (2008). A qualitative study on establishing and enforcing smoking rules in family cars. Nicotine *Tob Res,* 10(3):493-497.

Kellogg JH (1922). *Tobaccoism, or, how tobacco kills.* Battle Creek, Michigan, The Modern Medicine Publishing Company.

Kennett L. (1987). GI: *The American soldier in World War II.* New York, NY, Scribner.

Kessler G (2006). Civil Action #99-2496. USA vs. Philip Morris Inc.

Khuder SA, Milz S, Jordan T, *et al.* (2007). The impact of a smoking ban on hospital admissions for coronary heart disease. *Prev Med,* 45(1):3-8.

King G, Mallett R, Kozlowski L, *et al.* (2005). Personal space smoking restrictions among African Americans. *Am J Prev Med,* 28(1):33-40.

Kinne S, Kristal A, White E, *et al.* (1993). Work-site smoking policies: their population impact in Washington State. *Am J Public Health,* 83(7):1031-1033.

Klein EG, Forster JL, McFadden B, *et al.* (2007). Minnesota tobacco-free park policies: Attitudes of the general public and park officials. *Nicotine Tob Res,* 9(Suppl 1):S49-S55.

Klepeis NE, Ott WR, Repace JL (1999). The effect of cigar smoking on indoor levels of carbon monoxide and particles. *J Expo Anal Environ Epidemiol,* 9(6):622-635.

Klepeis NE, Ott WR, Switzer P (2007). Real-time measurement of outdoor tobacco smoke particles. *J Air Waste Manag Assoc,* 57(5):522-534.

Klerman L (2004). Protecting children: reducing their environmental tobacco smoke exposure. *Nicotine Tob Res,* 6(Suppl 2):S239-S253.

Kluger R (1996). *Ashes to ashes: America's hundred-year cigarette war, the public health, and the unabashed triumph of Philip Morris.* New York, NY, Alfred A. Knopf.

Kodl MM, Mermelstein R (2004). Beyond modeling: parenting practices, parental smoking history, and adolescent cigarette smoking. *Addict Behav,* 29(1):17-32.

Komro KA, McCarty MC, Forster JL, *et al.* (2003). Parental, family, and home characteristics associated with cigarette smoking among adolescents. *Am J Health Promot,* 17(5):291-299.

KPMG (1998). The impact of California's smoking ban on bars, taverns and night clubs: a survey of owners and managers. Washington, DC, The American Beverage Institute *(http://www.tobaccoscam.ucsf.edu/pdf/068-KPMG.pdf).*

KPMG (2001). Proposed smoking ban: impacts on Hong Kong hospitality businesses. Hong Kong Catering Industry Association *(http://www.tobaccoscam.ucsf.edu/pdf/089-HongKongHospitality.pdf).*

Kumar R, O'Malley P, Johnston L (2005). School tobacco control policies related to students' smoking and attitudes toward smoking: national survey results, 1999-2000. *Health Educ Behav,* 32(6):780-794.

Kunyk D, Els C, Predy G, *et al.* (2007). Development and introduction of a comprehensive tobacco control policy in a Canadian regional health authority. *Prev Chronic Dis,* 4:A30.

Kurahashi N, Inoue M, Liu Y, *et al.* (2008). Passive smoking and lung cancer in Japanese non-smoking women: a prospective study. *Int J Cancer,* 122(3):653-657.

Kuusimaki L, Peltonen K, Vainiotalo S (2007). Assessment of environmental tobacco smoke exposure of Finnish restaurant workers, using 3-ethenylpyridine as marker. *Indoor Air,* 17(5):394-403.

LaKind JS, Jenkins RA, Naiman DQ, *et al.* (1999). Use of environmental tobacco smoke constituents as markers for exposure. *Risk Anal,* 19(3):359-373.

Lal A, Siahpush M, Scollo M (2003). The economic impact of smoke-free policies on sales in restaurants and cafés in Victoria. *Aust N Z J Public Health,* 27(5):557-558.

Lal A, Siahpush M, Scollo M (2004). The economic impact of smoke-free legislation on sales turnover in restaurants and pubs in Tasmania. *Tob Control,* 13(4):454-455.

Lal A, Siahpush M (2008). The effect of smoke-free policies on electronic gaming machine expenditure in Victoria, Australia. *J Epidemiol Community Health,* 62(1):11-15.

Lam TH, Janghorbani M, Hedley AJ, *et al.* (2002). Public opinion on smoke-free policies in restaurants and predicted effect on patronage in Hong Kong. *Tob Control,* 11(3):195-200.

Laugesen M, Swinburn B (2000). New Zealand's tobacco control programme 1985-1998. *Tob Control,* 9(2):155-162.

Lawn S, Pols R (2005). Smoking bans in psychiatric inpatient settings? A review of the research. *Aust N Z J Psychiatry,* 39(10):866-885.

Lazcano-Ponce E, Benowitz N, Sanchez-Zamorano L, *et al.* (2007). Secondhand smoke exposure in Mexican discotheques. *Nicotine Tob Res,* 9(10):1021-1026.

Leaderer BP, Hammond SK (1991). Evaluation of vapour-phase nicotine and respirable suspended particle mass as markers for environmental tobacco smoke. *Environ Sci Technol,* 25(4):770-777.

Leatherdale ST, Smith P, Ahmed R (2008). Youth exposure to smoking in the home and in cars: how often does it happen and what do youth think about it? *Tob Control,* 17(2):86-92.

Lee CW, Kahende J (2007). Factors associated with successful smoking cessation in the United States, 2000. *Am J Public Health,* 97(8):1503-1509.

Lee K, Hahn E, Riker C, *et al.* (2007). Immediate impact of smoke-free laws on indoor air quality. *South Med J,* 100(9):885-889.

Lee LY, Gerhardstein DC, Wang AL, *et al.* (1993). Nicotine is responsible for airway irritation evoked by cigarette smoke inhalation in men. *J Appl Physiol,* 75(5):1955-1961.

Lee PN (1988). *Misclassification of smoking habits and passive smoking*. Berlin, Springer Verlag.

Lee PN (1998). Difficulties in assessing the relationship between passive smoking and lung cancer. *Stat Methods Med Res*, 7(2):137-163.

Lee PN, Chamberlain J, Alderson MR (1986). Relationship of passive smoking to risk of lung cancer and other smoking-associated diseases. *Br J Cancer*, 54(1):97-105.

Lee SC, Chan LY, Chiu MY (1999). Indoor and outdoor air quality investigation at 14 public places in Hong Kong. *Environ Int*, 22:443-450.

Lemstra M, Neudorf C, Opondo J (2008). Implications of a public smoking ban. *Can J Public Health*, 99(1):62-65.

Leung GM, Ho LM, Lam TH (2004). Secondhand smoke exposure, smoking hygiene, and hospitalization in the first 18 months of life. *Arch Pediatr Adolesc Med*, 158(7):687-693.

Levin ML, Goldstein H, Gerhardt PR (1950). Cancer and tobacco smoking. *JAMA*, 143:336-338.

Levy DT, Friend KB (2003). The effects of clean indoor air laws: what do we know and what do we need to know? *Health Educ Res*, 18(5):592-609.

Lewit EM, Hyland A, Kerrebrock N, *et al.* (1997). Price, public policy, and smoking in young people. *Tob Control*, 6(Suppl 2):S17-S24.

Li D, Wang M, Dhingra K, *et al.* (1996). Aromatic DNA adducts in adjacent tissues of breast cancer patients: clues to breast cancer etiology. *Cancer Res*, 56(2):287-293.

Li WM, Lee SC, Chan LY (2001). Indoor air quality at nine shopping malls in Hong Kong. *Sci Total Environ*, 273(1-3):27-40.

Lichtenstein E, Andrews J, Lee M, *et al.* (2000). Using radon risk to motivate smoking reduction: evaluation of written materials and brief telephone counseling. *Tob Control*, 9(3):320-326.

Lilla C, Verla-Tebit E, Risch A, *et al.* (2006). Effect of NAT1 and NAT2 genetic polymorphisms on colorectal cancer risk associated with exposure to tobacco smoke and meat consumption. *Cancer Epidemiol Biomarkers Prev*, 15(1):99-107.

Lissowska J, Brinton LA, Zatonski W, *et al.* (2006). Tobacco smoking, NAT2 acetylation genotype and breast cancer risk. *Int J Cancer*, 119(8):1961-1969.

Lissowska J, Brinton LA, Garcia-Closas M (2007). Re: more data regarding the effects of passive smoking on breast cancer risk among younger women. *Int J Cancer*, 120(11):2517-2518.

Little CC (1961). Some phases of the problem of smoking and lung cancer. *N Engl J Med*, 264:1241-1245.

Lo AC, Soliman AS, El-Ghawalby N, *et al.* (2007). Lifestyle, occupational, and reproductive factors in relation to pancreatic cancer risk. *Pancreas*, 35(2):120-129.

Lofroth G (1989). Environmental tobacco smoke: overview of chemical composition and genotoxic components. *Mutat Res*, 222(2):73-80.

Lombard HL, Doering CR (1980). Cancer studies in Massachusetts. 2. Habits, characteristics and environment of individuals with and without cancer. *CA Cancer J Clin*, 30(2):115-122.

Longo DR, Brownson R, Johnson J, *et al.* (1996). Hospital smoking bans and employee smoking behavior: Results of a national survey. *JAMA*, 275(16):1252-1257.

Longo DR, Johnson J, Kruse R, *et al.* (2001). A prospective investigation of the impact of smoking bans on tobacco cessation and relapse. *Tob Control*, 10(3):267-272.

Lopez MJ, Nebot M, Albertini M, *et al.* (2008). Secondhand smoke exposure in hospitality venues in Europe. *Environ Health Perspect*, 116:1469-1472.

Lubin JH (1999). Estimating lung cancer risk with exposure to environmental tobacco smoke. *Environ Health Perspect*, 107(Suppl 6):879-883.

Luk R, Ferrence R, Gmel G (2006). The economic impact of a smoke-free bylaw on restaurant and bar sales in Ottawa, Canada. *Addiction*, 101:738-745.

Lund KE (2006). The introduction of smoke-free hospitality venues in Norway. Impact on revenues, frequency of patronage, satisfaction and compliance. Oslo, Norway, Norwegian Institute for Alcohol and Drug Research (SIRUS) (*http://www.sirus.no/files/pub/375/SIRUSskrifter0206eng.pdf*).

Lund KE, Rise J (2004). Mediekampanje om roykfrie serveringssteder varen 2004 [with English language summary on p8]. Oslo, Norwegian Institute for Alcohol and Drug Research (SIRUS) (*http://www.sirus.no/*).

Lund KE, Helgason AR (2005). Environmental tobacco smoke in Norwegian homes, 1995 and 2001: changes in children's exposure and parent's attitudes and health risk awareness. *Eur J Public Health*, 15(2):123-127.

Lund KE, Lund M (2006). The impact of smoke-free hospitality venues in Norway. Eurohealth, 12(4):22-24 (*http://www.euro.who.int/Document/Obs/Eurohealth12_4.pdf*).

Lund M, Lindbak R (2007). Norwegian tobacco statistics 1973-2006. Oslo, Norwegian Institute for Alcohol and Drug Research (SIRUS) (*http://www.sirus.no/internett/forsiden?factory=index*).

Lund M, Lund K, Rise J, *et al.* (2005). Smoke-free bars and restaurants in Norway. Oslo, Norway, The Norwegian Institute for Alcohol and Drug Research (*http://www.globalink.org/documents/2005smokefreebarsandrestaurantsinNorway.pdf*).

Lundborg P (2007). Does smoking increase sick leave? Evidence using register data on Swedish workers. *Tob Control*, 16(2):114-118.

Lung SC, Wu MJ, Lin CC (2004). Customers' exposure to PM2.5 and polycyclic aromatic hydrocarbons in smoking/nonsmoking sections of 24-h coffee shops in Taiwan. *J Expo Anal Environ Epidemiol*, 14(7):529-535.

Lushchenkova O, Fernandez E, Lopez M, *et al.* (2008). [Secondhand smoke exposure in Spanish adult non-smokers following the introduction of an anti-smoking law]. *Rev Esp Cardiol*, 61(7):687-694.

Mackenzie CR, Campbell GD (1963). Cigarettes and disease. *S Afr Med J*, 37:974-975.

Maclure M, Katz RB, Bryant MS, *et al.* (1989). Elevated blood levels of carcinogens in passive smokers. *Am J Public Health*, 79(10):1381-1384.

MacMahon B, Trichopoulos D, Cole P, *et al.* (1982). Cigarette smoking and urinary estrogens. *N Engl J Med*, 307(17):1062-1065.

Madden D (2003). The cost of employee smoking in Ireland. Dublin, University College Dublin (*http://otc.ie/Uploads/Download%20David%20Maddens%20Presentation.pdf*).

Mandel LL, Alamar BC, Glantz SA (2005). Smoke-free law did not affect revenue from gaming in Delaware. *Tob Control,* 14(1):10-12.

Manor R (1997). Where there's smoke: there'll soon be a lounge, at Lambert Airport. *St. Louise Post*-Dispatch, A1-A6.

Mao Y, Hu J, Semenciw R, *et al.* (2002). Active and passive smoking and the risk of stomach cancer, by subsite, in Canada. *Eur J Cancer Prev,* 11(1):27-38.

Markowitz S (2000). The price of alcohol, wife abuse, and husband abuse. *South Econ J,* 67(2):279-303.

Marlatt GA, Curry S, Gordon JR (1988). A longitudinal analysis of unaided smoking cessation. *J Consult Clin Psychol,* 56(5):715-720.

Martin J, George R, Andrews K, *et al.* (2006). Observed smoking in cars: a method and differences by socioeconomic area. *Tob Control,* 15(5):409-411.

Martinez-Donate AP, Hovell MF, Hofstetter CR, *et al.* (2005). Smoking, exposure to secondhand smoke, and smoking restrictions in Tijuana, Mexico. *Rev Panam Salud Publica,* 18(6):412-417.

Martinez-Donate AP, Hovell MF, Hofstetter CR, *et al.* (2007). Correlates of home smoking bans among Mexican-Americans. *Am J Health Promot,* 21(4):229-236.

Maskarinec MP, Jenkins RA, Counts RW, *et al.* (2000). Determination of exposure to environmental tobacco smoke in restaurant and tavern workers in one US city. *J Expo Anal Environ Epidemiol,* 10(1):36-49.

Matanoski G, Kanchanaraksa S, Lantry D, *et al.* (1995). Characteristics of nonsmoking women in NHANES I and NHANES I epidemiologic follow-up study with exposure to spouses who smoke. *Am J Epidemiol,* 142(2):149-157.

Matt GE, Wahlgren DR, Hovell MF, *et al.* (1999). Measuring environmental tobacco smoke exposure in infants and young children through urine cotinine and memory-based parental reports: empirical findings and discussion. *Tob Control,* 8(3):282-289.

Matt GE, Quintana PJ, Hovell MF, *et al.* (2004). Households contaminated by environmental tobacco smoke: sources of infant exposures. *Tob Control,* 13(1):29-37.

Mauderly JL, Gigliotti AP, Barr EB, *et al.* (2004). Chronic inhalation exposure to mainstream cigarette smoke increases lung and nasal tumor incidence in rats. *Toxicol Sci,* 81(2):280-292.

Maziak W, Ali R, Fouad M, *et al.* (2008). Exposure to secondhand smoke at home and in public places in Syria: a developing country's perspective. *Inhal Toxicol,* 20(1):17-24.

Mcghee SM, Hedley AJ, Ho LM (2002). Passive smoking and its impact on employers and employees in Hong Kong. *Occup Environ Med,* 59(12):842-846.

McKee M, Gilmore A, Novotny T (2003). Smoke free hospitals. *Br Med J,* 326(7396):941-942.

McMillen RC, Winickoff JP, Klein JD, *et al.* (2003). US adult attitudes and practices regarding smoking restrictions and child exposure to environmental tobacco smoke: changes in the social climate from 2000-2001. *Pediatrics,* 112:e55-e60.

McMorrow MJ, Foxx RM (1983). Nicotine's role in smoking: an analysis of nicotine regulation. *Psychol Bull,* 93(2):302-327.

McMullen KM, Brownson R, Luke D, *et al.* (2005). Strength of clean indoor air laws and smoking related outcomes in the USA. *Tob Control,* 14(1):43-48.

McNabola A, Broderick B, Johnston P, *et al.* (2006). Effects of the smoking ban on benzene and 1,3-butadiene levels in pubs in Dublin. *J Environ Sci Health A Tox Hazard Subst Environ Eng,* 41(5):799-810.

Medical Research Council (MRC) (1957). Tobacco smoking and cancer of the lung. *Br Med J,* 1:1523-1524.

Menegaux F, Steffen C, Bellec S, *et al.* (2005). Maternal coffee and alcohol consumption during pregnancy, parental smoking and risk of childhood acute leukaemia. *Cancer Detect Prev,* 29(6):487-493.

Menegaux F, Ripert M, Hemon D, *et al.* (2007). Maternal alcohol and coffee drinking, parental smoking and childhood leukaemia: a French population-based case-control study. *Pediatr Perinat Epidemiol,* 21(4):293-299.

Menzies D, Nair A, Williamson P, *et al.* (2006). Respiratory symptoms, pulmonary function, and markers of inflammation among bar workers before and after a legislative ban on smoking in public places. *JAMA,* 296(14):1742-1748.

Mermelstein R, Lichtenstein E, McIntyre K (1983). Partner support and relapse in smoking-cessation programs. *J Consult Clin Psychol,* 51(3):465-466.

Merom D, Rissel C (2001). Factors associated with smoke-free homes in NSW: results from the 1998 NSW Health Survey. *Aust N Z J Public Health,* 25(4):339-345.

Messer K, Trinidad D, Al-Delaimy W, *et al.* (2008a). Smoking cessation rates in the United States: a comparison of young adult and older smokers. *Am J Public Health,* 98(2):317-322.

Messer K, Mills A, White M, *et al.* (2008b) The effect of smoke-free homes on smoking behavior in the United States. *Am J Prev Med,* 35(3):210-216.

Metzger KB, Mostashari F, Kerker B (2005). Use of pharmacy data to evaluate smoking regulations' impact on sales of nicotine replacement therapies in New York City. *Am J Public Health,* 95(6):1050-1055.

Michnovicz JJ, Hershcopf RJ, Naganuma H, *et al.* (1986). Increased 2-hydroxylation of estradiol as a possible mechanism for the anti-estrogenic effect of cigarette smoking. *N Engl J Med,* 315(21):1305-1309.

Miller C (2002). Evaluation of the South Australian smoke-free homes and cars project. In: The Cancer Council South Australia. Tobacco Control Research and Evaluation Report, 1998-2001. Adelaide, Tobacco Control Research Evaluation Unit, The Cancer Council South Australia *(http://www.cancersa.org.au/cms_resources/documents/TCRE/TCRE_Eval_Report_Vol1_Ch9.pdf).*

Mills CA, Porter MM (1950). Tobacco smoking habits and cancer of the mouth and respiratory system. *Cancer Res,* 10(9):539-542.

Ministry of Health (1990). Smoke-free law in New Zealand *(http://www.moh.govt.nz/smoke freelaw).*

Ministry of Health (2003). Il rapporto sull'impatto della legge 16 gennaio 2003, n. art.51 "Tutela della salute dei non fumatori" *(http://www.ministerosalute.it/resources/static/primopiano/255/conferenzaFumo.pdf).*

Ministry of Health (2007). New Zealand tobacco use survey 2006. Wellington, Ministry of Health.

Ministry of Health & Care Services (1973). Act No.14 of 9 March 1973 relating to prevention of the harmful effects of tobacco. Oslo, Norway *(http://www.regjeringen.no/en/dep/hod/Subjects/The-Department-of-Public-Health/Act-No-14-of-9-March-1973-relating-to-Prevention-of-the-Harmful-Effects-of-Tobacco.html?id=224962).*

Moher M, Ley K, Lancaster T (2005). Workplace interventions for smoking cessation (Review). *The Cochrane Library,* 2:1-79.

Moore L, Roberts C, Tudor-Smith C (2001). School smoking policies and smoking prevalence among adolescents: multilevel analysis of cross-sectional data from Wales. *Tob Control,* 10(2):117-123.

Moore M, Hrushow A (2004). Increasing compliance with California Smoke-free workplace law in San Francisco: Final evaluation report. San Francisco, CA

Moore RS, Lee JP, Antin TM, *et al.* (2006). Tobacco free workplace policies and low socioeconomic status female bartenders in San Francisco. *J Epidemiol Community Health,* 60(Suppl 2):51-56.

Morabia A, Bernstein M, Heritier S, *et al.* (1996). Relation of breast cancer with passive and active exposure to tobacco smoke. *Am J Epidemiol,* 143(9):918-928.

Morozumi R, Ii M (2006). The impact of smoke-free workplace policies on smoking behavior in Japan. *Appl Econ,* 13:549-555.

Moshammer H, Neuberger M, Nebot M (2004). Nicotine and surface of particulates as indicators of exposure to environmental tobacco smoke in public places in Austria. *Int J Hyg Environ Health,* 207(4):337-343.

Moskowitz JM, Lin Z, Hudes E (2000). The impact of workplace smoking ordinances in California on smoking cessation. *Am J Public Health,* 90(5):757-761.

Mudarri D (1994). *The costs and benefits of smoking restrictions: an assessment of the Smoke-Free Environment Act of 1993.* (H.R. 3434) Washington, DC, US Environmental Protection Agency.

Mulcahy M, Evans D, Hammond S, *et al.* (2005). Secondhand smoke exposure and risk following the Irish smoking ban: an assessment of salivary cotinine concentrations in hotel workers and air nicotine levels in bars. *Tob Control,* 14(6):384-388.

Muller FH (1939). Tabakmissbrauch und lungercarcinoma. Z Krebsforsch, 49:57-85.

Mumford EA, Levy DT, Romano EO (2004). Home smoking restrictions. Problems in classification. *Am J Prev Med,* 27(2):126-131.

Nagao M, Ushijima T, Wakabayashi K, *et al.* (1994). Dietary carcinogens and mammary carcinogenesis. Induction of rat mammary carcinomas by administration of heterocyclic amines in cooked foods. *Cancer,* 74(3 Suppl): 1063-1069.

Nagle AL, Schofield MJ, Redman S (1996). Smoking on hospital grounds and the impact of outdoor smoke-free zones. *Tob Control,* 5(3):199-204.

Nardini S, Pacifici R, Mortali C, *et al.* (2003). A survey on policies of smoking control in Italian hospitals. *Monaldi Arch Chest Dis,* 59(4):310-313.

National Cancer Institute (1999). *Health effects of exposure to environmental tobacco smoke: the report of the California Environmental Protection Agency.* Smoking and Tobacco Control Monograph 10. NIH Pub. No. 99-4645. Bethesda, MD, U.S. Department of Health and Human Services, National Institutes of Health, National Cancer Institute.

National Cancer Institute (2000). *State and local legislative action to reduce tobacco use.* Smoking and Tobacco Control Monograph 11. NIH Pub. No. 00-4804. Bethesda, MD, U.S. Department of Health and Human Services, National Institutes of Health, National Cancer Institute.

National Health and Medical Research Counciln (NHMRC) (1987). Effects of passive smoking on health. Report of the NHMRC working party on the effect of passive smoking on health. Canberra, Australian Government Publishing Service.

National Health and Medical Research Council (NHMRC) (1997). The health effects of passive smoking: A scientific information paper. Canberra, Australian Government Publishing Service.

National Health Service (2006). The smoking, health and social care (Scotland) Act 2005 (Commencement No.4), Order 2006 *(http://www.legislation.gov.uk/legislation/scotland/ssi2006/20060121.htm).*

National Libraries of Medicine (2007). The Reports of the Surgeon General: chronological listing by primary document type. National Libraries of Medicine *(http://profiles.nlm.nih.gov/NN/ListByDate.html).*

National Research Council (1986). Environmental tobacco smoke: measuring exposures and assessing health effects. Washington, DC, National Academy Press. *(http://www.nap.edu/openbook.php?isbn=0309037301).*

Navas-Acien A, Peruga A, Breysse P, *et al.* (2004). Secondhand tobacco smoke in public places in Latin America, 2002-2003. *JAMA,* 291(22):2741-2745.

Nebot M, Lopez M, Gorini G, *et al.* (2005). Environmental tobacco smoke exposure in public places of European cities. *Tob Control,* 14(1):60-63.

New Zealand Ministry of Health (2005). The smoke is clearing: Anniversary report. Wellington, New Zealand, Ministry of Health *(http://www.moh.govt.nz/publications).*

Nishino Y, Tsubono Y, Tsuji I, *et al.* (2001). Passive smoking at home and cancer risk: a population-based prospective study in Japanese nonsmoking women. *Cancer Causes Control,* 12(9):797-802.

Noonan G (1976). Passive smoking in enclosed public places. *Med J Aust,* 2(2):68-70.

Norman GJ, Ribisl KM, Howard-Pitney B, *et al.* (1999). Smoking bans in the home and car: Do those who really need them have them? *Prev Med,* 29(6 Pt 1):581-589.

Norman GJ, Ribisl KM, Howard-Pitney B, *et al.* (2000). The relationship between home smoking bans and exposure to state tobacco control efforts and smoking behaviors. *Am J Health Promot,* 15(2):81-88.

Norway Ministry of Health and Care Services (1973). Act No. 14 of 9 March 1973 relating to prevention of the harmful effects of tobacco *(http://www.regjeringen.no/en/dep/hod/Subjects/The-Department-of-Public-Health/Act-No-14-of-9-March-1973-relating-to-Prevention-of-the-Harmful-Effects-of-Tobacco.html?id=224962).*

Office of Tobacco Control (2005). Smoke-free workplaces in Ireland: a one-year review. Clane, Co Kildare, Ireland, Office of Tobacco Control *(http://www.otc.ie/Uploads/1_Year_Report_FA.pdf).*

Office of Tobacco Control (2007). Annual Report *(http://www.otc.ie/uploads/Annual_Report_2007.pdf).*

Okah FA, Choi WS, Okuyemi KS, et al. (2002). Effect of children on home smoking restriction by inner-city smokers. Pediatrics, 109(2):244-249.

Okah FA, Okuyemi K, McCarter K, et al. (2003). Predicting adoption of home smoking restriction by inner-city black smokers. Arch Pediatr Adolesc Med, 157(12):1202-1205.

Osthus S, Pape H, Lund K (2007). [Smoking restrictions and smoking prevalence in high schools]. Tidsskr Nor Laegeforen, 127(9):1192-1194.

Otsuka R, Watanabe H, Hirata K, et al. (2001). Acute effects of passive smoking on the coronary circulation in healthy young adults. JAMA, 286(4):436-441.

Ott WR (1999). Mathematical models for predicting indoor air quality from smoking activity. Environ Health Perspect, 107(Suppl 2):375-381.

Pakko MR (2006). Smoke-free law did affect revenue from gaming in Delaware. Tob Control, 15(1):68-69.

Palinkas LA, Pierce J, Rosbrook BP, et al. (1993). Cigarette smoking behavior and beliefs of Hispanics in California. Am J Prev Med, 9(6):331-337.

Pang D, McNally R, Birch JM (2003). Parental smoking and childhood cancer: results from the United Kingdom Childhood Cancer Study. Br J Cancer, 88(3):373-381.

Parrott S, Godfrey C, Raw M (2000). Costs of employee smoking in the workplace in Scotland. Tob Control, 9(2):187-192.

Patten CA, Gilpin E, Cavin S, et al. (1995). Workplace smoking policy and changes in smoking behavior in California: a suggested association. Tob Control, 4:36-41.

Payne TJ, Smith P, Sturges L, et al. (1996). Reactivity to smoking cues: mediating roles of nicotine dependence and duration of deprivation. Addict Behav, 21(2):139-154.

Pell JP, Haw S, Cobbe S, et al. (2008). Smoke-free legislation and hospitalizations for acute coronary syndrome. N Engl J Med, 359(5):482-491.

Penner M, Penner S (1990). Excess insured health care costs from tobacco-using employees in a large group plan. J Occup Med, 32(6):521-523.

Petrakis NL, Gruenke LD, Beelen TC, et al. (1978). Nicotine in breast fluid of nonlactating women. Science, 199(4326):303-305.

Petrakis NL, Miike R, King EB, et al. (1988). Association of breast fluid coloration with age, ethnicity, and cigarette smoking. Breast Cancer Res Treat, 11(3):255-262.

Phillips K, Bentley M, Howard D, et al. (1996). Assessment of air quality in Stockholm by personal monitoring of nonsmokers for respirable suspended particles and environmental tobacco smoke. Scand J Work Environ Health, 22(Suppl 1):1-24.

Phillips LE, Longstreth WT Jr, Koepsell T, et al. (2005). Active and passive cigarette smoking and risk of intracranial meningioma. Neuroepidemiology, 24(3):117-122.

Pickett MS, Schober SE, Brody DJ, et al. (2006). Smoke-free laws and secondhand smoke exposure in US non-smoking adults, 1999-2002. Tob Control, 15(4):302-307.

Pickett W, Northrup D, Ashley M (1999). Factors influencing implementation of the legislated smoking ban on school property in Ontario. Prev Med, 29(3):157-164.

Picone GA, Sloan F, Trogdon JG (2004). The effect of the tobacco settlement and smoking bans on alcohol consumption. Health Econ, 13(10):1063-1080.

Pierce JP, Gilpin EA (1995). A historical analysis of tobacco marketing and the uptake of smoking by youth in the United States: 1890-1977. Health Psychol, 14(6):500-508.

Pierce JP, Leon M (2008). Effectiveness of smoke-free policies. Lancet Oncol, 9(7):614-615.

Pierce JP, Dwyer T, DiGiusto E, et al. (1987). Cotinine validation of self-reported smoking in commercially run community surveys. J Chronic Dis, 40(7):689-695.

Pierce JP, Fiore M, Novotny T, et al. (1989). Trends in cigarette smoking in the United States. Educational differences are increasing. JAMA, 261(1):56-60.

Pierce JP, Naquin M, Gilpin E, et al. (1991). Smoking initiation in the United States: a role for worksite and college smoking bans. J Natl Cancer Inst, 83(14):1009-1013.

Pierce J, Evans D, Farkas A, et al. (1994). Tobacco use in California. An evaluation of the Tobacco Control Program 1989-1993. San Diego, CA, La Jolla, University of California.

Pierce JP, Choi WS, Gilpin EA, et al. (1996). Validation of susceptibility as a predictor of which adolescents take up smoking in the United States. Health Psychol, 15(5):355-361.

Pierce J, Gilpin E, Emery S, et al. (1998a). Tobacco control in California: Who's winning the war? An evaluation of the tobacco control program 1989-1996. San Diego, CA, La Jolla, University of California.

Pierce JP, Gilpin E, Emery S, et al. (1998b). Has the California tobacco control program reduced smoking? JAMA, 280(10):893-899.

Pierce JP, Gilpin E, Farkas AJ (1998c). Can strategies used by statewide tobacco control programs help smokers make progress in quitting? Cancer Epidemiol Biomarkers Prev, 7(6):459-464.

Pierce JP, Farkas AJ, Gilpin EA (1998d). Beyond stages of change: the quitting continuum measures progress towards successful smoking cessation. Addiction, 93(2):277-286.

Pierce JP, White MM, Messer K (2009). Changing age-specific patterns of cigarette consumption in the United States, 1992-2002: Association with smoke-free homes and state-level tobacco control activity. Nicotine Tob Res, 11(2):171-177.

Pikora T, Phang J, Karro J, et al. (1999). Are smoke-free policies implemented and adhered to at sporting venues? Aust N Z J Public Health, 23(4):407-409.

Pinilla J, Gonzalez B, Barber P, et al. (2002). Smoking in young adolescents: an approach with multilevel discrete choice models. J Epidemiol Community Health, 56(3):227-232.

Pion M, Givel M (2004). Airport smoking rooms don't work. Tob Control, 13(Suppl 1):i37-i40.

Pirkle JL, Flegal KM, Bernert JT, et al. (1996). Exposure of the US population to environmental tobacco smoke: the Third National Health and Nutrition Examination Survey, 1988 to 1991. JAMA, 275(16):1233-1240.

Pirkle JL, Bernert JT, Caudill SP, et al. (2006). Trends in the exposure of nonsmokers in the U.S. population to secondhand smoke: 1988-2002. Environ Health Perspect, 114(6):853-858.

Pizacani BA, Martin DP, Stark MJ, et al. (2003). Household smoking bans: which households have them and do they work? Prev Med, 36(1):99-107.

Pizacani BA, Martin DP, Stark MJ, et al. (2004). A prospective study of household smoking bans and subsequent cessation related behaviour: the role of stage of change. Tob Control, 13(1):23-28.

Porter RS, Gowda V, Kotchou K, et al. (2001). Tobacco use among adults: Arizona, 1996 and 1999. MMWR Morb Mortal Wkly Rep, 50(20):402-406.

Poulsen LH, Osler M, Roberts C, et al. (2002). Exposure to teachers smoking and adolescent smoking behaviour: analysis of cross sectional data from Denmark. Tob Control, 11(3):246-251.

Prabhat J, Chaloupka F (2000). Tobacco control in developing countries. Oxford, UK, Oxford University Press (http://www.sciencedirect. com/science?_ob=ArticleURL&_udi=B6VBF-45JPF9S-1&_user=382452&_rdoc=1&_ fmt=&_orig=search&_sort=d&view=c&_ acct=C000055308&_version=1&_urlVersion=0& _userid=382452&md5=0674ca2b4a6aa0dc70 ald70240e9641a).

Proescholdbell RJ, Chassin L, MacKinnon DP (2000). Home smoking restrictions and adolescent smoking. Nicotine Tob Res, 2(2):159-167.

Proescholdbell SK, Foley KL, Johnson J, et al. (2008). Indoor air quality in prisons before and after implementation of a smoking ban law. Tob Control, 17(2):123-127.

Pron GE, Burch JD, Howe GR, et al. (1988). The reliability of passive smoking histories reported in a case-control study of lung cancer. Am J Epidemiol, 127(2):267-273.

Pruss-Ustun A, Corvalan C, eds. (2006). Preventing disease through health environments. Towards an estimate of the environmental burden of disease. Geneva, World Health Organization.

Przewozniak K, Zatonski W (2002). Sharp decline in smoking prevalence in Polish female doctors: they reach world standards [Abstract]. Abstract book and programme of the 3rd European Conference on Tobacco or Health. Warsaw, Poland (http://eng.pw.edu.pl/).

Przewozniak K, Gumkowski J, Zagroba M, et al. (2007). ETS exposure in public places in Poland: A look at PM2.5 levels and implications for policy. Abstract book of the 4th European Conference on Tobacco or Health. Basel, Switzerland.

Przewozniak K, Gumkowski J, Zatonski W (2008). Passive smoking in Poland - exposure, health effects and prevention [In Polish with English language summary]. In: Proceedings of the National Conference on Environment and Health. Warsaw, Poland, Warsaw Technical University (http://eng.pw.edu.pl/).

Pyles MK, Mullineaux DJ, Okoli CT, et al. (2007). Economic effect of a smoke-free law in a tobacco-growing community. Tob Control, 16(1):66-68.

Rainio SU, Rimpela AH (2008). Home smoking bans in Finland and the association with child smoking. Eur J Public Health, 18(3):306-311.

Reeder A, Glasgow H (2000). Are New Zealand schools smoke-free? Results from a national survey of primary and intermediate school principals. N Z Med J, 113(1104):52-54.

Rees VW, Connolly GN (2006). Measuring air quality to protect children from secondhand smoke in cars. Am J Prev Med, 31(5):363-368.

Renaud T (2007). Smoking ban in public areas. Health Policy Monitor, (April):1-7.

Repace JL (2004). Respirable particles and carcinogens in the air of Delaware hospitality venues before and after a smoking ban. J Occup Environ Med, 46(9):887-905.

Repace JL, Lowrey AH (1980). Indoor air pollution, tobacco smoke, and public health. Science, 208(4443):464-472.

Repace JL, Lowrey AH (1990). Risk assessment methodologies for passive smoking-induced lung cancer. Risk Anal, 10(1):27-37.

Repace JL, Lowrey AH (1993). An enforceable indoor air quality standard for environmental tobacco smoke in the workplace. Risk Anal, 13(4):463-475.

Repace JL, Al-Delaimy W, Bernert J (2006a). Correlating atmospheric and biological markers in studies of secondhand tobacco smoke exposure and dose in children and adults. J Occup Environ Med, 48(2):181-194.

Repace JL, Hyde JN, Brugge D (2006b). Air pollution in Boston bars before and after a smoking ban. BMC Public Health, 6:266.

Reynolds P, Hurley S, Goldberg DE, et al. (2004). Active smoking, household passive smoking, and breast cancer: evidence from the California Teachers Study. J Natl Cancer Inst, 96(1):29-37.

Rigotti NA (1989). Trends in the adoption of smoking restrictions in public places and worksites. N Y State J Med, 89(1):19-26.

Rise J, Lund K (2005). Predicting children's level of exposure to environmental tobacco smoke based on two national surveys in Norway in 1995 and 2001. Addict Behav, 30(6):1267-1271.

Rissel C, McLellan L, Bauman A (2000). Factors associated with delayed tobacco uptake among Vietnamese/Asian and Arabic youth in Sydney, NSW. Aust N Z J Public Health, 24(1):22-28.

Roberts LM, Wakefield MA, Reynolds CS (1996). Children's exposure to environmental tobacco smoke in private vehicles. Med J Aust, 165(6):350.

Robinson J, Kirkcaldy A (2007). Disadvantaged mothers, young children and smoking in the home: mothers' use of space within their homes. Health Place, 13(4):894-903.

Roddam AW, Pirie K, Pike MC, et al. (2007). Active and passive smoking and the risk of breast cancer in women aged 36-45 years: a population based case-control study in the UK. Br J Cancer, 97(3):434-439.

Rodriguez D, Tscherne J, Udrain-McGovern J (2007). Contextual consistency and adolescent smoking: testing the indirect effect of home indoor smoking restrictions on adolescent smoking through peer smoking. Nicotine Tob Res, 9(11):1155-1161.

Rogers T, Feighery EC, Haladjian HH (2008). Current practices in enforcement of California laws regarding youth access to tobacco products and exposure to secondhand smoke. Sacramento, CA (http://www.publichealth. pitt.edu/docs/Land_conference_committee_ testimony_3-13-08.pdf).

Roseby R, Waters E, Polnay A, et al. (2004). Family and carer smoking control programs for reducing children's exposure to ETS (Cochrane Review). Cochrane Library, Chichester: John Wiley & Sons Ltd (http://www. thecochranelibrary.com).

Rosenlund M, Berglind N, Gustavsson A, et al. (2001). Environmental tobacco smoke and myocardial infarction among never-smokers in the Stockholm Heart Epidemiology Program (SHEEP). Epidemiology, 12(5):558-564.

Ross H (2006). Economics of smoke-free policies. In: Smokefree Partnership, ed. Lifting the smokescreen: 10 reasons for a smoke free Europe. Brussels, European Respiratory Society: 1-148.

Royal College of Physicians of London (1962). *Smoking and health. Summary of a report of the Royal College of Physicians of London on smoking in relation to cancer of the lung and other diseases.* London, Pitman Medical Publishing Co., Ltd.

Rubenstein D, Jesty J, Bluestein D (2004). Differences between mainstream and sidestream cigarette smoke extracts and nicotine in the activation of platelets under static and flow conditions. *Circulation,* 109(1):78-83.

Ruprecht A, Boffi R, Mazza R, *et al.* (2006). [A comparison between indoor air quality before and after the implementation of the smoking ban in public places in Italy]. *Epidemiol Prev,* 30(6):334-337.

Ryan P, Lee MW, North B, *et al.* (1992). Risk factors for tumors of the brain and meninges: results from the Adelaide Adult Brain Tumor Study. *Int J Cancer,* 51(1):20-27.

Saloojee Y, Dagli E (2000). Tobacco industry tactics for resisting public policy on health. *Bull World Health Organ,* 78(7):902-910.

Samanic C, Kogevinas M, Dosemeci M, *et al.* (2006). Smoking and bladder cancer in Spain: effects of tobacco type, timing, environmental tobacco smoke, and gender. *Cancer Epidemiol Biomarkers Prev,* 15(7):1348-1354.

Samet JM (2006). Smoking bans prevent heart attacks. *Circulation,* 114:1450-1451.

Sandler DP, Everson RB, Wilcox AJ (1985a). Passive smoking in adulthood and cancer risk. *Am J Epidemiol,* 121(1):37-48.

Sandler DP, Everson RB, Wilcox AJ, *et al.* (1985b). Cancer risk in adulthood from early life exposure to parents' smoking. *Am J Public Health,* 75(5):487-492.

Sandler DP, Comstock GW, Helsing KJ, *et al.* (1989). Deaths from all causes in non-smokers who lived with smokers. *Am J Public Health,* 79(2):163-167.

Sargent RP, Shepard RM, Glantz SA (2004). Reduced incidence of admissions for myocardial infarction associated with public smoking ban: before and after study. *Br Med J,* 328(7446):977-980.

Scherer G (1999). Smoking behavior and compensation: a review of the literature. *Psychopharmacology,* 145:1-20.

Schiaffino A, Fernandez E, Kunst A, *et al.* (2007). Time trends and educational differences in the incidence of quitting smoking in Spain (1965-2000). *Prev Med,* 45(2-3):226-232.

Schick S, Gvinianidze K, Tsereteli D, *et al.* (2008). Pilot study of compliance with healthcare facility smoking laws in Georgia. *Georgian Med News,* (154):47-52.

Schofield MJ, Edwards K (1995). Community attitudes to bans on smoking in licensed premises. *Aust J Public Health,* 19(4):399-402.

Schrek R, Baker LA, Ballard GP, *et al.* (1950). Tobacco smoking as an etiologic factor in disease: cancer. *Cancer Res,* 10:49-58.

Schulze A, Mons M (2005). Trends in cigarette smoking initiation and cessation among birth cohorts of 1926-1970 in Germany. *Eur J Cancer Prev,* 14(5):477-483.

Scientific Committee on Tobacco and Health (1998). Report of the Scientific Committee on Tobacco and Health. United Kingdom, The Stationary Office *(http://www.archive.official-documents.co.uk/).*

Scollo M, Lal A (2002). Summary of studies assessing the economic impact of smoke-free policies in the hospitality industry – includes studies produced to 31 August 2002. Melbourne, Australia, VicHealth Centre for Tobacco Control *(http://www.vctc.org.au/publ/reports/hospitality_paper_summary.pdf).*

Scollo M, Lal A (2005). Summary of studies assessing the economic impact of smoke-free policies in the Hospitality industry - includes studies produced to July 2005. Melbourne, VicHealth Centre for Tobacco Control *(http://www.vctc.org.au/tc-res/Hospitalitysummary.pdf).*

Scollo M, Lal A (2008). Summary of studies assessing the economic impact of smoke-free policies in the hospitality industry. Melbourne, Australia, VicHealth Centre for Tobacco Control *(http://www.vctc.org.au/tc-res/Hospitalitysummary.pdf).*

Scollo M, Lal A, Hyland A (2003). Review of the quality of studies on the economic effects of smoke-free policies on the hospitality industry. *Tob Control,* 12:13-20.

Scottish Executive (2004). A breath of fresh air for Scotland. Improving Scotland's health: the challenge. Tobacco Control Action Plan. Edinburgh, Scotland, Scottish Executive, St Andrew's House *(http://www.scotland.gov.uk/Publications/2004/01/18736/31541).*

Scottish Government (2005). Clearing the air. Enforcement protocol *(http://www.clearingtheairscotland.com/faqs/enforcement.html).*

Scottish Government (2008). Smoke-free legislation - National compliance data: summary *(http://www.clearingtheairscotland.com/latest/index.html).*

Scottish Parliament. (2004). Prohibition of smoking in regulated areas (Scotland) bill *(http://www.scottish.parliament.uk/business/bills/20-prohibitionSmoking/b20s2-introd.pdf).*

Scottish Parliament. (2006). Prohibition of smoking in certain premises (Scotland) regulations *(http://www.opsi.gov.uk/legislation/scotland/ssi2006/20060090.htm).*

Sebrie EM, Glantz SA (2007). "Accommodating" smoke-free policies: tobacco industry's Courtesy of Choice programme in Latin America. *Tob Control,* 16(5):e6.

Sebrie EM, Schoj V, Glantz SA (2008). Smoke free environments in Latin America: on the road to real change? *Prev Control,* 3:21-35.

Sellstrom E, Bremberg S (2006). Is there a "school effect" on pupil outcomes? A review of multilevel studies. *J Epidemiol Community Health,* 60(2):149-155.

Semple S, Maccalman L, Naji A, *et al.* (2007a). Bar workers' exposure to second-hand smoke: the effect of Scottish smoke-free legislation on occupational exposure. *Ann Occup Hyg,* 51(7):571-580.

Semple S, Creely K, Naji A, *et al.* (2007b). Secondhand smoke levels in Scottish pubs: the effect of smoke-free legislation. *Tob Control,* 16(2):127-132.

Semple S, Naji A, Haw S, *et al.* Care home workers' exposure to SHS: A short summary of findings. *Occup Environ Med,* in press.

Seo DC, Torabi MR (2007). Reduced admissions for acute myocardial infarction associated with a public smoking ban: matched controlled study. *J Drug Educ,* 37(3):217-226.

Shavers VL, Fagan P, Alexander L, *et al.* (2006). Workplace and home smoking restrictions and racial/ethnic variation in the prevalence and intensity of current cigarette smoking among women by poverty status, TUS-CPS 1998-1999 and 2001-2002. *J Epidemiol Community Health,* 60(Suppl 2):ii34-ii43.

Shelley D, Nguyen N, Yerneni R, et al. (2008). Tobacco use behaviors and household smoking bans among Chinese Americans. Am J Health Promot, 22(3):168-175.

Shields M (2005). The journey to quitting smoking. Health Rep, 16(3):19-36.

Shields M (2007). Smoking bans: influence on smoking prevalence. Health Rep, 18(3):9-24.

Shiffman S, Gnys M, Richards T, et al. (1996). Temptations to smoke after quitting: a comparison of lapsers and maintainers. Health Psychol, 15(6):455-461.

Shopland DR, Anderson CM, Burns DM (2006). Association between home smoking restrictions and changes in smoking behaviour among employed women. J Epidemiol Community Health, 60(Suppl 2):ii44-ii50.

Shrubsole MJ, Gao YT, Dai Q, et al. (2004). Passive smoking and breast cancer risk among non-smoking Chinese women. Int J Cancer, 110(4):605-609.

Siahpush M, Scollo M (2001). Trends in public support for smoking bans in public places in Australia. Aust N Z J Public Health, 25(5):473.

Siahpush M, Borland R, Scollo M (2003). Factors associated with smoking cessation in a national sample of Australians. Nicotine Tob Res, 5(4):597-602.

Siegel M (2002). The effectiveness of state-level tobacco control interventions: a review of program implementation and behavioral outcomes. Annu Rev Public Health, 23:45-71.

Siegel M, Albers A, Cheng D, et al. (2005). Effect of local restaurant smoking regulations on progression to established smoking among youths. Tob Control, 14(5):300-306.

Siegel M, Albers A, Cheng D, et al. (2008). Local restaurant smoking regulations and the adolescent smoking initiation process: results of a multi-level contextual analysis among Massachusetts youths. Arch Pediatr Adolesc Med, 162(5):477-483.

Skeer M, Land M, Cheng D, et al. (2004). Smoking in Boston bars before and after a 100% smoke-free regulation: an assessment of early compliance. J Public Health Manag Pract, 10(6):501-507.

Skogstad M, Kjaerheim K, Fladseth G, et al. (2006). Cross shift changes in lung function among bar and restaurant workers before and after implementation of a smoking ban. Occup Environ Med, 63(7):482-487.

Slattery ML, Robison LM, Schuman KL, et al. (1989). Cigarette smoking and exposure to passive smoke are risk factors for cervical cancer. JAMA, 261(11):1593-1598.

Slattery ML, Edwards S, Curtin K, et al. (2003). Associations between smoking, passive smoking, GSTM-1, NAT2, and rectal cancer. Cancer Epidemiol Biomarkers Prev, 12(9):882-889.

Slattery ML, Curtin K, Giuliano AR, et al. (2008). Active and passive smoking, IL6, ESR1, and breast cancer risk. Breast Cancer Res Treat, 109(1):101-111.

Sly PD, Pronczuk J (2007). Guest editorial: susceptibility of children to pollutants. Paediatr Respir Rev, 8(4):273-274.

Sly PD, Deverell M, Kusel MM, et al. (2007). Exposure to environmental tobacco smoke in cars increases the risk of persistent wheeze in adolescents. Med J Aust, 186(6):322.

Smith SJ, Deacon JM, Chilvers CE (1994). Alcohol, smoking, passive smoking and caffeine in relation to breast cancer risk in young women. UK National Case-Control Study Group. Br J Cancer, 70(1):112-119.

Smoke Free Partnership (2006). Lifting the smokescreen: 10 reasons for a smokefree Europe (http://www.european-lung-foundation.org/uploads/Document/WEB_CHEMIN_282_1142435970.pdf).

Sobel R (1978). They satisfy: the cigarette in American life. Garden City, NJ, Anchor Press/Doubleday.

Sobti RC, Kaur S, Kaur P, et al. (2006). Interaction of passive smoking with GST (GSTM1, GSTT1, and GSTP1) genotypes in the risk of cervical cancer in India. Cancer Genet Cytogenet, 166(2):117-123.

Soliman S, Pollack H, Warner K (2004). Decrease in the prevalence of environmental tobacco smoke exposure in the home during the 1990s in families with children. Am J Public Health, 94(2):314-320.

Sorahan T, Lancashire RJ (2004). Parental cigarette smoking and childhood risks of hepatoblastoma: OSCC data. Br J Cancer, 90(5):1016-1018.

Spencer N, Blackburn C, Bonas S, et al. (2005). Parent reported home smoking bans and toddler (18-30 month) smoke exposure: a cross-sectional survey. Arch Dis Child, 90(7):670-674.

Stayner L, Bena J, Sasco AJ, et al. (2007). Lung cancer risk and workplace exposure to environmental tobacco smoke. Am J Public Health, 97(3):545-551.

Stephen GA, McRill C, Mack M, et al. (2003). Assessment of respiratory symptoms and asthma prevalence in a U.S.-Mexico border region. Arch Environ Health, 58(3):156-162.

Stephens T, Pederson L, Koval J, et al. (1997). The relationship of cigarette prices and no-smoking bylaws to the prevalence of smoking in Canada. Am J Public Health, 87(9):1519-1521.

Stephens T, Pederson L, Koval J, et al. (2001). Comprehensive tobacco control policies and the smoking behaviour of Canadian adults. Tob Control, 10(4):317-322.

Stephens YD, English G (2002). A statewide school tobacco policy review: process, results, and implications. J Sch Health, 72(8):334-338.

Stillman F, Navas-Acien A, Ma J, et al. (2007). Second-hand tobacco smoke in public places in urban and rural China. Tob Control, 16(4):229-234.

Study Group on Smoking and Health (1957). Smoking and health: joint report of the study group on smoking and health. Science, 1129-1133.

Sumida H, Watanabe H, Kugiyama K, et al. (1998). Does passive smoking impair endothelium-dependent coronary artery dilation in women? J Am Coll Cardiol, 31(4):811-815.

Sweda L (2004). Lawsuits and secondhand smoke. Tob Control, 13(Suppl 1):i61-i66.

Szabo E, White V, Hayman J (2006). Can home smoking restrictions influence adolescents' smoking behaviors if their parents and friends smoke? Addict Behav, 31(12):2298-2303.

Tan AS, Arulanandam S, Chng CY, et al. (2000). Overview of legislation and tobacco control in Singapore. Int J Tuberc Lung Dis, 4(11):1002-1008.

Tang H, Cowling D, Lloyd J, et al. (2003). Changes of attitudes and patronage behaviors in response to a smoke-free bar law. Am J Public Health, 93(4):611-617.

Tang H, Cowling D, Stevens C, et al. (2004). Changes of knowledge, attitudes, beliefs, and preference of bar owner and staff in response to a smoke-free bar law. Tob Control, 13(1):87-89.

Tauras JA (2005). Can public policy deter smoking escalation among young adults? *J Policy Anal Manage*, 24(4):771-784.

Tauras JA, Chaloupka FJ (1999a). Price, clean indoor air laws, and cigarette smoking: evidence from longitudinal data for young adults, National Bureau of Economic Research. NBER Working Paper Series. Working Paper #6937 *(http://www.nber.org/)*.

Tauras JA, Chaloupka FJ (1999b). Determinants of smoking cessation: an analysis of young adult men and women, National Bureau of Economic Research. NBER Working Paper Series. Working Paper #726. *(http://www.nber.org/)*.

Tay SK, Tay KJ (2004). Passive cigarette smoking is a risk factor in cervical neoplasia. *Gynecol Oncol*, 93(1):116-120.

Taylor AE, Johnson DC, Kazemi H (1992). Environmental tobacco smoke and cardiovascular disease. A position paper from the Council on Cardiopulmonary and Critical Care, *American Heart Association. Circulation*, 86(2):699-702.

Taylor R, Najafi F, Dobson A (2007). Meta-analysis of studies of passive smoking and lung cancer: effects of study type and continent. *Int J Epidemiol*, 36(5):1048-1059.

The Scotland Office (1999). Devolution. *(http://www.scotlandoffice.gov.uk/devolution/)*.

Thompson B, Coronado G, Chen L, *et al.* (2006). Preferred smoking policies at 30 Pacific Northwest colleges. *Public Health Rep*, 121:586-593.

Thomson GW, Wilson N (2004). Public attitudes about tobacco smoke in workplaces: the importance of workers' rights in survey questions. *Tob Control*, 13(2):206-207.

Thomson G, Wilson N (2006). One year of smokefree bars and restaurants in New Zealand: Impacts and responses. *BMC Public Health*, 6(64):1-9.

Thomson G, Wilson N, Howden-Chapman P (2006). Population level policy options for increasing the prevalence of smokefree homes. *J Epidemiol Community Health*, 60(4):298-304.

Tobacco Control Research and Evaluation (TCRE) (2007). Community support for smoke-free cars legislation, findings from new South Australian research. Adelaide, Tobacco Control Research and Evaluation Program *(http://www.cancersa.org.au/aspx/home.aspx)*.

Tominz R, Murolo G, Montina G, *et al.* (2006). [Exposure to passive smoking in local health units of northern Italy before and after the enforcement of the smoking ban]. *Epidemiol Prev*, 30(6):338-342.

Tong EK, Nguyen TT, Vittinghoff E, *et al.* (2008). Smoking behaviors among immigrant Asian Americans: rules for smoke-free homes. *Am J Prev Med*, 35(1):64-67.

Travers M, Cummings K, Hyland A, *et al.* (2004). Indoor air quality in hospitality venues before and after the implementation of a Clean Indoor Air Law - Western New York, 2003. *MMWR Morb Mortal Wkly Rep*, 53(44):1038-1041.

Travers MJ, Hyland A, Higbee C, *et al.* (2007). Tobacco smoke pollution exposure in hospitality venues around the U.S. and the effect of smokefree air policies. In: Proceedings of 13th annual meeting 21-24 February 2007, Austin TX. Madison, WI, Society for research on nicotine and tobacco. POS2-156: 114.

Trichopoulos D, Kalandidi A, Sparros L, *et al.* (1981). Lung cancer and passive smoking. *Int J Cancer*, 27(1):1-4.

Trichopoulos D, Kalandidi A, Sparros L (1983). Lung cancer and passive smoking: conclusion of Greek study. *Lancet*, 2(8351):677-678.

Trimble CL, Genkinger JM, Burke AE, *et al.* (2005). Active and passive cigarette smoking and the risk of cervical neoplasia. *Obstet Gynecol*, 105(1):174-181.

Trinidad DR, Gilpin EA, Pierce JP (2005). Compliance and support for smoke-free school policies. *Health Educ Res*, 20(4):466-475.

Trotter L, Wakefield M, Borland R (2002). Socially cued smoking in bars, nightclubs, and gaming venues: a case for introducing smoke-free policies. *Tob Control*, 11(4):300-304.

Tsai FC, Smith KR, Vichit-Vadakan N, *et al.* (2000). Indoor/outdoor PM10 and PM2.5 in Bangkok, Thailand. *J Expo Anal Environ Epidemiol*, 10(1):15-26.

Tsai HT, Tsai Y, Yang SF, *et al.* (2007). Lifetime cigarette smoke and second-hand smoke and cervical intraepithelial neoplasm--a community-based case-control study. *Gynecol Oncol*, 105(1):181-188.

Tyrrell I (1999). Deadly enemies: tobacco and its opponents in Australia. Sydney, Australia, UNSW Press *(http://books.google.fr/books?id=np8GnBIHkcAC&pg=PR5&lpg=PR3&dq=%22deadly+enemies+tobacco+and+its+opponents+in+australia%22&psp=1&output=html&sig=SfCuBlmkQwtDC5c_ME6uYS45QXE)*.

U.S. Department of Health Education and Welfare (USDHEW) (1964). Smoking and health: report of the Advisory Committee to the Surgeon General of the Public Health Service. Washington, DC, U.S. Public Health Service. Publication No. 1103.

U.S. Department of Health Education and Welfare (USDHEW) (1972). The health consequences of smoking. A report of the Surgeon General: 1972. Washington, DC, U.S. Public Health Service. Publication No. (HSM) 72-7516 *(http://profiles.nlm.nih.gov/NN/B/B/P/M/_/nnbbpm.pdf)*.

U.S. Department of Health and Human Services (USDHHS) (1982). The health consequences of smoking: cancer. A report of the Surgeon General. Rockville, MD, U.S. Department of Health and Human Services, Center for Disease Control and Prevention, National Center for Chronic Disease Prevention and Health Promotion, Office on Smoking and Health *(http://profiles.nlm.nih.gov/NN/B/C/D/W/_/nnbcdw.pdf)*.

U.S. Department of Health and Human Services (USDHHS) (1986). The health consequences of involuntary smoking: a report of the Surgeon General. Rockville, MD, U.S. Department of Health and Human Services, Center for Disease Control and Prevention, National Center for Chronic Disease Prevention and Health Promotion, Office on Smoking and Health *(http://www.surgeongeneral.gov/library/secondhandsmoke/report/)*.

U.S. Department of Health and Human Services (USDHHS) (1988). The health consequences of nicotine addiction. A report of the Surgeon General. Rockville, MD, U.S. Department of Health and Human Services, Center for Disease Control and Prevention, National Center for Chronic Disease Prevention and Health Promotion, Office on Smoking and Health. CDC - 88-8406 *(http://www.surgeongeneral.gov/library/secondhandsmoke/report/)*.

U.S. Department of Health and Human Services (USDHHS) (1989). Reducing the health consequences of smoking, 25 years of progress. Rockville, MD, U.S. Department of Health and Human Services, Center for Disease Control and Prevention, National Center for Chronic Disease Prevention and Health Promotion, Office on Smoking and Health.

U.S. Department of Health and Human Services (USDHHS) (1990). The health benefits of smoking cessation: a report of the Surgeon General. Rockville, MD, U.S. Department of Health and Human Services, Center for Disease Control and Prevention, National Center for Chronic Disease Prevention and Health Promotion, Office on Smoking and Health (http://profiles.nlm.nih.gov/NN/B/B/C/T/_/nnbbct.pdf).

U.S. Department of Health and Human Services (USDHHS) (2000). Healthy people 2010. Volume 1, 2nd ed. Rockville, MD, U.S. Department of Health and Human Services, Center for Disease Control and Prevention, National Center for Chronic Disease Prevention and Health Promotion, Office on Smoking and Health. (http://www.healthypeople.gov/Document/tableofcontents.htm#volume1).

U.S. Department of Health and Human Services (USDHHS) (2001). Women and smoking: a report of the Surgeon General. Rockville, MD, U.S. Department of Health and Human Services, Center for Disease Control and Prevention, National Center for Chronic Disease Prevention and Health Promotion, Office on Smoking and Health (http://www.cdc.gov/tobacco/data_statistics/sgr/sgr_2001/#full).

U.S. Department of Health and Human Services (USDHHS) (2004). The health consequences of smoking: a report of the Surgeon General. Atlanta, GA, U.S. Department of Health and Human Services, Center for Disease Control and Prevention, National Center for Chronic Disease Prevention and Health Promotion, Office on Smoking and Health.

U.S. Department of Health and Human Services (USDHHS) (2006). Control of secondhand smoke exposure. In: The health consequences of involuntary exposure to tobacco smoke: a report of the surgeon general. Atlanta, GA, U.S. Department of Health and Human Services, Center for Disease Control and Prevention, National Center for Chronic Disease Prevention and Health Promotion, Office on Smoking and Health.

U.S. Environmental Protection Agency (EPA) (1992). Respiratory health effects of passive smoking: lung cancer and other disorders. Washington, DC, Office of Health and Environmental Assessment, Office of Research and Development, U.S Environmental Protection Agency. Publication No. EPA/600/6-90/006F.

Valente P, Forastiere F, Bacosi A, et al. (2007). Exposure to fine and ultrafine particles from secondhand smoke in public places before and after the smoking ban, Italy 2005. Tob Control, 16(5):312-317.

van Walbeek C, Blecher H, van Graan M (2007). Effects of the tobacco products control amendment Act of 1999 on restaurant revenues in South Africa--a survey approach. S Afr Med J, 97(3):208-211.

Viehbeck SM, McDonald PW (2004). An examination of the relationship between municipal smoke-free bylaw strength and the odds of being a former smoker. Can J Public Health, 96(1):42-44.

Villeneuve PJ, Johnson KC, Mao Y, et al. (2004). Environmental tobacco smoke and the risk of pancreatic cancer: findings from a Canadian population-based case-control study. Can J Public Health, 95(1):32-37.

Vineis P (2008). Personal communication to E. Khaykin and J. Samet.

Vineis P, Hoek G, Krzyzanowski M, et al. (2007). Lung cancers attributable to environmental tobacco smoke and air pollution in non-smokers in different European countries: a prospective study. Environ Health, 6:1-7.

Wakefield MA, Chaloupka F (2000). Effectiveness of comprehensive tobacco control programmes in reducing teenage smoking in the USA. Tob Control, 9(2):177-186.

Wakefield MA, Wilson D, Owen N, et al. (1992). Workplace smoking restrictions, occupational status, and reduced cigarette consumption. J Occup Med, 34(7):693-697.

Wakefield MA, Roberts L, Owen N (1996). Trends in prevalence and acceptance of workplace smoking bans among indoor workers in South Australia. Tob Control, 5(3):205-208.

Wakefield MA, Chaloupka F, Kaufman N, et al. (2000a). Effect of restrictions on smoking at home, at school, and in public places on teenage smoking: cross sectional study. Br Med J, 321(7257):333-337.

Wakefield MA, Banham D, Martin J, et al. (2000b). Restrictions on smoking at home and urinary cotinine levels among children with asthma. Am J Prev Med, 19(3):188-192.

Wakefield MA, Siahpush M, Scollo M, et al. (2002). The effect of a smoke-free law on monthly restaurant retail turnover in South Australia. Aust N Z J Public Health, 26(4):375-382.

Wald NJ, Nanchahal K, Thompson SG, et al. (1986). Does breathing other people's tobacco smoke cause lung cancer? Br Med J (Clin Res Ed), 293(6556):1217-1222.

Walsh RA, Tzelepis F (2003). Support for smoking restrictions in bars and gaming areas: review of Australian studies. Aust N Z J Public Health, 27(3):310-322.

Walsh RA, Paul CL, Tzelepis F (2000). Overwhelming support for smoking bans. Aust N Z J Public Health, 24(6):640-641.

Wamboldt FS, Balkissoon RC, Rankin AE, et al. (2008). Correlates of household smoking bans in low-income families of children with and without asthma. Fam Process, 47(1):81-94.

Wang Z, Tang L, Sun G, et al. (2006). Etiological study of esophageal squamous cell carcinoma in an endemic region: a population-based case control study in Huaian, China. BMC Cancer, 6:287.

Waring MS, Siegel JA (2007). An evaluation of the indoor air quality in bars before and after a smoking ban in Austin, Texas. J Expo Sci Environ Epidemiol, 17(3):260-268.

Warren CW, Riley L, Asma S, et al. (2000). Tobacco use by youth: a surveillance report from the Global Youth Tobacco Survey project. Bull World Health Organ, 78(7):868-876.

Wartenberg D, Calle EE, Thun MJ, et al. (2000). Passive smoking exposure and female breast cancer mortality. J Natl Cancer Inst, 92(20):1666-1673.

Wasserman J, Manning W, Newhouse J, et al. (1991). The effects of excise taxes and regulations on cigarette smoking. J Health Econ, 10(1):43-64.

Weber MD, Bagwell DA, Fielding JE, et al. (2003). Long term compliance with California's Smoke-Free Workplace Law among bars and restaurants in Los Angeles County. Tob Control, 12(3):269-273.

Weiss B (1989). Behavior as an endpoint for inhaled toxicants. In: McClellan RO, Henderson RF, eds. Concepts in inhalation toxicology. New York, Hemisphere Publishing: 475-493.

Weiss ST (1986). Passive smoking and lung cancer. What is the risk? Am Rev Respir Dis, 133(1):1-3.

Wewers ME, Uno M (2002). Clinical interventions and smoking ban methods to reduce infants' and children's exposure to environmental tobacco smoke. *J Obstet Gynecol Neonatal Nurs*, 31(5):592-598.

Whincup PH, Gilg JA, Emberson JR, *et al.* (2004). Passive smoking and risk of coronary heart disease and stroke: prospective study with cotinine measurement. *Br Med J*, 329(74 59):200-205.

White JR, Froeb HF (1980). Small-airways dysfunction in nonsmokers chronically exposed to tobacco smoke. *N Engl J Med*, 302(13):720-723.

WHO (1970). WHA23.32 Health consequences of smoking. Smoking and Health, WHO Chronicle 24,365. Geneva, Switzerland, World Health Organization.

WHO (1975). Smoking and its effects on health. Report of a WHO expert committee. Technical report series 568. Geneva, Switzerland, World Health Organization *(http://whqlibdoc.who.int/trs/WHO_TRS_568.pdf)*.

WHO (1986). WHA39.14 Tobacco or health. Resolution WHA39.14. Geneva, Switzerland, World Health Organization.

WHO (1990). WHA 43.16 Tobacco or health. Resolution WHA43.16. Geneva, Switzerland, World Health Organization.

WHO (1999). International consultation on environmental tobacco smoke (ETS) and child health. Geneva, Switzerland, World Health Organization *(http://www.who.int/tobacco/research/en/ets_report.pdf)*.

WHO (2005). WHO Framework Convention on Tobacco Control. Geneva, Switzerland, World Health Organization *(http://www.who.int/tobacco/framework/WHO_FCTC_english.pdf)*.

WHO (2007a). Guidelines for Article 8 of the Framework Convention on Tobacco Control. Geneva, Switzerland, World Health Organization.

WHO (2007b). Protection from exposure to secondhand tobacco smoke: policy recommendations. Geneva, Switzerland, World Health Organization *(http://www.who.int/tobacco/resources/publications/wntd/2007/who_protection_exposure_final_25June2007.pdf)*.

WHO (2008). WHO report on the global tobacco epidemic: the MPOWER package. Geneva, Switzerland, World Health Organization *(http://www.who.int/tobacco/mpower/mpower_report_full_2008.pdf)*.

Wilkinson JD, Arheart KL, Lee DJ (2006). Accuracy of parental reporting of secondhand smoke exposure: The National Health and Nutrition Examination Survey III. *Nicotine Tob Res*, 8(4):591-597.

Wilson N, Thomson G, Edwards R (2007). Lessons from Hong Kong and other countries for outdoor smokefree areas in New Zealand? *N Z Med J*, 120:U2624.

Winkelstein ML, Tarzian A, Wood RA (1997). Parental smoking behavior and passive smoke exposure in children with asthma. *Ann Allergy Asthma Immunol*, 78(4):419-423.

Wipfli H, Avila-Tang E, Navas-Acien A, *et al.* (2008). Secondhand smoke exposure among women and children: evidence from 31 countries. *Am J Public Health*, 98(4):672-679.

Wold B, Currie C, Roberts C, *et al.* (2004a). National legislation on school smoking restrictions in eight European countries. *Health Promot Int*, 19(4):482-488.

Wold B, Torsheim T, Currie C, *et al.* (2004b). National and school policies on restrictions of teacher smoking: a multilevel analysis of student exposure to teacher smoking in seven European countries. *Health Educ Res*, 19(3):217-226.

Wong S (2002). York region no-smoking by-law #A-0285-2000-105. Ontario, Canada, Ontario Campaign for Action on Smoking *(http://www.york.ca/services/public+health+and+safety/tobacco+free+living/york+region+no-smoking+by-law.htm)*.

Wong GC, Berman B, Hoang T, *et al.* (2002). Children's exposure to environmental tobacco smoke in the home: comparison of urine cotinine and parental reports. *Arch Environ Health*, 57(6):584-590.

Wong GC, Bernaards CA, Berman BA, *et al.* (2004). Do children with asthma and their parents agree on household ETS exposure? Implications for asthma management. *Patient Educ Couns*, 53(1):19-25.

Woodruff TJ, Rosbrook B, Pierce J, *et al.* (1993). Lower levels of cigarette consumption found in smoke-free workplaces in California. *Arch Intern Med*, 153(12):1485-1493.

Woodward A, Laugesen M (2001). How many deaths are caused by second hand cigarette smoke? *Tob Control*, 10(4):383-388.

Wu AH (1999). Exposure misclassification bias in studies of environmental tobacco smoke and lung cancer. *Environ Health Perspect*, 107(Suppl 6):873-877.

Wu MT, Lee L, Ho C, *et al.* (2003). Lifetime exposure to environmental tobacco smoke and cervical intraepithelial neoplasms among nonsmoking Taiwanese women. *Arch Environ Health*, 58(6):353-359.

Wynder EL, Graham EA (1950). Tobacco smoking as a possible etiologic factor in bronchiogenic carcinoma; a study of 684 proved cases. *J Am Med Assoc*, 143(4):329-336.

Wynder EL, Graham EA, Croninger AB (1953). Experimental production of carcinoma with cigarette tar. *Cancer Res*, 13(12):855-864.

Wynder WL (1961). An appraisal of the smoking-lung-cancer issue. *N Engl J Med*, 264:1235-1240.

Yang G, Fan L, Tan J, *et al.* (1999). Smoking in China: findings of the 1996 National Prevalence Survey. *JAMA*, 282(13):1247-1253.

Yang T, Wu Y, Abdullah A, *et al.* (2007). Attitudes and behavioral response toward key tobacco control measures from the FCTC among Chinese urban residents. *BMC Public Health*, 7(1):248.

Yañez E (2002). Clean indoor air and communities of color: challenges and opportunities. Washington, DC, The Praxis Project *(http://www.thepraxisproject.org/tools/CIA_and_CoC.pdf)*.

You RX, Thrift AG, McNeil J, *et al.* (1999). Ischemic stroke risk and passive exposure to spouses' cigarette smoking. Melbourne Stroke Risk Factor Study (MERFS) Group. *Am J Public Health*, 89(4):572-575.

Young D, Borland R, Siahpush M, *et al.* (2007). Australian smokers support stronger regulatory controls on tobacco: findings from the ITC Four-Country Survey. *Aust N Z J Public Health*, 31(2):164-169.

Yousey YK (2006). Household characteristics, smoking bans, and passive smoke exposure in young children. *J Pediatr Health Care*, 20(2):98-105.

Yu MC, Garabrant DH, Huang TB, *et al.* (1990). Occupational and other non-dietary risk factors for nasopharyngeal carcinoma in Guangzhou, China. *Int J Cancer*, 45(6):1033-1039.

Yuan JM, Wang XL, Xiang YB, *et al.* (2000). Non-dietary risk factors for nasopharyngeal carcinoma in Shanghai, China. *Int J Cancer*, 85(3):364-369.

Yurekli AA, Zhang P (2000). The impact of clean indoor-air laws and cigarette smuggling on demand for cigarettes: an empirical model. *Health Econ*, 9(2):159-170.

Zeegers MP, Goldbohm RA, van den Brandt PA (2002). A prospective study on active and environmental tobacco smoking and bladder cancer risk (The Netherlands). *Cancer Causes Control*, 13(1):83-90.

Zhang X, Shu X, Yang G, *et al.* (2005). Association of passive smoking by husbands with prevalence of stroke among Chinese women nonsmokers. *Am J Epidemiol*, 161(3): 213-218.

Zheng W, McLaughlin J, Chow W, *et al.* (1993). Risk factors for cancers of the nasal cavity and paranasal sinuses among white men in the United States. *Am J Epidemiol*, 138(11):965-972.

Working procedures

Starting in 2006, the series of International Agency for Research on Cancer (IARC) Handbooks of Cancer Prevention added tobacco control as a new area of prevention for their reviews. When appropriate, in addition to cancer, other health outcomes preventable by avoiding tobacco use or exposure to secondhand smoke (SHS) may be included for evaluation in a Handbook.

The Working Procedures described herein are largely taken from the Handbooks of Cancer Prevention devoted to Chemoprevention and Screening, and from the IARC Monograph Preamble (updated in January 2006).

The text that follows is organised in two principal parts. The first addresses the general scope, objectives, and structure of the Handbooks with emphasis on tobacco control. The second describes the scientific procedures for evaluating cancer-preventing agents and tobacco control policy interventions.

The term "exposure" appears repeatedly in these procedures, borrowed from the IARC Monographs devoted to the evaluation of carcinogenicity. Epidemiological studies conducted to assess the association between exposure to a given hazard and disease outcome, are based on the meaning of the term "exposure" implying increased risk to an undesired health effect. However, in this series of Handbooks, dedicated to the evaluation of the preventive effects of compounds, biological or pharmaceutical products, behaviours, programmes, and policy interventions, the traditional meaning of the term "exposure" is unfitting. Therefore in several instances the term "intervention," which lacks a hazardous connotation, is preferred. Examples of interventions with expected benefits in the area of tobacco control are tobacco use cessation, banning of smoking in public places, and taxation on tobacco products.

Part one: General principles

General scope

The prevention and control of cancer are the strategic objectives of IARC. Cancer prevention may be achieved at the individual level by avoiding cancer-causing agents (e.g. not using tobacco products), and at the population level by adopting programmes or legislation to reduce or eliminate exposure to cancer-causing agents (e.g. removing exposure to SHS through banning smoking in public and workplaces).

The Handbooks on tobacco control will evaluate the strength of the available evidence on the effects of interventions intended to prevent or reduce tobacco use, tobacco supply, and, when possible, tobacco-associated morbidity and mortality. The aim of the Handbook series is to provide the scientific community, policymakers, and governing bodies of IARC member states, as well as other countries with evidence-based assessments of these interventions at the individual and population levels, with the ultimate goal of assisting in the global implementation of tobacco control provisions within national and international programmes aimed at reducing tobacco-related morbidity and mortality.

Objectives

The objective is to prepare and publish, in the form of Handbooks, critical reviews and consensus evaluations of evidence on the effects of interventions focusing on tobacco control, with the help of an internationally formed Working Group (WG) of experts. The Handbooks may also indicate where additional research efforts are needed, specifically when data immediately relevant to an evaluation are not available. The evaluations in the Handbooks are scientific and qualitative judgments of peer-reviewed, published data, conducted during a week-long meeting of peer review and discussions by the WG.

Topic for the Handbook

The topic to be evaluated in a Handbook is selected approximately 12 months prior to the meeting by the head of the Lifestyle, and Cancer Group, after consultation with IARC scientists involved in tobacco research. A Handbook may cover a single topic or a group of related topics in the area of tobacco control.

Meeting participants

Soon after the topic of a Handbook is chosen, international scientists with relevant expertise are identified by IARC staff (usually through literature searches), in consultation with other experts. Each participant serves as an independent scientist and not as a representative of any organisation, government, or industry. Every effort is made to achieve a balanced group of experts in terms of gender, geographic origin, expertise, and diversity of scientific opinion.

Five categories of participants may attend Handbook meetings: WG members, Invited Specialists, Representatives of national and international health agencies, Observers, and the IARC Secretariat. Participants in the first two groups generally have published significant research related to the topic being reviewed or in tobacco control in particular. All participants are listed, with their addresses and principal affiliations, at the beginning of each Handbook volume. A description of each participant type, and their responsibilities, is listed below.

1. *The Working Group* is responsible for the critical reviews and evaluations that are developed during the meeting. WG members are selected based on knowledge and experience pertinent to the topic evaluated and absence of real or apparent conflicts of interest. The tasks of the WG are: (i) to ascertain that all appropriate data have been collected; (ii) to select the data relevant for the evaluation on the basis of scientific merit; (iii) to prepare accurate summaries of the data to enable the reader to follow the reasoning of the WG; (iv) to critically evaluate the results of epidemiological, clinical, and other type of studies; (v) to prepare recommendations for research and for public health action; and (vi) if the topic being reviewed so permits, to make an overall evaluation of the evidence of a protective effect or reduced risk associated with the exposure or intervention focus of the evaluation.

2. *Invited Specialists* are experts who also have critical knowledge and experience, but have a real or apparent conflict of interest. These experts are invited, when necessary, to assist in the WG by contributing their unique knowledge and experience during subgroup and plenary discussions. They may also contribute text on the intervention being evaluated. Invited Specialists do not serve as meeting chair or subgroup chair, redact summaries, or participate in the evaluations.

3. *Representatives* of national and international health agencies may attend meetings because their agencies are interested in the topic of a Handbook. Representatives do not serve as meeting chair or subgroup chair, draft any part of a Handbook, or participate in the evaluations.

4. *Observers* with relevant scientific credentials may be admitted to a meeting by IARC in limited numbers. Priority will be given to achieving a balance of Observers from constituencies with differing perspectives. They are invited to observe the meeting and should not attempt to influence it. Observers serve as sources of first-hand information from the meeting to their sponsoring organisations. They can play a valuable role in ensuring that all published information and scientific perspectives are considered. Observers will not serve as meeting chair or subgroup chair, draft any part of a Handbook, or participate in the evaluations. At the meeting, the chair and subgroup chairs may grant Observers the opportunity to speak, generally after they have heard a discussion.

5. The *IARC Secretariat* consists of scientists who have relevant expertise and are designated by IARC to attend a meeting. They serve as rapporteurs and participate in all discussions. When requested by the meeting chair or subgroup chair, they may also draft text or prepare tables and analyses.

The WHO Declaration of Interest form is sent to each prospective participant at the first contact, with the preliminary letter presenting the Handbook meeting. Before an official invitation is extended, each potential participant, including the IARC Secretariat, completes the WHO

Declaration of Interest form to report financial interests, employment and consulting, and individual and institutional research support related to the topic of the meeting. IARC assesses the declared interests to determine whether there is a conflict that warrants some limitation on participation. WG members are selected based on the absence of real or apparent conflicts of interest. If a real or apparent conflict of interest is identified, then the expert is asked to attend as an Invited Specialist. The declarations are updated and reviewed again at the opening of the meeting, approximately eight months later. Interests related to the subject of the meeting are disclosed to the meeting participants and in the published volume (Cogliano *et al.*, 2004).

Data for the Handbooks

The Handbooks review all pertinent studies on the intervention to be evaluated. Only those data considered relevant to evaluate the evidence are included and summarised. Those judged inadequate or irrelevant to the evaluation may be cited but not summarised. If a group of similar studies is not reviewed, the reasons are indicated.

With regard to reports of basic scientific research, epidemiological studies, and clinical trials, only studies that have been published or accepted for publication in the openly available scientific literature are reviewed. In certain instances, government agency reports that have undergone peer review and are widely available can be considered. Exceptions may be made ad hoc to include unpublished reports that are in their final form and publicly available, if their inclusion is considered pertinent to making an evaluation. Abstracts from scientific meetings, and other reports that do not provide sufficient detail upon which to base an assessment of their quality are generally not considered.

Inclusion of a study does not imply acceptance of the adequacy of the study design or of the analysis and interpretation of the results, and limitations identified by the WG are clearly outlined in square brackets (i.e. [ ]). The reasons for not giving further consideration to an individual study are also indicated in square brackets. Important aspects of a study, directly impinging on its interpretation, are brought to the attention of the reader. In general, numerical findings are indicated as they appear in the original report; units are converted when necessary for easier comparison. The WG may conduct additional analyses of the published data and use them in their assessment of the evidence. These analyses and their results are outlined in square brackets or in italics in the Handbook.

Working procedures

Chair of the meeting

The chair of the Handbook meeting is identified among leading international experts soon after the topic of a Handbook is chosen. The chair will help develop an outline for the Handbook early on and aid in identifying prospective experts to form the WG. The chair participates on conference calls with WG members and Invited Specialists in preparing for the meeting, provides early feedback on working papers, directs the meeting, and helps resolve queries emerging on the working papers once the meeting is over.

Literature to be reviewed

After the topic of the Handbook is chosen, pertinent studies are identified by IARC from recognised sources of information, such as PubMed, and made available to WG members and Invited Specialists to prepare the working papers for the meeting. Meeting participants are invited to supplement the IARC literature searches with their own searches. Studies cited in the working papers are available at the time of the meeting.

Working papers

Working papers are due about six to eight months after original contact of invited experts. The first version of the working papers is compiled and formatted by IARC staff about two months prior to the meeting, or as soon as they are received, and made available ahead of time through IARC's internet to all WG members, Invited Specialists, and the IARC Secretariat. Reception of working papers ahead of the established deadline is encouraged, as it allows review of their content, facilitating identification of information gaps from the start. When possible, or when deemed necessary, working papers may be discussed early on among experts to expedite the review process to be accomplished during the meeting. Conference calls will be scheduled after reception of all working papers and prior to the meeting, with the aim of identifying areas deserving additional work by experts before the meeting.

Acknowledgement of significant contributions to the chapters by colleagues of the invited experts, either at their home institution or elsewhere, can be included in the Handbook under an acknowledgement paragraph to be shown following the listing of the meeting participants.

Meeting

The meeting participants convene at IARC for seven to eight days to discuss and finalise the texts of the working papers that will constitute the Handbook and to formulate the evaluations. The WG members and Invited Specialists are grouped into subgroups according to their area of expertise. Subgroups meet during the first three to four days to review in detail the last versions of their working papers, develop a joint subgroup draft, and write summaries. During the last few days the participants meet in plenary session to review the subgroup working papers and summaries and to develop the consensus evaluations. Scheduling of plenary and subgroup time may change from one Handbook meeting to another.

Post-meeting

After the meeting, the draft Handbook is verified by consulting the original literature, edited, and prepared for publication by IARC staff. The aim is to publish Handbooks within 12 months of the meeting. If applicable, summaries reporting the results of

the evaluation may be available on the IARC website (http://www.iarc.fr) soon after the meeting, and a short report may be published in the international literature.

Part two: Scientific review of the evidence and evaluation

Scientific review

The evidence forming the foundation of the evaluation results from the studies reviewed. The validity of these studies will be examined critically to determine the weight they contribute to the assessment. This entails judging the appropriateness of study design, data collection (including adequate description of the intervention and follow-up), data analysis, and ultimately, deciding if chance, bias, confounding, or lack of statistical power may account for the observed results. The experts will ascertain how the limitations of the studies affect the results and conclusions reported. The criteria that follow apply to epidemiological and clinical studies, and therefore may not be as relevant to studies where other quality criteria would be indicated (e.g. those assessing the impact of economic policies or when health outcomes are not contemplated).

Quality of studies considered

It is necessary to take into account the possible roles of bias, confounding, and chance in the interpretation of epidemiological studies. Bias is the operation of factors in the study design or execution that leads erroneously to a stronger or

weaker association than in fact exists between the exposure/intervention being evaluated and the outcome. Confounding is a form of bias that occurs when the association with the disease is made to appear stronger or weaker than it truly is, as a result of an association between the apparent causal factor and another factor that is associated with either an increase or decrease in the incidence of the disease. The role of chance is related to biological variability and the influence of sample size on the precision of estimates of effect.

In evaluating the extent to which these factors have been taken into account in an individual study, the Handbook considers a number of aspects of design and analysis as described in the report of the study.

First, the study population, disease (or diseases), and exposure/intervention should have been well-defined by the authors. Cases of disease in the study population should have been identified independently of the intervention of interest, and the intervention assessed in a way that was not related to disease status.

Second, in the study design and analysis, the authors should have taken into account other variables that can influence the risk of disease or impact of an intervention and that may have been related to the intervention of interest. Potential confounding by such variables should have been dealt with either in the design of the study, such as by matching, or in the analysis, by statistical adjustment. In cohort studies, comparisons with local rates of the disease may or may not be more appropriate than those with national rates. Internal comparisons of disease frequency among individuals at different levels of the intervention are also desirable in cohort studies, since they minimise the potential for confounding related to difference in risk factors between an external reference group and the study population.

Third, the authors should have reported the basic data on which the conclusions are founded, even if sophisticated statistical analyses were employed. The numbers of exposed and unexposed cases and controls in a case-control study, and the numbers of cases observed and expected in a cohort study should have been provided. Further tabulations by time since exposure began, and other temporal factors, are also important. In a cohort study, data on all cancer sites and all causes of death should have been given to reveal the possibility of reporting bias. In a case-control study, the effects of investigated factors other than the exposure of interest should have been reported.

Finally, the statistical methods used to obtain estimates of relative risk, absolute rates of cancer, confidence intervals, and significance tests, and to adjust for confounding should have been clearly stated by the authors.

Aspects that are particularly important in evaluating experimental studies are: the selection of participants, the nature and adequacy of the randomisation procedure, evidence that randomisation achieved an adequate balance between groups, the exclusion criteria used before and after randomisation, compliance with the intervention in the intervention group, and 'contamination' with the intervention in the control group.

Other considerations are the means by which the endpoint was determined and validated, the length and completeness of follow-up of the groups, and the adequacy of the analysis.

Detailed analyses of both relative and absolute risks in relation to temporal variables, such as age at first exposure, time since first exposure, duration of exposure, cumulative exposure, peak exposure (when appropriate), and time since exposure ceased, will be reviewed and summarised when available.

Independent, population-based studies of the same exposure or intervention may lead to ambiguous results. Combined analyses of data from multiple studies may be a means of resolving this ambiguity. There are two types of combined analysis: the first combines summary statistics, such as relative risks, from individual studies (meta-analysis); the second involves a pooled analysis of the raw data from the individual studies (pooled analysis).

Advantages of combined analyses include better precision due to increased sample size, as well as the opportunity to explore potential confounders, interactions, and modifying effects that may explain heterogeneity among studies in more detail. A disadvantage of combined analyses is the possible lack of compatibility of data from various studies due to differences in subject recruitment, data collection procedures, measurement methods, and effects of unmeasured covariates that may differ between studies.

Meta-analyses may be conducted by the WG during the course of preparing a Handbook and are

identified as original calculations by placement of the results in square brackets or in italics. These may be de novo analyses or updates of previously conducted analyses that incorporate the results from new studies. Whenever possible, however, such analyses are preferably conducted preceding the Handbook meeting. Publication of the results of such meta-analyses prior to, or concurrently with, the Handbook meeting is encouraged for purposes of peer review. The same criteria for data quality that would be applied to individual studies must be applied to combined analyses, and such analyses must take into account heterogeneity between studies.

Criteria for causality

After the quality of each study has been summarised and assessed, a judgment is made concerning the strength of evidence that the intervention in question reduces the risk of disease or is protective for humans. Hill (1965) lists areas for evaluating the strength of epidemiological associations used in the review of human data when assessing carcinogenesis. These criteria, in many instances, will apply to the assessment included in a Handbook:

• Consistency of observed associations across studies and populations;
• Magnitude of the reported association;
• Temporal relationship between exposure/intervention and change in disease;
• Exposure-response biologic gradient;
• Biological plausibility;

• Coherence of results across other lines of evidence; and

• Analogy present in related exposures and their effects on health.

If the results are inconsistent among investigations, possible explanations are sought (e.g. differences in level of exposure/ intervention). Results of studies judged to be of high quality are given more weight than those of studies judged to be less methodologically sound. When several studies show little or no indication of an association between an intervention and cancer prevention, the judgment may be made that, in the aggregate, they show evidence of lack of effect. The possibility that bias, confounding, or misclassification of exposure or outcome could explain the observed results should be considered and excluded when reasonable certainty exists.

Assessing studies reporting the impact of tobacco control policy interventions not necessarily contemplating health outcomes

Evaluating the outcomes of population level tobacco control policy involves three interrelated questions: (1) Does the policy have an impact? (causality); if so, (2) Under what conditions? (moderation); and (3) How (mediation)?

The choice of design elements will depend on which questions are considered to be a part of the evaluation effort. It is important to ensure that the appropriate concepts are chosen, and, that for each, measures are identified that are

suitable to answer the evaluation question.

In the absence of a randomised trial, there are two study design strategies that can be employed for the rigorous evaluation of the effects of policies. First is the use of measurements both before and after the policy's implementation. These measurements can be taken from either units (usually, but not limited to, individuals; the same logic would apply if the measures were of households, schools, or other venues) that are either the same (as in a cohort design) or different, but drawn from the same sampling process (as in a repeat cross-sectional design). The second design strategy is the use of a quasi-experimental design, in which one group that is exposed to a policy is compared to a similar unexposed group, as discussed above. Combining these two strategies in a single study yields a two-group, pre-post design, which offers a higher degree of internal validity than either feature alone. The utility of longitudinal designs is strengthened if there are multiple data collections before and/or after policy implementation, allowing more precise specification of effects (e.g. taking into account temporal trends that were occurring before the implementation of the policy).

A distinction between study designs and study features is worth noting. In addition to the two design considerations stated above, there are two study feature strategies that contribute to increasing an evaluation study's internal validity. The first is the measurement of policy-specific variables that are theorised to be affected initially after the policy is

implemented. A second strategy is the measurement of policy-specific variables for policies that have not changed; such variables act as another form of control. Recommendations for measures pertinent to the evaluation of each WHO Framework Convention on Tobacco Control policy domain are provided in Handbook Volume 12 (IARC, 2008).

Combining the two design and two study feature strategies, along with the inclusion of other explanatory variables (covariates) that might help explain differences between two jurisdictions, creates a powerful research design, allowing more confident inferences to be made about the causal effects of policies and/or combinations of policies.

Evaluation efforts should be informed by knowledge of the nature of the policy being evaluated, and the goals of the evaluation study should be clearly stated. Evaluation planning should be guided by understanding what threats to internal validity may be present in the study of a given policy situation, and then adding design elements and other measures to reduce or eliminate those threats.

Knowledge of the mediational pathways that are theorised to explain how policy affects behaviour and environment (or environmental risk) should lead to an appropriate study design, the inclusion of appropriate constructs and measures, and the selection of analytic tools that are well-suited to estimating the causal impact of policies by providing an explanatory pathway and helping to eliminate alternative explanations.

The utility of longitudinal designs is strengthened if there are multiple data collections before and/or after policy implementation, as this allows more precise specification of effects (e.g. taking into account temporal trends that were occurring before the implementation of the policy). The role of time series analysis on aggregate sales/consumption data that demonstrate the effect of price on consumption is a good example of the power of multiple measurements.

Both repeated cross-sectional and longitudinal (cohort) designs are useful for assessing the impact of a given policy. The use of cohort designs provides an additional capability for tracking the impact of policies within individuals, allowing stronger tests of mediational pathways.

Addition of samples from other populations to either or both intervention and control arms, also adds strength to the evaluation design, as does having varying levels of intensity of the intervention.

Similarly, parallel assessment of alternative explanations for observed changes in outcomes (e.g. possibly being due to other policies or industry counter-actions) adds strength over assessing these effects in separate studies.

The existence of studies with complementary strengths and weaknesses is particularly useful in triangulating the results of a corpus of evaluation studies to see if a consistent pattern emerges.

The use of probability sampling in an evaluation study increases its external validity - the extent to which the findings of a policy evaluation study can be generalised to draw conclusions about the impact of the policy on the larger population.

At a broader level, the design of

an evaluation study should be guided by knowledge of how prior evaluation studies in the same policy domain have been conducted. An analysis of the similarity or differences in policy impact across similar studies can yield powerful conclusions about the overall impact of a policy.

Summary of the data reviewed (evidence)

This section summarises the results of the evidence presented in the preceding sections in a Handbook in a concise manner. Traditionally, this section does not include citation of literature, as do preceding sections presenting and discussing the evidence.

Evaluation of the evidence

An evaluation of the strength of the evidence for disease prevention or reduction in morbidity and mortality is made using standard terms described in previous volumes of the Handbooks of Cancer Prevention (e.g. Volume 11). In evaluating the strength of the evidence on the effects of tobacco control interventions directed at the population, disease prevention or health outcomes may not always be a measurable endpoint. Also, it is conceivable that not every exposure/intervention reviewed in a Handbook of tobacco control will permit a formal evaluation of the evidence, as traditionally done in other Handbooks of Cancer Prevention and in the Monographs.

The following criteria are proposed when evaluating the weight of the evidence on the effects of tobacco control interventions:

Sufficient evidence: The WG considers that an association has been observed in studies in which chance, bias, and confounding can be ruled out with reasonable confidence. The association is highly likely to be causal. A statement that there is *sufficient evidence* should be followed by a separate sentence that identifies the nature and magnitude of the observed effect.

Strong evidence: There is consistent evidence of an association between the intervention under consideration and a given effect, but evidence of causality is limited by the fact that chance, bias, or confounding have not been ruled out with reasonable confidence. However, explanations other than causality are unlikely.

Limited evidence: There is some evidence of association between the intervention under consideration and a given effect, but alternative explanations are possible.

Inadequate/no evidence: There are no available methodologically sound studies showing an association. The available studies are of insufficient quality, consistency, or statistical power to permit a conclusion regarding the presence or absence of a causal association between the intervention and a given effect. Alternatively, this category is used when no data are available.

Evidence suggesting lack of effect: There are several methodologically adequate studies that are mutually consistent in not showing an association between the intervention and a given effect.

Overall evaluation

The overall evaluation, usually in the form of a narrative, will include a summary of the body of evidence considered as a whole, and summary statements made about the strength of the evidence for policy effects, including changes in tobacco use, changes in health risks, and incidental effects.

IARC WGs make every effort to achieve a consensus evaluation. Consensus reflects broad agreement among WG members, but not necessarily unanimity. The chair may elect to poll WG members to determine the diversity of scientific opinion on issues where consensus is not readily apparent.

Recommendations

After reviewing the data and deliberating on them, the WG may formulate recommendations, where applicable, for further research and public health action.